CONTRACEPTIVE STEROIDS

Pharmacology and Safety

REPRODUCTIVE BIOLOGY

Series Editor: Sheldon J. Segal
The Rockefeller Foundation
New York, New York

THE ANTIPROGESTIN STEROID RU 486 AND HUMAN FERTILITY CONTROL
Edited by Etienne-Emile Baulieu and Sheldon J. Segal

CONTRACEPTIVE STEROIDS: Pharmacology and Safety
Edited by A. T. Gregoire and Richard P. Blye

GOSSYPOL: A Potential Contraceptive for Men
Edited by Sheldon J. Segal

IMMUNOLOGICAL APPROACHES TO CONTRACEPTION AND PROMOTION OF FERTILITY
Edited by G. P. Talwar

CONTRACEPTIVE STEROIDS

Pharmacology and Safety

Edited by

A. T. Gregoire

Food and Drug Administration
Rockville, Maryland

and

Richard P. Blye

National Institutes of Health
Bethesda, Maryland

PLENUM PRESS • NEW YORK AND LONDON

Library of Congress Cataloging in Publication Data

Contraceptive steroids.

(Reproductive biology)
Based on the proceedings of the Workshop on Animal Testing Requirements for New Generation Steroidal Contraceptives, which included a meeting of the Fertility and Maternal Health Drug Advisory Committee, held Apr. 27–29, 1983 at the National Institutes of Health and sponsored by the Food and Drug Administration and others.
Includes bibliographies and index.
1. Contraceptive drugs—Side effects—Congresses. 2. Steroid drugs—Side effects—Congresses. 3. Contraceptive drugs—Toxicology—Congresses. 4. Steroid drugs—Toxicology—Congresses. 5. Pharmacology, Experimental—Congresses. I. Gregoire, A. T. II. Blye, Richard P. III. Workshop on Animal Testing Requirements for New Generation Steroidal Contraceptives (1983: National Institutes of Health) IV. United States. Food and Drug Administration. Fertility and Maternal Health Drug Advisory Committee. V. Series. [DNLM: 1. Animal Testing Alternatives—congresses. 2. Contraceptives—adverse effects—congresses. 3. Contraceptives—pharmacodynamics—congresses. 4. Steroids—pharmacodynamics—congresses. QV 177 C764 1983]
RG137.4.C66 1986 613.9′432 86-20448
ISBN 0-306-42393-6

Based on the proceedings of a Workshop and Meeting of the Fertility and Maternal Health Drugs Advisory Committee, sponsored by the Food and Drug Administration and the National Institutes of Health in cooperation with the Population Council, the World Health Organization, and the Agency for International Development, held April 27–29, 1983, at the National Institutes of Health, Bethesda, Maryland

A Division of Plenum Publishing Corporation
233 Spring Street, New York, N.Y. 10013

Printed in the United States of America

This book is dedicated to the pharmacologists and physiologists working in university, industrial, private, and governmental laboratories throughout the world, whose aggregate labors provide the foundation for new drug development.

PREFACE

One of the United States Food and Drug Administration's most difficult tasks is the assessment of risk-benefit ratios for a broad spectrum of therapeutic and prophylactic drugs. Furthermore, it is now widely recognized that no drug, chemical or even natural substance is completely devoid of risk. Nowhere has this issue been the subject of more controversy than with steroidal contraceptive drugs. Regulated as a special class of products because of their prophylactic use in healthy individuals for prevention of pregnancy rather than for treatment of disease, steroid contraceptives drugs undergo more extensive animal safety tests than any other pharmaceutical agent. This view also contemplates the availability of alternative contraceptive measures posing fewer risks, but the use of less effective methods must take into consideration the hazards associated with pregnancy itself.

In April 1983, the Food and Drug Administration and the National Institutes of Health in cooperation with the World Health Organization, the Population Council, and the Agency for International Development sponsored a three-day workshop to evaluate current guidelines for preclinical safety studies of contraceptive drugs in light of our extensive knowledge of the side effects of marketed products. The meeting included presentations by experts in the fields of comparative metabolism, pharmacokinetics, pharmacology, carcinogenicity, toxicology, coagulation, lipid metabolism, epidemiology and pathology at a meeting of the Fertility and Maternal Health Drugs Advisory Committee of the National Center for Drugs and Biologics, Food and Drug Administration. Representatives of drug regulatory agencies from several foreign countries and the United States also addressed the Committee. Following the presentations and general discussion, the Advisory Committee addressed the following six questions:

1. How can the knowledge of steroid pharmacokinetics, metabolism, and steroid hormone action be utilized in the design of meaningful animal safety studies?

2. Should guidelines for preclinical animal safety studies be amended to allow earlier Phase I clinical pharmacology studies?

3. How can the current long term animal safety requirements be modified to consider the drug's chemical structure, pharmacology, and mode of administration for extrapolation to humans?

4. Should dose levels in animal safety studies consider an end organ's responsiveness? How can the results of these studies be extrapolated and predictive of potential human adverse reactions, e.g., thromboembolic and other vascular disorders?

5. What research should be undertaken to make data interpretation and evaluation predictive of potential clinical problems?

6. What are the alternatives to long term animal studies that the FDA can rely on for the assessment of safety of steroid contraceptives?

All participants received the questions in advance of the workshop. Some speakers chose to provide answers directly while others addressed only those issues pertinent to the field of expertise in their presentation. However, the Committee's responses to these questions form the basis for their recommendations to the Food and Drug Administration on animal testing requirements for new generation steroidal contraceptives.

The transcript of the discussion has been extensively edited. We are grateful to the participants of this workshop and for the preparation of manuscripts which constitute a major portion of these proceedings.

A.T. Gregoire Richard P. Blye

ACKNOWLEDGEMENT

Grateful acknowledgement is extended to Joan McDonald, Doris Cross, Penny Colbert, Wanda Hill, Melanie Wilson and Arnita Smith, Center for Population Research, NIH, for their assistance in preparing draft copies of manuscripts as well as transcriptions of the discussions. The editors also appreciate the technical assistance of Carol Knoth and Kathryn Kruse, FDA librarians, for their research in the verification of references.

Organization and preparation of the final copies of all manuscripts and discussions for publication were accomplished by Joan McDonald. Without her patience and untiring efforts, completion of this volume would not have been possible.

CONTENTS

SECTION II

CONTRACEPTIVE STEROIDS AND CARCINOGENICITY

Moderator: M.B. Lipsett

SECTION III

EFFECTS OF CONTRACEPTIVE STEROIDS ON COAGULATION AND LIPID METABOLISM

Moderator: H. Berendes

SECTION IV

PANEL OF INTERNATIONAL DRUG REGULATORY AGENCIES

Moderator: S. Sobel

SECTION V

DISCUSSION AND ADVISORY COMMITTEE RECOMMENDATIONS

Moderator: W. Andrews

OPENING REMARKS

Solomon Sobel and William Andrews

DR. SOBEL: On behalf of the Food and Drug Administration and the National Institute of Child Health and Human Development, I wish to welcome our distinguished participants to the Workshop on Animal Testing Requirements for New Generation Steroidal Contraceptives.

This workshop has been convened to address issues of practical concern. At the October 1982 meeting of the FDA's Fertility and Maternal Health Drugs Advisory Committee, we posed questions concerning the appropriate preclinical testing of steroidal contraceptives. It was decided to defer answers to those questions to a workshop of this nature. In addition to routine animal studies, the Food and Drug Administration requires long-term testing in dogs and monkeys. With the advent of modifications of contraceptive steroids which are closely related to those already approved for marketing, the Agency is striving to develop policies to facilitate the development and clinical introduction of these modified drugs. Specifically, we must evaluate steroids that fall into various categories such as (1) parenteral forms of previously evaluated and marketed steroids as components of oral contraceptives; (2) new esters of parenteral steroids, the parent compounds of which have already undergone or are undergoing long-term evaluation in animal models; (3) new delivery systems for parenteral steroids, such as silastic implants, polymeric microspheres, vaginal rings, and others.

One of the aims of this workshop is to seek ways to adapt and modify animal models, through application of principles of pharmacokinetics, comparative pharmacology, etc. Through these approaches, we hope to facilitate preclinical testing of a new generation of contraceptive steroids. It is not our intention to abandon current models, but rather to adapt them in meaningful ways to give us more information and to eliminate unnecessary duplicative testing. Also, we will attempt to enter new areas of investigation as far as the predictability of certain clinical events, such as thromboembolic disease.

Our long-term animal studies thus far have addressed issues of carcinogenicity, teratogenicity, organ toxicity, and effects on target endocrine organs. It has become apparent to us over the years since the clinical introduction of oral contraceptives that important clinical problems such as hypercoagulability, alteration of blood lipids and vascular effects have not been well addressed by our animal testing systems. During the workshop, we will attempt to address methods for increasing the sensitivity and predictability of our models in these areas.

I realize I have outlined difficult tasks. However, I am confident that we will achieve at least some of our aims during the next several days of this workshop.

Again, let me say welcome and express the thanks of our Agencies for your presence and participation.

DR. ANDREWS: On behalf of the Fertility and Maternal Health Drugs Advisory Committee of the FDA, I would like to add my word of welcome. Our Committee is delighted to have this opportunity to meet and work with our colleagues from the NIH, the World Health Organization, and distinguished participants from other institutions. The issues before us were raised a few months ago. It was the consensus of the Committee at that time, after a half day presentation, that we did not have enough time or information to offer firm recommendations. I would hope that during the next three days the distinguished array of speakers will provide this information and at the end of this session we will be able to provide the FDA with firm recommendations.

ORAL CONTRACEPTIVES AND THE OCCURRENCE OF DISEASE

Clinical Overview

Bruce Stadel

National Institutes of Health
National Institute of Child Health and Human Development
Bethesda, Maryland

INTRODUCTION

During the past two decades, numerous clinical, epidemiological, and laboratory studies have been conducted in an effort to clarify the effects of oral contraceptives (OCs) on the health of women. These studies have shown that, in addition to preventing unwanted pregnancy, OCs influence the occurrence of various diseases. For some of these diseases the influence is beneficial, while for others it is adverse. During the 1960s to the mid-1970s, research on OCs and health was focused primarily on the major adverse effects such as an increased risk of cardiovascular disease[1]. Subsequently, important beneficial effects have also been described such as a decreased risk of pelvic inflammatory disease[2]. The major reason for this progression from risks to benefits is that case reports of unusual illnesses in OC users have stimulated the early investigation of adverse effects. For beneficial effects, there are no case reports, and more systematic research is necessary. This demonstrates the importance of a comprehensive approach for evaluation of the overall benefits and risks of OCs.

The purpose of this review is to summarize current information about the major effects of OCs on the occurrence of disease in women, and to recommend ways in which this information may be useful in designing animal studies for evaluating the beneficial and adverse effects of new steroid contraceptive formulations. The review is subject, however, to certain limitations. First, this article is based almost entirely upon studies that have been conducted in Britain, the United States, and similar countries. All of the information presented here should be regarded as coming from these countries unless otherwise specified, and it should be noted that this information may not be directly relevant to other areas of the world. Second, many of the findings in this article pertain to the aggregate effect of OCs as they were used during the 1960s - 1970s: A large proportion of these were combined OCs containing a 19-nortestosterone progestogen with 50 mcg. of mestranol (ME) or ethinyl estradiol (EE)[3,4]. Although some important data are available for other OC formulations, and for the separate effects of the progestogens and estrogens in OCs, the extent of these data is limited. Thus, many of the findings presented here do not take account of the trend toward use of OCs containing less than 50 mcg. of EE or ME which began during the late 1970s[3]. Likewise, these findings do not reflect recent changes in the way that women and their physicians assess the benefits and risks of OCs at the time OCs are prescribed. Finally, the scope of this review precludes any detailed discussion of methodological issues, although a few comments will be made about the estimation of disease risk from epidemiological studies.

Most information about the beneficial and adverse effects of OCs on the occurrence of disease comes from case-control studies and cohort studies[5]. Case-control and cohort studies provide estimates of two measures of the benefits and risks of OCs: Relative risk and attributable risk. Relative risk, which is the ratio of the incidence of a disease in OC users to the incidence in non-users, is very useful for identifying the benefical and adverse effects of OCs, but can be misleading as an indicator of risk in the usual sense. Attributable risk, which is the difference in the incidence of a disease between OC users and non-users, is a better indicator of the overall importance of an effect of OCs on the occurrence of disease, and will be emphasized here whenever possible. Because of sampling variation and other methodological problems, the estimates of both relative and attributable risk in this review are only approximate. Nevertheless, they do serve to illustrate major findings.

ADVERSE EFFECTS

OCs have been observed to increase the risk of a variety of diseases, including conditions which are as diverse in origin as photosensitivity[4], chicken pox[4], and gallbladder disease[6*]. In terms of attributable risk, however, the most important adverse effect of OCs that has been clearly demonstrated is an increased risk of cardiovascular disease[1], while the most important area of uncertainty has been the effect of OCs on the risk of breast cancer and certain other forms of neoplasia[7]. OCs and the risk of neoplasia will be considered first.

NEOPLASIA

The forms of neoplasia that have been of greatest concern with regard to the question of increased risk in OC users are cancer of the breast and reproductive tract (endometrium, ovary, and cervix), hepatocellular adenoma, malignant melanoma and pituitary adenoma. The reasons for the emphasis on these forms of neoplasia have been in part theoretical and in part empirical. On the theoretical side, for example, it is well-established that the etiology of breast cancer in women who are not using OCs is related to stimulation with endogenous sex hormones[8]. It has therefore been considered possible that OCs might increase risk. An example on the empirical side is the process by which it was established that OCs increase the risk of hepatocellular adenoma. The first suggestion of this increased risk was the appearance of case reports of hepatocellular adenoma in long-term OC users[9]. Subsequently, case control studies of hepatocellular adenoma in women of reproductive age were conducted, and it was found that OC use, especially long-term use, was much more common in the hepatocellular adenoma cases than in the controls[10].

---

*To be precise, OCs appear to accelerate the development of gallbladder disease in susceptible women, rather than to increase the overall lifetime risk[6].

Breast, Endometrial, and Ovarian Cancer

During the past five years, the Centers for Disease Control has been conducting a comprehensive, population-based, case-control study of OCs and the risk of breast, endometrial, and ovarian cancer under an Intraagency Agreement with the National Institute of Child Health and Human Development (and with additional support from the National Cancer Institute). This large study, which is called the Cancer and Steroid Hormones (CASH) Study, is designed to rigorously test numerous hypotheses that have been raised by previous studies, including the hypotheses that OCs increase the risk of breast cancer in longterm OC users[11,12], in women with a family history of breast cancer[13], in women with a history of benign breast disease[11,14,15] and in women with a history of OC use prior to first childbirth[12,14].

The preliminary results from the CASH Study were published in March 1983, and are reassuring. There is no evidence that OCs increase the risk of breast cancer either in OC users generally, in long-term OC users or in women with a family history of breast cancer, a history of benign breast disease, or a history of OC use prior to first childbirth[16]. Furthermore, the CASH Study strongly supports previous studies which have suggested that combined OCs decrease the risk of endometrial cancer[17] and that OCs decrease the risk of ovarian cancer[18]. These latter two findings will be considered further under beneficial effects.

Cervical Cancer

There have been numerous case-control and cohort studies of OCs and the risk of cervical cancer and its precursor, cervical dysplasia, although most of the data about cancer pertain to carcinoma *in situ* rather than to invasive cancer[7,19-23]. These studies have provided useful information about the major risk factors for cervical cancer and dysplasia such as relatively high sexual activity and have shown that the question of whether OCs increase risk must be addressed in the context of these other factors. The question itself, however, has only been partially resolved. The major reason for this lack of resolution is that virtually all studies in this area have had substantial limitations with regard to one or another of several important methodological issues, such as the variation that exists among pathologists in the classification of cervical dysplasia and carcinoma *in situ*[23], or the breadth and depth of information that is necessary to investigate possible interactions between OCs and established or probable risk factors for cervical cancer and dysplasia such as sexual activity, cigarette smoking, and nutritional status[20,21,24,5]. Thus only tentative conclusions can be drawn at the present time. These are as follows: OCs do not dramatically increase the risk of cervical dysplasia or cancer[3,19]; OCs may increase the risk to a limited extent, however, especially in long-term OC users[22] or in women with characteristics such as high sexual activity[20] or low nutritional folate status[24,25]. Future research on OCs and cervical cancer or dysplasia that is designed to overcome the methodological limitations of previous studies should be able to resolve these issues.

Hepatocellular Adenoma

In contrast to the uncertainty about OCs and cervical cancer or dysplasia, it is very clear that OCs increase the risk of hepatocellular adenoma, which can cause serious intraabdominal hemorrhage[10,26]. The increased risk of hepatocellular adenoma in OC users appears to be directly related to the duration of OC use, the age of the OC user, and the estrogen/progestogen content of OCs[10]. In one well-designed case control study, for example, the relative risk of hepatocellular adenoma in women who had used OCs for a total of three years or more at some time in their lives as compared to women who had used OCs for one year or less, was estimated to be over 100[10]. Hepatocellular adenoma rarely occurs in women who have not used OCs and the attributable risk is therefore small. In women who have used OCs for five years or longer as compared to women who have used OCs for two years or less, the attributable risk has been estimated at only about two cases per 100,000 OC users per year[10]. This illustrates the importance of relying upon attributable risk, rather than relative risk, for evaluating the overall benefits and risks of OCs.

Malignant Melanoma

Several case-control and cohort studies have provided information about OCs and the risk of malignant melanoma and these studies are in general agreement that OCs do not dramatically increase the risk[27-31]. This conclusion is also supported by evidence that the ratios for incidence and mortality rates from malignant melanoma in women of reproductive age as compared to men did not change following the introduction of OCs[32]. Certain studies, however, do suggest that OCs may increase the risk of malignant melanoma to a limited extent, especially in long-term OC users who have a history of OC use that occurred many years in the past[27,29,30]. This is not a consistent finding in all pertinent studies[31] and therefore should be regarded as tentative. If the finding is real, one possible explanation is that long-term use of high estrogen OCs (i.e., OCs containing >50 mcg. of EE or ME) may increase the risk of malignant melanoma to some extent, and that some studies which involve long-term OC use that occurred many years in the past may pertain in large part to high estrogen OCs, which were used extensively during the 1960s[3].

Pituitary Adenoma

Recently, a large and well-designed case-control study has provided convincing evidence that OCs do not increase the risk of pituitary adenoma or the amenorrhea/galactorrhea syndrome. This absence of an increased risk pertains to OC users generally, and also to long-term users[33]. The results from this study support the following conclusions about previous evidence suggesting that OCs might increase the risk of pituitary adenoma or amenorrhea/galactorrhea. The large increase that occurred during the 1970s in the incidence of diagnosed pituitary adenoma in young women was primarily related to improvements in diagnostic technology and only coincidentally related to the increasing use of OCs[34]. The coincidence of increasing OC use and improved diagnostic technology also explains the results of uncontrolled clinical studies and the one small case-control study, not rigorously designed, which have appeared to relate the development of pituitary adenoma or amenorrhea/galactorrhea to the prior use of OCs[35,36]. The administration of pharmacologic doses of OCs to mice and rats, which has been shown to increase the occurrence of pituitary adenoma, is not an appropriate animal model for evaluating the risk of pituitary adenoma or amenorrhea/galactorrhea in women using OCs at clinically prescribed doses[37].

CARDIOVASCULAR DISEASE

There is overwhelming evidence that OCs increase the risk of cardiovascular disease, primarily the risk of venous thromboembolism, myocardial infarction, and stroke. To a large extent, however, it has been found that the risk of serious illness or death from cardiovascular disease that is attributable to OCs is concentrated in certain groups of women such as those about 35 years of age or older and who smoke cigarettes heavily. In other groups of women, the attributable risk appears to be small, and OCs can be used with reasonable safety[1].

Venous Thromboembolism

OCs have been shown to increase both the risk of overt venous thromboembolism (VTE)[38] and the occurrence of subclinical thrombosis that is extensive enough to be detected by procedures such as ^{125}I-fibrinogen uptake[39,40] and plasma fibrinogen chromatography[41]. In previously healthy, nonpregnant women of reproductive age who are not using OCs, the overall incidence of (overt) superficial or deep VTE has been found to be about one new case per 1,000 women per year. In comparable women who are using OCs, the corresponding incidence is about 3 cases per 1,000 women per year[42,43]. In relation to these findings about VTE, results from plasma fibrinogen chromatographic studies have suggested that the overall incidence of subclinical thrombosis in women (previously healthy, etc.) who are not using OCs is about one episode per woman per year, and that the corresponding incidence in women who are using OCs is about three episodes per woman per year[41]. The most plausible explanation for these findings is that OCs increase the size of intravascular clots that are formed in response to thrombotic stimuli[44], thereby causing a similar relative increase in the risk of VTE and in the incidence of subclinical thrombosis that is extensive enough to be detected by plasma fibrinogen chromatography.

Current and Past OC Use

The risk of VTE has been found to increase during the first month or so of OC use, to then remain constant for as long as three years of continuous use, and to decrease within about one month after OCs are discontinued to the level of risk in women who have never used OCs[42,45,46]. There are few data for more than three years of continuous use. Furthermore, the occurrence of subclinical thrombosis, as detected by plasma fibrinogen chromatography, has been found to increase during the first month or so of OC use, and then to remain constant for up to eight years of continuous use[41]. These findings indicate that it is only current (or very recent) OC use that increases the risk of VTE, and that the increased risk of VTE in current OC users* does not disappear with continuing use.

Relative and Attributable Risk

Numerous case-control studies have provided estimates of the relative risk of VTE in current OC users as compared to nonusers.** These estimates are about three for idiopathic superficial venous thrombosis (i.e., for first episodes of superficial VT in previously healthy women) in the range of 4-11 for idiopathic deep VT or pulmonary embolism (PE) and in the range

---

*"Current (or very recent) OC users," or "women using OCs," are defined as women who have used OCs within the past month.

** "Nonusers," or "women not using OCs," are defined as women who have not used OCs within the past month, regardless of prior usage.

Table 1. Oral Contraceptives and Risk of Venous Thromboembolic Disease.

Category of venous thrombo-embolic disease	Incidence*		Relative* risk	Attributable* risk
	Current OC User	Nonuser		
	Cases per 10,000 women per year			Cases per 10,000 current OC users per year
Idiopathic†				
Superficial leg vein[42]	19	8	2	11
Deep leg vein, other sites, or pulmonary embolism ††[42,43]	11	3	4	8
In women with predisposing conditions				
Postoperative venous thrombosis[38]	61§	30§	2	31§
In women with any predisposing condition, ¶ venous thrombosis or pulmonary embolism‖[55]	Unknown	Unknown	2	Unknown

* All estimates are rounded to the nearest integer.
† First episodes of venous thromboembolic disease in previously healthy women.
†† The estimates are averages from the references cited.
§ Incidence per 10,000 surgical procedures.
¶ E.g., preexisting vascular disease, metabolic disorder, surgery or trauma.
‖ Eighty-eight per cent of the cases were venous thrombosis or pulmonary embolism; 12 per cent were arterial thrombosis.

of 1.5-6 for VT or PE in women with previous medical, surgical, or traumatic conditions that predispose to the development of VTE[45-56].

Case-control studies provided the first clear evidence that OCs increase the risk of VTE[45, 47-50] and such studies have been very important for examining the effect of OCs on the risk of VTE in relation to other risk factors. In terms of attributable risk, however, the most valuable source of information about OCs and the risk of VTE is the experience of the two cohort studies that were begun in Britain in 1968[38,42,43,57,58].

Estimates of the incidence of VTE in current OC users and in non-users and estimates of the relative and attributable risk, are presented in Table 1. With one exception[55], these estimates are derived from the cohort studies in Britain[38,42,43]. All of the estimates pertain to VTE that occurred during the late 1960's to mid-1970's.

The figures in Table 1 illustrate three major findings. The risk of idiopathic VT or PE that is attributable to OCs is about 19 cases per 10,000 current OC users per year. About one-half of these cases involved superficial leg VT only, while the other one-half involved deep leg VT, VT at other sites, or PE[42,43]. In relation to these figures, it should be noted that the risk of death from VTE that is attributable to OCs is extremely small. The cohort studies in Britain began in 1968 with over

60,000 women, about one-half of whom were using OCs. During over 450,000 women-years of followup, only five fatalities from VTE have been observed (three fatalities from PE in current OC users and two in past users)[57,58].

The relative risk of postoperative VT in current OC users as compared to nonusers, is about two[38]. This figure is lower than the relative risk of idiopathic deep VT or PE which is about four[42,43]. The attributable risk of postoperative VT, however, is higher than the attributable risk of idiopathic deep VT or PE. Using the figures in Table 1, and assuming that the average postoperative period is about three months, the risk of postoperative VT that is attributable to OCs is about 10 cases per 10,000 current OC users per month. In contrast, the risk of idiopathic deep VT or PE that is attributable to OCs is only about one case per 10,000 current OC users per month[38,2,43]. This again emphasizes the importance of relying upon attributable risk for evaluating the overall benefits and risks of OCs.

In women with previous medical, surgical, or traumatic conditions that predispose to VTE, the relative risk of VT or PE, in current OC users as compared to nonusers, is about two[55]. This figure is similar to the relative risk of postoperative VT (also about two)[38]. Although the risk of VT or PE that is attributable to OCs in women with medical, surgical, or traumatic predisposing conditions has not been established, it is prudent to assume that this attributable risk is substantially higher than the attributable risk of idiopathic deep VT or PE.

Estrogen/Progestogen Content of OCs

A direct relationship has been observed between the risk of VTE in current OC users and the estrogen content of the OCs being used[42,54,59,60]. The most important finding in this regard is that the risk of fatal or nonfatal PE in women using OCs containing 50-80 mcg of either ethinyl estradiol (EE) or mestranol (ME) appears to be only about one-third to one-half as large as the risk in women using OCs containing 100-150 mcg of EE or ME[59]. There is also some evidence that the risk of fatal PE in women using OCs containing 30 mcg of EE is lower than the risk in women using OCs containing 50 mcg of EE[60], but more data are needed before the importance of this finding can be established.

No clear relationship has been observed between the risk of PE or other deep VTE in current OC users and the progestogen content of the OCs being used[59]. It has been found, however, that the risk of idiopathic superficial leg VT in women using OCs containing either 1,3, or 4 mg of norethindrone acetate with 50 mcg of EE is directly related to the amount of norethindrone acetate in the OCs being used[42]. Also, one progestogen-only OC (containing ethynodiol diacetate) has been found to increase the occurrence of subclinical thrombosis as detected by plasma fibrinogen chromatography[41]. These findings suggest that the progestogenic components of at least some OCs are capable of increasing the occurrence of small thrombi that either remain subclinical or, at most, become large enough to occlude superficial veins. It is the estrogenic component of OCs, however, that has been found to increase the risk of developing a thrombus that is large enough to occlude a deep vein or form a pulmonary embolus.

OCs In Relation to Other Risk Factors

Several studies have provided information about OCs and the risk of

VTE in relation to other known or hypothesized risk factors for VTE. The findings from these studies which indicate that the risk of VTE that is attributable to OCs is higher for post-operative VTE than for idiopathic deep VTE, and is probably also higher for VTE in women with other medical, surgical, or traumatic conditions that predispose to VTE, were presented in Table 1 and the related discussion[38,42,43,55]. Consideration will now be given to the risk of idiopathic VTE that is attributable to OCs in relation to factors other than the obvious medical, surgical, or traumatic predisposing conditions.

The risk of idiopathic superficial or deep VTE that is attributable to OCs has been found to be unrelated to age, socioeconomic status, or parity[42,45,46]. Furthermore, although there has been some controversy in the past about cigarette smoking and body weight, it does not currently appear that the risk of idiopathic superficial or deep VTE that is attributable to OCs is related in any substantial way to either mild obesity ($\leq$ 15% overweight for age and height)[45,56] or cigarette smoking[42,50,61].

Whereas the risk of idiopathic VTE that is attributable to OCs has been found to be unrelated to age, economic status, etc., there is evidence that this attributable risk is related to ABO blood type. In a collaborative study that was carried out in the United States, Britain and Sweden, the relative risk of idiopathic deep VTE in women who were not using OCs was found to be about two in women with blood types A, B or AB as compared to women with blood type O. In women who were using OCs, the relative risk in women with blood types A, B, or AB as compared to women with blood type O was about 3[62]. These findings indicate both that there is a genetic susceptibility to idiopathic VTE which is related to ABO blood type, and that OCs magnify this genetic susceptibility, such that the risk of idiopathic deep VTE that is attributable to OCs is probably only about four cases per 10,000 current OC users per year in women with blood type O, but about 12 cases per 10,000 current OC users per year in women with blood types A, B, or AB[42,43,62].

Pathogenesis of VTE in OC Users

OCs have been observed to induce a variety of changes in the circulatory system which are believed to increase the occurrence of thrombosis, including endothelial proliferation[63], a decrease in the rate of venous blood flow[64], and an increase in the coagulability of blood that involves numerous alterations in the platelet, coagulation, and fibrinolytic systems[65-68]. Most of these changes are similar to changes that are seen in the latter part of pregnancy, and appear to be stimulated by the estrogenic component of OCs. Because subclinical thrombosis has been found to occur far more frequently than VTE, the effects of OCs on the circulatory system that are most responsible for increasing the risk of VTE are probably those that involve a decrease in the ability to control the progression of intravascular coagulation by inactivating the enzyme thrombin (or certain of its antecedents)[44], or to dissolve fibrin clots that threaten to obstruct circulation by activating the enzyme plasmin (fibrinolysin) from its precursor, plasminogen[69].

The most important inhibitor of thrombin in plasma is antithrombin III (AT III), an enzyme which inactivates both thrombin and certain of the enzymes involved in the generation of thrombin, including activated factor X (Xa), which plays the critical role of converting prothrombin to thrombin[44,70,71]. The amount of AT III in plasma can be directly measured by quantitative assays and the activity of AT III in plasma can be indirectly measured by assays of the rate at which a test specimen of plasma inactivates a known quantity of thrombin or Xa[44,71]. In studies of individuals with a genetic deficiency of AT III, it has been found that the risk of VTE is increased[70,72,73] and that both the amount and the activity of AT III in plasma are considerably lower than below normal[44]. In studies of women using OCs, the findings have been somewhat different. The amount of AT III in plasma is normal or nearly normal, but the activity of AT III is decreased[44,71,74]. This decrease in the activity of AT III in current OC users appears to develop within the first month or so of OC use[74], to be unrelated to the duration of use[44], and to disappear within about one month after OCs are discontinued[74]. When current OC users and nonusers have been compared, it has been observed that the activity of AT III is decreased to the range of 60 percent of normal or lower in about 16 percent of current OC users, as compared to only about 2 percent of nonusers[44]. This is an important finding, because there is evidence that a decrease in the activity of AT III to the range of 50 percent of normal or lower leads to a substantial increase in the risk of VTE.[72] When women using different OC formulations have been compared, it has been further observed that the activity of AT III is decreased in direct relation to the estrogen content of the OCs being used. For example, a greater decrease in the activity of AT III has been found in women using OCs containing 75-150 mcg of EE or ME than in women using OCs containing only 50 mcg of EE or ME[75]. Also, no decrease in the activity of AT III has been observed in women using various progestogen-only OCs (with one exception)[76]. Finally, it has been found that the amount of AT III in plasma is lower in women with blood types A, B, and AB than in women with blood type O[77], although the question of whether OCs induce a critical decrease in the activity of AT III (i.e., to the range of 50 percent of normal or lower) more frequently in women with blood types A, B, or AB than in women with blood type O remains to be answered.

The capacity of blood to dissolve fibrin clots arises from the conversion of circulating plasminogen to plasmin (fibrinolysin), an enzyme which degrades both fibrin and fibrinogen[69]. Plasminogen is converted to plasmin by plasminogen activators, which are released from endothelial cells[69]. The amount of plasminogen activators that is present in endothelium can be measured by histochemical procedures and the ability to increase the spontaneous fibrinolytic activity of blood through accelerated release of plasminogen activators from endothelium can be measured by comparing the fibrinolytic activity of blood before and after venous occlusion[69]. In studies of individuals with a history of venous or arterial thromboembolic disease, it has been found that both the spontaneous fibrinolytic activity of blood and the fibrinolytic response to venous occlusion tend to be lower than normal[69,79-81]. Because of this, it may seem paradoxical that EE has been found to increase both the spontaneous fibrinolytic activity of blood and the fibrinolytic response to venous occulsion (medroxyprogesterone acetate does not appear to have these effects; other progestogens have not been studied)[69]. These effects of EE, however, have been shown to be accompanied by a decrease in the amount of plasminogen activators in endothelium[82]. Thus, the increased fibrinolytic activity that has been observed during exposure to EE and during OC use[66], probably represents an increase in the release of plasminogen activators from endothelium in response to increased intravascular coagulation, a response that may not be adequate in some women. This concept is supported by studies of women who have developed VTE during OC use. After OCs have been discontinued and recovery from VTE has occurred, the proportion of these women with lower than normal amounts of plasminogen activators in vein biopsy specimens, and with lower than normal fibrinolytic responses to venous occlusion, has been found to be larger than the corresponding proportion of women with similar characteristics (not using OCs, about the same age) who do not have a history of VTE[81,83]. The implication of this finding is that women who develop VTE during OC use are women who have an inherently lower than normal capacity to increase fibrinolytic activity in response to the increased intravascular coagulation that occurs during OC use.

Summary

Current information about OCs and the risk of VTE supports the following conclusions: Current OC use increases the risk of VTE. This increased risk does not persist in past OC users. In previously healthy women, the overall risk of superficial or deep VTE that is attributable to OCs is about two cases per 1000 current OC users per year. The risk of both superficial and deep VTE in current OC users is directly related to the estrogen content of the OCs being used, while only the risk of superficial VTE is (directly) related to the progestogen content. The risk of VTE that is attributable to OCs is higher in women with blood types A, B, or AB than in women with blood type O. The pathogenesis of VTE in current OC users involves an increase in the size of intravascular clots that are formed in response to thrombotic stimuli, and this increase in the size of intravascular clots is the result of estrogen-induced decreases in the activity of AT III and in the amount of plasminogen activators content in endothelium.

Myocardial Infarction and Stroke

In terms of the overall benefits and risks of OCs, the increased risk of VTE that was described previously appears to be an important source of mild illness (superficial VT) or moderate illness (deep VTE) that is attributable to OCs, but a very infrequent source of illness that is serious enough to result in death (from PE)[57,58]. In contrast, there is strong evidence that the increased risk of myocardial infarction (MI), thrombotic stroke, and hemorrhagic stroke that has been observed in current OC users is an important source of serious illness or death that is attributable to OCs in certain groups of women. In other women, fortunately, the attributable risk appears to be small[1]. This can be illustrated by the following two observations. First, vital statistics and numerous studies in Britain, the United States and similar countries have shown that the risk of MI and stroke (thrombotic and hemorrhagic) in nonpregnant women of reproductive age increases with age and is increased by the presence of risk factors other than age such as heavy cigarette smoking (MI, hemorrhagic stroke) and hypertension (MI, thrombotic stroke, hemorrhagic stroke)[3,84-93]. Second, studies of OCs and the risk of MI and stroke have usually found that the relative risk of MI or stroke, in current OC users as compared to nonusers, is similar in women of different ages and in women with and without risk factors such as heavy cigarette smoking[84,86,87,89-94]. The consequence of these two observations is that the risk of MI and stroke that is attributable to OCs is concentrated in older women (especially in women about 35 years of age or older) and in women who smoke cigarettes heavily or who have other risk factors for MI or stroke.

Current and Past OC Use

Most studies of OCs and the risk of MI have found that the pattern of risk in relation to current OC use is similar to the pattern that was described for VTE, i.e., the risk of MI is increased in current OC users, decreases within about one month after OCs are discontinued and, in current OC users, is unrelated to duration of use. Only one study of OCs and the risk of MI, however, has been large enough to thoroughly examine the effects of past OC use and duration of use on the risk of MI[95]. In this case-control study of 556 women who were hospitalized with first episodes of MI in the Northeastern United States from 1976-79 (and 2036 controls), there were three main findings. First, in women 25-49 years of age, the relative risk of MI, in current OC users as compared to never users, was about 3-4, and did not appear to be related to the duration of use. Second, the relative risk of MI in short term past OC users* (<5 years duration of use) as compared to never users was not increased (i.e., was not significantly greater than 1). Third, however, the relative risk of MI in long-term past OC users (≥5 years duration of use) as compared to never users was about 2 and this increased risk of MI in long-term past OC users appeared to persist up to 10 years after OCs had been discontinued[95].

The risk of thrombotic stroke has been found in numerous studies to be increased in current OC users but has not been observed to be increased in past OC users[45,48,50,94,96]. In contrast, two studies have provided evidence that the risk of subarachnoid hemorrhage (the most common form of hemorrhagic stroke in women of reproductive age) is increased in both current and past OC users[57,93]. These findings, however, are based upon a total of 37 cases of subarachnoid hemorrhage, all of which occurred before 1976 and all but three of which occurred in women 35 years of age or older[57,93]. In two larger studies of subarachnoid hemorrhage that occurred in women 15-44 years of age in 1976 (134 cases) and 1978 (158 cases), only borderline evidence of an increased risk in current or past OC users was found[97,98]. Although the results of the two studies of subarachnoid hemorrhage that occurred before 1976 appear to be in conflict with the two studies of subarachnoid hemorrhage that occurred during or after 1976, this conflict is probably more apparent than real. During the 1970s there were important changes in the pattern of OC use in relation to formulation (e.g., a decrease in the use of OCs containing >50 mcg of EE or ME)[3] and in the pattern of OC use in relation to age (e.g., a decrease in use by older women)[99]. Because of these changes, it is reasonable to conclude that the OC formulations that were most widely used before 1976 probably did increase the risk of subarachnoid hemorrhage in current and past OC users about 35 years of age or older. When women 15-44 years of age are merged together in an overall analysis of risk, however, the OC formulations that were most widely used during and after 1976 probably did not increase the risk of subarachnoid hemorrhage substantially in either current or past OC users.

Relative and Attributable Risk

Estimates of the incidence of MI and stroke (thrombotic and hemorrhagic combined) in current OC users and in nonusers, and estimates of the relative and attributable risk, are presented in Table 2. The estimates for MI are

*"Past OC users" are defined as women who have used OCs, but not within the past month.

Table 2. Oral Contraceptives and Risk of Myocardial Infarction and Stroke.

Category of disease and age (Years)	Incidence*		Relative* Risk	Attributable* Risk
	Current OC User	Nonuser		
	Cases per 100,000 women per year			Cases per 100,000 current OC users per year
Myocardial Infarction†[84,86,70]				
30-39	11	4	3	7
40-44	89	22	4	67
Stroke†† (thrombotic and hemorrhagic combined), women of reproductive age generally[99,100]	47	10	5	37

*All estimates are rounded to the nearest integer.
†The estimates are derived from data about non-fatal and fatal M.I. in the references cited. About one-half of the MI cases were fatal. The attributable risk is concentrated in cigarette smokers and in women with other risk factors (see Table 4).
††The estimates are averages from the references cited. About 5-10% of the strokes were fatal: Most of the fatalities were due to subarachnoid hemorrhage. The attributable risk is concentrated in women about 35 years of age and older and in women with other risk factors.

based upon case-control studies of nonfatal and fatal MI that occurred in Britain during the late 1960s to mid-1970s[84,86,87]. The estimates for stroke are based upon the cohort studies in Britain, and pertain to about the same period of time[4,57,58,100]. Studies in the United States and other countries have yielded similar results but provide less information about attributable risk[89-96].

The figures in Table 2 illustrate two major findings. The relative risk of MI in current OC users as compared to nonusers is similar in women 30-39 years of age and 40-44 years of age (i.e., about 3-4)[84,86,87]. The incidence of MI in nonusers, however, increases from about 4 cases per 100,000 women per year in women 30-39 years of age to about 22 cases per 100,000 women per year in women 40-44 years of age[84,86,87]. Thus, the risk of MI that is attributable to OCs increases from only about 7 cases per 100,000 current OC users per year in women 30-39 years of age to about 67 cases per 100,000 current OC users per year in women 40-44 years of age. About one-half of the MI cases that are attributable to OCs were fatal[84,86,87].

In women of reproductive age the risk of stroke that is attributable to OCs is about 37 cases per 100,000 current OC users per year (about 5-10% of these strokes were fatal[4,100]. Most of the fatalities were due to subarachnoid hemorrhage)[57,58]. Although estimates of the risk of stroke that is attributable to OCs in women of different ages are not available, it is known that the incidence of stroke in women in countries such as Britain and the United States increases markedly between the ages 25-34 and 35-44[3], while the relative risk of stroke, in current OC users as compared to nonusers, does not appear to decrease[94]. Because of this, the risk of stroke that is attributable to OCs is undoubtedly much lower than 37 cases per 100,000 current OC users per year in women less than 35 years of age, and correspondingly higher in women about 35 years of age or older.

Table 3. Oral Contraceptives and Risk of Mortality from All Circulatory Diseases.

Mortality Rates*			Relative Risk*		Attributable Risk*	
Current OC User	Past OC User	Never-User	Current OC User vs. Never-user	Past OC User vs. Never-user	Current OC User vs. Never-user	Past OC User vs. Never-user
Deaths per 100,000 women per year					Deaths per 100,000 women per year	
29	31	7	4	4	22	24

*All estimates are rounded to the nearest integer, and refer to women of reproductive age generally: The source is reference 57. Most of the deaths were from ischemic heart disease or subarachnoid hemorrhage. The attributable risk is concentrated in women about 35 years of age or older and in cigarette smokers.

This pattern of attributable risk is similar to the pattern for MI.

Little information is available about the overall risk of MI and stroke (i.e., nonfatal and fatal combined) that is attributable to past OC use. Estimates are available, however, of death rates from all circulatory disease combined in current OC users, past OC users, and never users[57]. These estimates are presented in Table 3. It appears that, in women of reproductive age generally, the risk of death from all circulatory disease combined that is attributable to OCs is in the range of 22-24 deaths per 100,000 women per year for both current and past OC users[57]. It should be noted, however, that 37 of the 65 deaths upon which this figure is based (and the majority of the excess deaths in current and past OC users) were due to ischemic heart disease or subarachnoid hemorrhage. Furthermore, the deaths were concentrated in women about 35 years of age or older (54 of the 65), and the deaths in current and past OC users were concentrated in women who smoked cigarettes[57]*.

Estrogen/Progestogen Content of OCs

In current OC users, the risk of MI and stroke (most data pertain to thrombotic stroke) appears to be directly related to both the estrogen and the progestogen content of the OCs being used, although information about this is fragmentary[59,60]. If the progestogen content of OCs is ignored and if older (1970) and more recent (1980) findings are combined, it appears that a decrease in the estrogen content of OCs from 100-150 mcg of EE or ME to 30 mcg is accompanied by a substantial decrease in the risk of MI and stroke in current OC users. This decrease might be as

* Subsequent to the preparation of this article, the author became aware of a recent study which does provide information about the overall risk of MI, stroke, and other arterial disease that is attributable to past OC use (i.e., the risk of nonfatal and fatal arterial disease combined). This study provides further evidence of an increased risk of arterial disease in past OC users that is concentrated in women about 35 years of age or older and in women who smoke cigarettes heavily. The reference is: Royal College of General Practitioners' Oral Contraception Study. Incidence of arterial disease among oral contraceptive users. J Roy Coll Gen Pract. 1983; 33: 75-82.

large as 80 percent[59,60]. Some of the decrease, however, may be related to changes in the progestogen content of OCs. There is evidence that the risk of MI and stroke is about 1.5-2 times greater in women using OCs containing 3-4 mg of norethindrone acetate with 50 mcg of EE than in women using OCs containing only 1-2 mg of norethindrone acetate with 50 mcg of EE (similar findings have also been observed for norgestrel)[60]. Little information is available about the estrogen/progestogen content of OCs and the risk of MI and subarachnoid hemorrhage in past OC users.

OCs and Other Risk Factors

The major factors other than age that have been found to increase the risk of MI in women of reproductive age in Britain and the United States who are not using OCs are cigarette smoking (especially $\geq$ 15 per day), a history of preeclamptic toxemia or hypertension, type II hyperlipoproteinemia and diabetes mellitus[84,85,88-91] and for thrombotic stroke, hypertension[92] and for hemorrhagic stroke, cigarette smoking and hypertension[92,93]. In general, OCs have been found to magnify the increased risk of MI and stroke that occur in the presence of these other risk factors, in the same way that OCs have been found to magnify the increasing risk of MI or stroke that occurs with increasing age[84,89-93]. Cigarette smoking, however, appears to be far more prevalent than other risk factors for MI and stroke in women of reproductive age in countries such as Britain and the United States[84,88,90,92]. One study in the United States shows that 40 percent of all women 20-49 years of age who were admitted to hospitals during 1976-79 for reasons other than cardiovascular disease smoked $\geq$ 15 cigarettes per day, whereas fewer than 15% had a history of preeclamptic toxemia, hypertension, hyperlipoproteinemia or diabetes mellitus[88,90]. Because of this, the risk of MI and stroke that is attributable to OCs in women with risk factors other than age is primarily a risk that is attributable to OCs in women who smoke cigarettes.

The data in Table 2 merge the risk of MI and stroke that is attributable to OCs in women who do smoke cigarettes with the risk in women who do not smoke cigarettes. In Table 4, the risk of MI that is attributable to current OC use in women who smoked cigarettes heavily ($\geq$ 15 per day) is separated from the attributable risk in non-smokers or light smokers ($<$ 15 per day). The data are from the same sources as those in Table 2[84,86,87]. In Table 4, it can be seen that the relative risk of MI, in current OC users as compared to non-users, is similar for younger and older women and for women who do and do not smoke cigarettes heavily. The risk of MI that is attributable to OCs, however, increases from only about 4 cases per 100,000 current OC users per year in women 30-39 years of age who do not smoke cigarettes heavily to about 185 cases per 100,000 current OC users per year in women 40-44 years of age who smoke cigarettes heavily[84,86,87]. Furthermore, the information that is available about current OC use, age, cigarette smoking, and the risk of subarachnoid hemorrhage or other hemorrhagic stroke is indicative of a pattern of risk that is similar to the pattern for MI[57,92,93]. Little information is available about the risk of MI and stroke that is attributable to past OC use in women with risk factors other than age.

Pathogenesis of MI and Stroke in OC Users

The studies of OCs and the risk of MI indicate that the effects of OCs on the circulatory system that are most responsible for increasing

Table 4. Oral Contraceptives, Cigarette Smoking, and Risk of Myocardial Infarction.

Age (Years)	Cigarettes Smoked Daily	Incidence*		Relative* Risk	Attributable* Risk
		Current OC User	Non-user		
		Cases per 100,000 women per year			Cases per 100,000 current OC users per year
30-39	0-14	6	2	3	4
	>15	30	11	3	19
40-44	0-14	47	12	4	35
	>15	246	61	4	185

*All estimates are rounded to the nearest integer. The estimates are derived from the data in references 84, 86, 87 with the formula:

$$I_{total}=[I_{0-14}][P_{0-14}] + RR_{>15 vs. 0-14} [I_{0-14}][I-P_{0-14}],$$

where I_{total} denotes the incidence in current OC users or non-users (from Table 2), I_{0-14} the incidence in smokers of 0-14 cigarettes per day, P_{0-14} the proportion of controls who smoke 0-14 cigarettes per day, and $RR_{>15 \text{ vs. } 0-14}$ the relative risk in smokers of >15 cigarettes per day as compared to smokers of 0-14.

the risk of MI probably involve two components. Effects of current OC use that are unrelated to duration of use and that disappear when OCs are discontinued, and effects of past OC use that are directly related to duration of use and that persist after OCs are discontinued.

Postmortem examinations of women who have died from MI while using OCs indicate that MI in current OC users is more likely to be thrombotic than atheromatous in origin[86]. The effects of current OC use that seem most likely to increase the risk of coronary thrombosis are of two types. First, there is evidence that platelet hyperactivity is important in the pathogenesis of coronary (or other arterial) thrombosis[70], and OCs have been found to accelerate platelet aggregation[68,101] and to increase platelet prothrombin converting (factor III) activity[68,102]. Second, fibrin deposition is necessary for platelet aggregation to become irreversible[70], and the effects of OCs on the activity of AT III[44,71] and the amount of plasminogen activators in endothelium[69,82] which were described previously appear to enhance the formation and accumulation of fibrin. The estrogenic component of OCs is believed to be primarily responsible for accelerating platelet aggregation[68] and for decreasing the activity of AT III[75,76] and the amount of plasminogen activators in endothelium[69,82]. Information about the separate effects of estrogens and progestogens on platelet prothrombin-converting activity is not available. It is probable that these effects of OCs are all effects of current OC use that are unrelated to duration of use and that disappear when OCs are discontinued, although this pattern has been described only for a decrease in the activity of AT III[44]. How these effects of current OC use magnify the increasing risk of MI that occurs with increasing age, or in the presence of risk factors for MI other than age, has not been established. An attractive possibility, however, is that age, cigarette smoking, and other risk factors for MI increase the occurrence of subclinical thrombosis in coronary arteries, and that the effects of current OC use increase the probability that subclinical coronary thrombosis will progress to coronary occlusion.

Information from postmortem examinations of women who have died from MI after long-term past OC use is not available. The most likely source of an increased risk of MI in long-term past OC users, however, is accelerated atherogenesis, and OCs have been observed to have potentially deleterious effects on each of the three major factors that have been found to influence the risk of atherosclerotic cardiovascular disease (blood pressure, an increase appears to accelerate atherogenesis; glucose tolerance, a decrease appears to accelerate atherogenesis; and high-density lipoprotein cholesterol concentration, a decrease appears to accelerate atherogenesis)[4,103-111]. Although all of these effects of OCs appear to be effects of current OC use that disappear when OCs are discontinued, any cumulative effect (i.e., related to duration of use) that they have on atherosclerosis seems likely to persist after discontinuation.

OCs have been found to elevate blood pressure in most women[107,108]. On average, the elevation in blood pressure in current OC users is small (about 1-2 mm Hg diastolic, 5 mm Hg systolic), but does apparently lead to a 3-6 fold increase in the risk of overt hypertension[4,107]. The risk of (overt) hypertension that is attributable to OCs has been observed to increase with increasing age (becoming substantial only in women about 35 years of age or older)[107], with increasing duration of use[4] and in direct relation to the amount of norethindrone acetate in OCs containing this progestogen[103]. It seems plausible that factors such as a family history of hypertension or a history of renal disease may also increase the risk of hypertension that is attributable to OCs, but this has not been established.

OCs have been found to decrease glucose tolerance in most women[108-109]. On average, the decreased glucose tolerance in current OC users appears to be small (an increase of about 11 mg per deciliter in 1-hour serum glucose), to be unrelated to duration of use, and to be only additive to the effects of other risk factors for decreased glucose tolerance such as age, obesity and a family history of diabetes[108]. Nevertheless, the level of glucose tolerance in current OC users does appear to be shifted to the level in non-users who are about 7-8 years older[108]. The decreased glucose tolerance in current OC users has been found to be directly related to the estrogen content of the OCs being used[109,110]. Of particular importance is the finding that OCs containing relatively small amounts of estrogen (e.g., 35 mcg of EE) do not decrease glucose tolerance to any appreciable extent[110]. Finally, it has been observed that estrogens given without progestogen do not decrease glucose tolerance[109], indicating that decreased glucose tolerance in current OC users represents an interplay between the estrogenic and progestogenic components of OCs.

The progestogenic components of OCs have been found to decrease HDL-C concentration, whereas the estrogenic components have been found to increase HDL-C concentration[104,111]. Thus, the net effect of different OC formulations on HDL-C concentration appears to depend entirely upon the specific estrogen/progestogen content. A study in the United States has provided information about the effects of 13 different OC formulations on HDL-C concentration. Of the 13 OC formulations, five were combined formulations containing 50 mcg of EE or ME (i.e., the type of OC formulation that was extensively used in Britain, the United States and similar countries during the late 1960s to mid-1970s)[104]. Two of these five OC formulations were found to decrease HDL-C concentration (mean decrease of about 10 mg per deciliter, or 16 percent), whereas the other three were found to have no effect on HDL-C concentration[104]. Of the two OC formulations that were found to decrease HDL-C concentration, one contained norethindrone acetate (2.5 mg) and the other contained norgestrel (0.5 mg); these progestogens appear to have strong anti-estrogenic effects, and thus may overpower the tendency of the estrogenic component of OCs to increase HDL-C concentration[104].

The studies of OCs and the risk of stroke indicate that the effect of OCs on the circulatory system that are most important for increasing the risk of thrombotic stroke are probably effects of current OC use that are unrelated to duration of use and that disappear when OCs are discontinued (e.g., accelerated platelet aggregation). For subarachnoid hemorrhage, however, it is likely that effects of past OC use that are directly related to duration of use and that persist when OCs are discontinued are also important (e.g., any cumulative effect of sustained blood pressure elevation)[57,93]. The distinction that has been made here between the effects of current and past OC use on the risk of MI and stroke is somewhat artificial, however. It seems likely that the effects of current OC use on blood pressure, glucose tolerance, and HDL-C concentration described above increase the risk of arterial thrombosis in addition to (probably) accelerating atherogenesis. Evidence that the risk of MI and stroke in current OC users is directly related to the amount of norethindrone acetate or norgestrel in OCs containing these progestogens suggests that this may be so[60].

<u>Summary</u>

Current information about OCs and the risk of MI and stroke supports the following conclusions. Current OC use increases the risk of MI, thrombotic stroke and hemorrhagic stroke (primarily subarachnoid hemorrhage), and some increase in the risk of MI and subarachnoid hemorrhage persists in long-term past OC users. The risk of MI and stroke that is attributable to current OC use is strongly influenced by age and by the presence of other risk factors, such as cigarette smoking. For example, the risk of MI that is attributable to OCs is only about 4 cases per 100,000 current OC users per year in women 30-39 years of age who do not smoke cigarettes heavily, but increases to about 185 cases per 100,000 current OC users per year in women 40-44 years of age who smoke cigarettes heavily. The risk of MI and subarachnoid hemorrhage that is attributable to past OC use is probably also concentrated in women about 35 years of age or older who smoke cigarettes heavily. The risk of MI and stroke in current OC users is directly related to both the estrogen and the progestogen content of the OCs being used. Little information is available about the estrogen/progestogen content of OCs and the risk of MI and stroke in past OC users; the pathogenesis of MI and stroke in OC users involves both effects of current OC use that are unrelated to duration of use and that disappear when OCs are discontinued (e.g., accelerated platelet aggregation, a decrease in the activity of AT III, a decrease in the amount of plasminogen activators in endothelium), and effects of past OC use that are directly related to duration of use and that persist when OCs are discontinued (e.g., any cumulative effects of sustained blood pressure elevation, decreased glucose tolerance, and decreased HDL-C concentration).

BENEFICIAL EFFECTS

There are 8 diseases for which a decreased risk in OCs users has been described; benign breast disease, functional ovarian cysts, iron deficiency anemia, pelvic inflammatory disease, ectopic pregnancy, rheumatoid arthritis, endometrial cancer and ovarian cancer[2]. In the United States, it has recently been estimated that the aggregate decrease in the risk of these diseases that is attributable to OCs prevents about 500-600 hospitalizations per 100,000 current and past OC users per year[2]. This is a rough estimate, but it does clearly suggest that the "attributable benefit" in OC users is substantial. Of the eight diseases described above, benign breast disease is the prototype, and will be considered in the greatest detail.

Benign Breast Disease

The major forms of benign breast disease (BBD) in countries such as Britain and the United States are fibrocystic disease (or chronic cystic mastitis) and fibroadenoma[112-114]. In addition, there is a miscellaneous group of "other" BBD (fat necrosis, acute mastitis, nipple discharge, etc.)[115]. In general, fibroadenoma and the various types of "other" BBD appear to be well-defined entities[114,115]. Fibrocystic disease, however, encompasses a spectrum of disorders which differ in important ways (e.g., the amount of epithelial proliferation or atypia), and there is no universally accepted system for classifying the specific types of fibrocystic disease[112,116]. Furthermore, conditions such as fibrocystic disease and fibroadenoma can occur together[112,113]. Thus, it is not surprising that information about the occurrence of BBD, the malignant potential of different forms or specific types is somewhat inconsistent in certain areas. What is surprising, perhaps, is the overall consistency with which OCs have been shown to decrease the risk of BBD[4,15,103,112,114-126]. Consideration will first be given to information about the occurrence and characteristics of BBD in general, and then to the evidence that OCs decrease the risk of BBD.

Occurrence/Characteristics of BBD

The physical manifestations of BBD, and the interpretation of those manifestations by women and their physicians, can vary widely[112]. Thus, little information is available about the incidence of "any" BBD (i.e., regardless of manifestations), although a few autopsy studies in the United States do suggest that most women develop some histologically evident BBD during their lives[112]. Estimates are available, however, of the incidence of BBD diagnosed by biopsy or by clinical observation. Estimates of this type are presented in Table 5, which pertains to the incidence of fibrocystic disease, fibroadenoma, and "mixed" lesions (fibrocystic disease with fibroadenoma) diagnosed by biopsy in the Greater Boston area of the United States during 1968-69 (Greater Boston Study)[113], and the incidence of fibrocystic disease and fibroadenoma diagnosed by biopsy, breast lumps observed clinically but not biopsied (most of these were probably fibrocystic disease), and "other" diagnosed BBD in the Oxford/Family Planning Association Study in Britain during 1968-79 (Oxford/FPA Study)[114]. These two studies provide more comprehensive information about the incidence of BBD than other studies and are emphasized here for this reason. It should be noted, however, that the data from both studies merge the incidence of BBD in OC users with the incidence in nonusers, and thus may somewhat under-represent the incidence that would be observed in the

Table 5. Incidence of Benign Breast Disease.

Age (Years)	Incidence*							
	Fibrocystic Disease†		Fibroadenoma†		Mixed Lesions† (Fibrocystic/ Fiberoadenoma)	Unbiopsied Breast Lumps††	"Other" Diagnosed BBD§
	Greater Boston[113]	Oxford/ FPA[114]	Greater Boston	Oxford/ FPA	Greater Boston	Oxford/FPA	Oxford/FPA
	Cases per 100,000 women per year						
15-19	7	-¶	15	-¶	5	-¶	-¶
25-29	145	127	133	39	23	210	35
35-39	213	173	48	66	27	274	63
45-49	310	228	33	76	21	417	76
55-59	50	-¶	0	-¶	2	-¶	-¶

* All estimates are rounded to the nearest integer.
† Diagnosed by biopsy.
†† Observed clinically.
§ Conditions such as fat necrosis, acute mastitis, nipple discharge, etc.
¶ No estimates available.

absence of OCs (see OCs and Risk of BBD). No estimates of OC use are available for the Greater Boston Study specifically, but it has been estimated that about 22 percent of married women in the United States generally were using OCs in 1970[127]. In contrast, 57 percent of the 17,032 women in the Oxford/FPA Study were using OCs when they were enrolled during 1968-74[100]. Thus, it is likely that the data about the incidence of BBD from the Oxford/FPA Study pertain somewhat more to OC users than the data from the Greater Boston Study.

The data in Table 5 illustrate three major findings. The incidence of BBD is low prior to the age of 20. Subsequently, however, the incidence increases rapidly with age and remains high until after the age of 50, when a sharp decline occurs. In the Oxford/FPA study, the combined incidence of fibrocystic disease, fibroadenoma, unbiopsied breast lumps, and "other" diagnosed BBD in women 25-29 years of age is about 411 cases per 100,000 women per year. In women 45-49 years of age this incidence is increased to about 797 cases per 100,000 women per year, or almost 1 case per 100 women per year[114].

The incidence of fibrocystic disease is somewhat higher in the Greater Boston Study than in the Oxford/FPA Study, but the pattern of increasing incidence with increasing age until after the age of 50 is similar in the two studies[113,114]. In contrast, the incidence of fibroadenoma in the Greater Boston Study peaks in women 25-29 years of age at about 133 cases per 100,000 women per year and then declines rapidly with increasing age, while the incidence of fibroadenoma in the Oxford/FPA Study is only about 39 cases per 100,000 per year in women 25-29 years of age and then increases somewhat with age (this increase, however, is not statistically significant). The major finding about the incidence of fibroadenoma in Table 5 is the absence in the Oxford/FPA Study of the large peak in incidence in women 25-29 years of age that is present in the Greater Boston Study:

This finding may in part reflect the more frequent OC use by women in the Oxford/FPA Study than by women in the Greater Boston Study[100,113,114,127].

In the Oxford/FPA study, the incidence of unbiopsied breast lumps is higher than the combined incidence of fibrocystic disease and fibroadenoma at all ages (overall, about 27% higher)[114]. This finding is indicative of a trend that is characteristic of many diseases, i.e., the more obvious cases represent only a fraction of the total. Thus, the incidence of "any" BBD in countries such as Britain and the United States is probably much higher than indicated by the figures in Table 5 for BBD diagnosed by biopsy or observed clinically.

A variety of studies in Britain and the United States have provided information about the risk of BBD in relation to factors other than age (or OCs) such as race, menstrual/reproductive history, and so forth. In addition, numerous other studies have provided information about the malignant potential of BBD[112]. Although many of the specific findings in these areas are somewhat inconsistent, two of the more general findings are well-established and are important for interpreting the decreased risk of BBD in OC users.

Numerous studies have shown that the risk of breast cancer is increased in women with a family history of the disease, and that the risk increases with decreasing age at menarche, increasing age at first childbirth, and increasing age at menopause[128]. The pattern of risk for BBD (most data pertain to fibrocystic disease), however, does not appear to be closely related to the pattern for breast cancer: The clearest findings are that the risk of BBD is unrelated to age at menarche, and is unrelated or at most weakly related to age at first childbirth[112]. There is some evidence that nulliparity, low parity, and late menopause may increase the risk of BBD, but these are inconsistent findings[112]. Finally, a clear increase in the risk of BBD has not been observed in women with a family history of breast cancer, although it has been suggested that some increase in risk may occur with certain types of family history[112]. These findings support the conclusion that a large portion of BBD is not closely related to breast cancer; certain types, however, may be more closely related.

Although a large portion of BBD does not appear to be closely related to breast cancer, there is strong evidence that a history of BBD is a risk factor for breast cancer. Most estimates of the relative risk of breast cancer, in women with prior BBD (diagnosed by biopsy) as compared to women with no prior BBD, are in the range of 2-5[112,128]. These findings highlight the importance of certain studies which have shown that the risk of breast cancer in women with a history of BBD is concentrated in women who have had certain forms or specific types of BBD[112]. Because of variation in the criteria that have been employed for classifying different forms or specific types of BBD, these studies are somewhat difficult to interpret, but it does appear that the risk of breast cancer is increased in women with a history of fibrocystic disease or "mixed" lesions, but may not be increased in women with a history of fibroadenoma alone, and the risk of breast cancer in women with a history of fibrocystic disease is higher for fibrocystic disease with epithelial proliferation or atypia than for fibrocystic disease without these characteristics[112].

OCs and Risk of BBD

The evidence that OCs decrease the risk of BBD is impressive. Of 16 studies in Britain, the United States, and other countries which are pertinent to this issue, 14 clearly show a decreased risk of BBD in OC users, including eight case-control studies[15,46,114-122], four cohort studies[4,100,123,124], and two sectional studies*[128,129]. In the aggregate, these 15 studies provide convincing evidence that OCs decrease the risk of fibrocystic disease and fibroadenoma diagnosed by biopsy and breast lumps observed clinically but not biopsied (most of these are probably fibrocystic disease). These findings are particularly clear in the recent and comprehensive Oxford/FPA Study, which also suggests that OCs may decrease the risk of "other" BBD to some extent[114].

Most information about the risk of BBD in relation to current OC use vs. past use, time since last use and duration of use supports the following conclusions. The decreased risk of fibrocystic disease, fibroadenoma and unbiopsied breast lumps in OC users occurs primarily in current or moderately recent (i.e., within about one year) OC users who have used OCs for about two years or longer. The risk of fibrocystic disease and unbiopsied breast lumps is not decreased in women who have used OCs for less than about two years. The risk of fibroadenoma may be decreased in these women, but this is an inconsistent finding. There is little or no persistent decrease in the risk of fibrocystic disease, fibroadenoma or unbiopsied breast lumps in past OC users who have discontinued OCs for more than about one year[4,15,46,100,103,114-126].

Estimates of the relative risk of BBD in ever users and current users of OCs as compared to never users are presented in Table 6. These estimates are derived from the Oxford/FPA Study[114], and pertain to fibrocystic disease and fibroadenoma diagnosed by biopsy, and to breast lumps observed clinically but not biopsied. Most other studies have yielded similar results but are less comprehensive.

The figures in Table 6 illustrate three major findings. In ever users of OCs as compared to never users, the overall relative risk of BBD, when duration of use is disregarded, is about 0.7 for fibrocystic disease, 0.4 for fibroadenoma and 0.6 for unbiopsied breast lumps[114]. When duration of use is taken into account, however, it is seen that the relative risk in women who have used OCs for $<$ 2 years is about 1.3 for fibrocystic disease and about 0.8 for unbiopsied breast lumps, while the relative risk in women who have used OCs for $\geq$ 2 years is about 0.6 for fibrocystic disease and about 0.5 for unbiopsied breast lumps. The relative risk of fibroadenoma in women who have used OCs for $<$ 2 years is about 0.4, which is essentially the same as the relative risk of about 0.3 in women who have used OCs for $\geq$ 2 years[114].

In current or moderately recent OC users as compared to never users, the overall relative risk of BBD, when duration of use is disregarded, is about 0.5 for fibrocystic disease, 0.3 for fibroadenoma and 0.5 for unbiopsied breast lumps[114]. When duration of use is taken into account, the relative risk of fibrocystic disease, in current OC users as compared

*The one cohort study which does not clearly demonstrate a decreased risk of BBD in OC users does show a trend in that direction[130]. The one case-control study which does not show any decreased risk involved OC users whose median duration of use was only about 6-7 months[129]. This duration of use appears to be too short to decrease the risk of BBD (see Current and Past OC use.).

Table 6. Oral Contraceptives and Relative Risk of Benign Breast Disease.

OC Use	Relative Risk*		
	Fibrocystic Disease†	Fibroadenoma††	Unbiopsied Breast Lumps††
Never-use	1.0 (reference)	1.0 (reference)	1.0 (reference)
Ever-use, all durations	0.7	0.4	0.6
< 2 Years	1.3	0.4	0.8
≥ 2 Years	0.6§	0.3§	0.5§
Current or moderately recent use (discontinued < 1 year), all durations	0.5§	0.3§	0.5§
Current use, < 2 years	1.3	--¶	--¶
≥ 2 years	0.4§	--¶	--¶
Past use (discontinued ≥ 1 year), all durations	1.1§	0.8§	0.6§ (0.8 for ≥ 2 years)

* All estimates are rounded to one decimal point. The estimates are derived from the data in reference 114.
† Diagnosed by biopsy.
†† Observed clinically.
§ The estimates are averages of the year-by-year data in reference

to never users, is about 1.3 in women who have used OCs for < 2 years, while the relative risk in women who have used OCs for ≥ 2 years is about 0.4[114]. Corresponding figures are not available for the relative risk of fibroadenoma and unbiopsied breast lumps in current OC users according to duration of use.

In past OC users who have discontinued OCs for ≥ 1 year as compared to never users, the relative risk of BBD is about 1.1 for fibrocystic disease, 0.8 for fibroadenoma and 0.6 for unbiopsied breast lumps (this increases to 0.8 for ≥ 2 years)[114].

Because the incidence of BBD in countries such as Britain and the United States is high (Table 5), a decrease of 50 percent or more in the risk of BBD in current (or moderately recent) OC users means that the attributable benefit is large. In the United States, it has been estimated that OCs prevent about 235 hospitalizations for BBD per 100,000 current OC users per year*[2].

Both of the cohort studies in Britain show that the risk of BBD in users of combined OCs containing 1-4 mg of norethindrone acetate with 50

*All estimates of attributable benefit in this article pertain to the United States.

mcg of EE is decreased in direct relation to the amount of norethindrone acetate in the OCs used[103,114]. The Oxford/FPA Study* provides the more detailed analysis, which indicates that this finding pertains specifically to fibrocystic disease, and not to fibroadenoma, unbiopsied breast lumps, or "other" BBD[114]. For fibrocystic disease, however, the finding is strong. When ever users of OCs are grouped according to the formulation used longest, used first, and used last, the relative risk of fibrocystic disease, in ever users of (combined) OCs containing 1, 2.5-3, or 4 mg of norethindrone acetate with 50 mcg of EE as compared to never users of OCs, is in the range of 0.8-1.2 for OCs containing 1.0 mg of norethindrone acetate; 0.4-0.5 for OCs containing 2.5-3 mg, and 0.0-0.3 for OCs containing 4.0 mg (all estimates are rounded to the nearest decimal point)[114].

The previous discussion shows that a history of BBD (especially fibrocystic disease) increases the risk of breast cancer and that OCs decrease the risk of BBD (including fibrocystic disease). It is clear, however, that OCs do not decrease the risk of breast cancer as suggested by these findings. The most plausible explanation for this apparent paradox is probably that OCs decrease the risk of the large portion of BBD that is not closely related to breast cancer but do not decrease the risk of the specific types that are more closely related. The first study to provide information about OCs and the risk of different histopathological types of fibrocystic disease clearly supports this concept[116] but the one subsequent study of the same issue does not provide similar support[131]. More information about OCs and the risk of specific histopathological types of BBD is needed.

Summary

Current information about OCs and the risk of BBD supports the following conclusions. Current or moderately recent OC use that is about two years in duration or longer decreases the risk of BBD, including the risk of fibrocystic disease, fibroadenoma, and unbiopsied breast lumps. This decreased risk of BBD does not persist in past OC users who have discontinued OCs for more than about 1 year. OCs prevent an estimated 235 hospitalizations for BBD per 100,000 current OC users per year. The risk of fibrocystic disease in OC users decreases as the progestogen content of the OCs being used increases (this is not evident for fibroadenoma or unbiopsied breast lumps). OCs may decrease the risk of BBD to a greater extent for the large portion of BBD that is not closely related to breast cancer than for the specific types that are more closely related, although findings in this area are inconsistent.

Functional Ovarian Cysts

There is definite evidence that OCs decrease the risk of functional ovarian cysts, including follicular, granulosa lutein and theca lutein cysts[4,100,132]. This decreased risk has been observed in current OC users, but not in past users[4], and is apparently related to the suppression of ovulation that occurs during OC use. It has been estimated that OCs prevent about 35 hospitalizations for functional ovarian cysts per 100,000 current OC users per year[2].

Iron Deficiency Anemia

*The Oxford/FPA Study that is referred to here is a case-control analysis of data from the Oxford/FPA cohort study.

There is also firm evidence that OCs decrease the risk of iron deficiency anemia. This decreased risk has been observed in both current and past OC users[4]. In current OC users the explanation seems clear; a decrease in menstrual blood loss. An increase in iron reserves probably accounts for the persistence of a decreased risk in past users[4]. It has been estimated that OCs prevent about 320 episodes of iron deficiency anemia (regardless of hospitalization) per 100,000 current OC users per year[2]; no estimate is available for past users. This figure pertains to the United States. In countries where the prevalence of iron deficiency anemia is higher, the attributable benefit in OC users may be correspondingly higher.

Pelvic Inflammatory Disease

Until recently, the emphasis in most studies of contraception and the risk of pelvic inflammatory disease (PID) was on the increased risk that is evident in women using intrauterine devices (IUDs)[133]. In 1980, however, a reanalysis of 16 major studies in this area appeared which also emphasizes findings about OCs[134]. In this reanalysis, 11 studies are examined which provide estimates of the relative risk of PID in OC users as compared to women using other contraceptive methods (including the IUD). All of these estimates are in the range of 0.2-0.8, with a median of 0.4. Seven of the 11 studies also provide estimates of the relative risk of PID in OC users as compared to women using no contraceptive method. All but one of these estimates are in the range of 0.3-0.9, with a median of 0.6. On average, these findings indicate that the risk of PID in OC users is about 40 percent lower than the risk in women using no contraceptive method and is about 60 percent lower than the risk in women using other contraceptive methods[134].

The findings described above are persuasive but are somewhat general in nature. In 1981, however, a rigorous and detailed analysis of OCs and the risk of PID appeared which both confirms the general finding of a decreased risk in OC users and provides information about the risk of PID in relation to current vs. past OC use and duration of use[135]. This analysis is based upon the Women's Health Study, a comprehensive case-control study of contraception and the risk of PID, ectopic pregnancy and other gynecologic/ obstetric disorders which was carried out during the late 1970's at 16 hospitals in 9 cities across the United States[136]. In general, the cases and controls in the Women's Health Study were women 18-44 years of age who were hospitalized during 1976-78 and who were menstruating, sexually active, not surgically sterile (and with partners not sterile) and not recently pregnant at the time of hospitalization[136]. In the analysis of OCs and the risk of PID specifically, the cases comprise 648 women hospitalized with first episodes of PID and the controls comprise 2516 women with no history of PID who were hospitalized for conditions such as trauma, nose and throat ailments, respiratory tract infections, and so forth[135]. The results of this analysis are described below.

The overall relative risk of PID, in current OC users as compared to women using no contraceptive method, is about 0.5. In past OC users, however, the corresponding relative risk is about 1.0[135]. In current OC users as compared to women using no contraceptive method, the relative risk of PID is about 0.3 for OC use that is $>$ one year in duration, but is about 1.1 for OC use that is $\leq$ one year in duration[135]. In PID cases and controls with a prior history of PID (analyzed separately), the overall relative risk of PID in current OC users as compared to women using no contraceptive method is 0.5[135].

These findings demonstrate that the risk of PID in current OC users who have used OCs for more than one year is about 70 percent lower than the risk in women using no contraceptive method. The risk of PID is not decreased, however, in current OC users who have used OCs for less than about one year and is not decreased in past OC users[135]. There are two plausible explanations for this decreased risk of PID in current OC users. First, there is evidence that OCs make cervical mucus more tenacious, apparently by compacting the glycoprotein filaments. This may cause the mucus to become a mechanical or chemical barrier to organisms in the lower genital tract. Second, menstrual blood flow is generally less in OC users than in nonusers which may decrease the amount of medium that is available for bacterial growth[135].

In terms of the overall benefits and risks of OCs, the finding that OCs decrease the risk of PID is of major importance. First, because the incidence of PID in the United States and many other countries is high, the attributable benefit is large: It has been estimated that OCs prevent about 600 first episodes of PID (regardless of hospitalization) per 100,000 current OC users per year and that about 156 of these episodes involve hospitalization[2]. Second, in general, the risk of PID is concentrated in young women. A previous analysis of the Women's Health Study shows that the relative risk of PID, in women < 25 years of age as compared to women ≥ 25 years of age, is about 2[136]. This means that the attributable benefit of a decreased risk of PID in OC users is concentrated in precisely those women for whom the risk of cardiovascular disease that is attributable to OCs is the least.

Ectopic Pregnancy

There is unequivocal evidence that OCs greatly decrease the risk of ectopic pregnancy. The Women's Health Study, for example, shows that the relative risk of ectopic pregnancy in current OC users as compared to women using no contraceptive method is about 0.1, which means that current OC use decreases the risk of ectopic pregnancy by about 90 percent[136]. This decreased risk has not been observed in past OC users[136] and is obviously related to the suppression of ovulation that occurs during current OC use. The attributable benefit is large. It has been estimated that OCs prevent about 117 hospitalizations for ectopic pregnancy per 100,000 current OC users per year[2].

Rheumatoid Arthritis

Three studies have suggested that OCs may decrease the risk of rheumatoid arthritis, primarily in current OC users, but possibly in past users also[137-139]. These findings, however, should be regarded as tentative for two reasons. First, there is one other study of OCs and the risk of rheumatoid arthritis which shows no decreased risk in OC users[140]. Second, each of the four studies described here has important methodological limitations which restrict the value of the findings. Further research in this area is needed.

Endometrial and Ovarian Cancer

In the United States, it has recently been estimated that on an annual basis about 39,000 women are diagnosed as new endometrial cancer cases and about 3,000 die from the disease, and about 18,000 women are diagnosed as new ovarian cancer cases and about 11,400 die from the disease[141]. These estimates of morbidity and mortality highlight the importance of recent studies which demonstrate that combined OCs decrease the risk of endometrial cancer[17,142-144], OCs decrease the risk of ovarian cancer[18,145,146], and a decrease in the risk of endometrial and ovarian cancer persists for many years in past OC users[17,18]. These benefits of OCs are particularly clear in the March 1983 results from the Cancer and Steroid Hormones (CASH) Study[17,18] which will be emphasized here. Previous studies have yielded similar results but provide less detailed information.

The CASH Study is a population-based, case-control study of OCs and the risk of breast, endometrial, and ovarian cancer which has been carried out over the past five years in eight geographic areas of the United States which have population-based cancer registries. The cases comprise women identified from the cancer registries who were 20-54 years of age and received a histological diagnosis of primary breast, endometrial or ovarian cancer during December 1, 1980 - December 31, 1983. All accessible cases were interviewed within six months of diagnosis. The controls comprise women selected at random from the same eight geographic areas as the cases by means of the Waksberg method of random digit telephone dialing. The controls were also 20-54 years of age and were identified and interviewed at about the same time as the cases. Cases and controls were interviewed in their homes by means of a structured questionnaire designed to elicit information about contraceptive use, reproductive history, general medical and surgical history, demographic and social characteristics[16-18].

The final analyses of the CASH Study are still in progress and are scheduled for completion in 1984. Preliminary results are available however and appeared in March 1983[16-18]. For endometrial and ovarian cancer, these preliminary results pertain to cases diagnosed during December 1, 1980 - September 30, 1981[17-18]. The major findings about the relative risk of endometrial and ovarian cancer in OC users and about attributable benefits follows.

Relative Risk

In women who are not using OCs, there is strong evidence that the risk of endometrial cancer is increased in the presence of factors such as obesity, nulliparity and late menopause. These risk factors reflect hormonal states which involve increased estrogenic stimulation of the endometrium relative to the level of progestogenic stimulation and this "unopposed" estrogenic stimulation results in an increased risk of endometrial cancer[17]. In women who are using OCs, however, the pituitary-gonadal axis is suppressed, and estrogen/progestogen stimulation of the endometrium is determined largely by the composition of the OCs used. Based upon 187 cases of endometrial cancer and 1320 controls, the CASH Study shows several interesting findings in ever users of OCs as compared to never users.

The overall relative risk of endometrial cancer is about 0.5 in users of combined OCs, whereas the overall relative risk in users of sequential OCs is about 2.1[17]. With regard to duration of OC use, the relative risk of endometrial cancer in users of combined OCs is about 1.1 for $<$ 1 year of use, about 0.4 for 1-5 years, and about 0.6 for $>$ 5 years[17]. With regard to years since last OC use, the relative risk of endometrial cancer in users of combined OCs is about 0.6 for $<$ 5 years since last use, about 0.6 for 5-9 years and about 0.8 for $\geq$ 10 years[17]. With regard to parity, the relative risk of endometrial cancer in users of combined OCs is about 0.4 in nulliparous women, about 0.8 for parity 1-2 and about 1.0 for parity $\geq$ 3[17].

These findings support the following conclusions. Combined OCs decrease the risk of endometrial cancer while sequential OCs increase the risk. These conclusions are commensurate with the progestogen dominance of most combined OCs and the estrogen dominance of sequential OCs. In women who have used combined OCs for about one year or longer, the overall risk of endometrial cancer is decreased by about 40-60 percent. In past users of combined OCs, there is a persistent decrease in the risk of endometrial cancer for as long as 10 years after OCs have been discontinued and the decreased risk of endometrial cancer in users of combined OCs is concentrated almost entirely in nulliparous women, i.e., in women who would otherwise be at comparatively high risk[17].

In women who are not using OCs, the most impressive finding about the risk of ovarian cancer is that the risk increases as parity decreases[18]. There is evidence to support two explanations for this finding. In some women, hormonal or gonadal disorders may both decrease fertility (and thereby parity) and increase ovarian cancer risk and pregnancy itself appears to decrease the risk of ovarian cancer[18]. In women who are using OCs, some hormonal or gonadal disorders may be suppressed, and pregnancy is mimicked to a certain extent. Based upon 179 cases of ovarian cancer and 1642 controls, the CASH Study shows several findings in ever users of OCs as compared to never users. The overall relative risk of ovarian cancer in OC users is about 0.6. (Most of the data pertain to combined OCs)[18]. With regard to duration of OC use, the relative risk of ovarian cancer in OC users is about 1.0 for $<$ 3 months of use, about 0.7 for 3-11 months, about 0.8 for 1-2 years, about 0.5 for 3-4 years and about 0.4 for $\geq$ 5 years.[18] With regard to years since last OC use, the relative risk of ovarian cancer in OC users is about 1.0 for $<$ 1 year since last use (this estimate probably pertains to short-term OC users, see 2 above), about 0.6 for 1-4 years, about 0.5 for 5-9 years and about 0.5 for $\geq$ 10 years[18]. With regard to parity, the relative risk of ovarian cancer in OC users is about 0.3 in nulliparous women, about 0.8 for parity 1-2 and about 0.7 for parity $\geq$ 3[18].

These findings support the following conclusions. OCs decrease the risk of ovarian cancer. Because OCs mimic pregnancy to a certain extent, this finding is commensurate with evidence that pregnancy itself decreases ovarian cancer risk. In women who have used OCs for about three years or longer, the risk of ovarian cancer is decreased by about 50-60 percent. In past OC users, there is a persistent decrease in the risk of ovarian cancer for over 10 years after OCs have been discontinued. The decreased risk of ovarian cancer in OC users is concentrated in nulliparous women, who would otherwise be at comparatively high risk[18].

Attributable Benefit

The attributable benefits in OC users which have been discussed previously (i.e., for BBD, PID, etc.) pertain almost entirely to current OC users, of whom there are an estimated 8.5 million in the United States. In contrast, the attributable benefits for endometrial and ovarian cancer which are described below pertain to both current and past OC users, as represented by the ever users of OCs in the CASH Study and there are an estimated 39 million ever users of OCs (mostly combined OCs)[2].

Based upon the CASH Study, it has been estimated that OCs prevent about 5 hospitalizations for endometrial cancer per 100,000 ever users of combined OCs per year. For the United States as a whole, this corresponds to the prevention of about 2,000 hospitalizations for endometrial cancer per year[2].

Based upon the CASH Study, it has also been estimated that OCs prevent about five hospitalizations for ovarian cancer per 100,000 ever users of OCs per year. For the United States as a whole, this corresponds to the prevention of about 1700 hospitalizations for ovarian cancer per year[2].

CONCLUSIONS AND RECOMMENDATIONS

This overview of current information about OCs and the occurrence of disease supports the following general conclusions about OCs as they have been used by women during the past two decades and the following recommendations about the design of animal studies for evaluating new steroid contraceptive formulations.

1. Conclusion

The major adverse effect of OCs in women is an increased risk of cardiovascular disease. This increased risk occurs primarily in current OC users but there is some persistent risk in long-term past users. The risk is directly related to both the progestogen and estrogen content of OCs and the attributable risk is concentrated in women with other risk factors such as age and cigarette smoking. The pathogenesis of this risk involves OC-induced changes in factors such as AT III activity (the estrogens in OCs decrease AT III activity) and plasma lipids/lipoproteins (e.g., the progestogens in some OC formulations decrease HDL-C concentration to a greater extent than is counterbalanced by the estrogens).

Recommendation

Animal studies of new steroid contraceptive formulations should include evaluation of cardiovascular disease risk as a major component. This evaluation should focus primarily on the effects of current OC use, but also obtain information about the effects of long-term past use, compare the effects of new steroid contraceptive formulations with the effects of one or more widely used OC formulations such as an OC containing 1 mg. of norethindrone with 35 mcg. of EE and employ animal species which are as similar as possible to women with regard to cardiovascular disease risk factors such as age. Consideration should also be given to exposing a portion of the animals to cigarette smoke and evaluation of factors such as AT III activity and plasma lipids/lipoproteins prior to, during, and after OC exposure.

2. Conclusion

The adverse effects of OCs on the risk of neoplasia are limited and there are important beneficial effects. Long-term OC use definitely does increase the risk of hepatocellular adenoma but the attributable risk is small. Long-term OC use may also increase the risk of cervical cancer and dysplasia or the risk of malignant melanoma to a limited extent. OCs do not increase the risk of pituitary adenoma. Thus far, extensive studies indicate that OCs probably do not increase the risk of breast cancer, either overall, in long-term OC users, or in women with a family history of breast cancer, a history of BBD, or a history of OC use prior to first childbirth. Combined OCs decrease the risk of endometrial cancer, preventing about 5 hospitalizations per 100,000 ever users of combined OCs per year. OCs decrease the risk of ovarian cancer, preventing about four hospitalizations for ovarian cancer per 100,000 ever users of OCs per year.

In relation to this conclusion from current information about OCs and the risk of neoplasia, it should be noted that several major studies of OCs and other steroid contraceptives and the risk of breast, reproductive tract, and other cancer are currently in progress. Two of these studies are particularly important. The CASH Study, which is scheduled for completion in 1984, and which will provide much more detailed information about OCs and the risk of breast, endometrial and ovarian cancer in the United States than is currently available and the World Health Organization Collaborative Study of Neoplasia and Steriod Contraceptives, which will provide essential information about the controversial issue of depo-medroxyprogesterone acetate and the risk of breast cancer.

Recommendation

Information from the CASH Study, the WHO Study and other major studies about OCs, DMPA and the risk of neoplasia should be used to evaluate the relevance of different animal species for predicting the effects of new steroid contraceptive formulations on the risk of neoplasia in women. For example, an appropriate animal species should, when exposed to appropriate doses of widely used OC formulations, exhibit no increase in the incidence of pituitary adenoma, a decrease in the incidence of endometrial cancer (combined OCs) and a decrease in the incidence of ovarian cancer. The WHO Study will be of particular value for evaluating the relevance to women of the increased incidence of breast cancer that occurs in beagle dogs exposed to depo-medroxyprogesterone acetate.

3. Conclusion

The major beneficial effects of OCs, other than a decreased risk of endometrial cancer (combined OCs) and ovarian cancer, are a decreased risk of BBD, PID and ectopic pregnancy. OCs also decrease the risk of functional ovarian cysts, iron deficiency anemia and may decrease the risk of rheumatoid arthritis. In the aggregate, the beneficial effects of OCs prevent about 500-600 hospitalizations per 100,000 current and past OC users per year.

Recommendation

Animal studies of new steroid contraceptive formulations should include the evaluation of beneficial effects on the risk of disease in addition to the evaluation of adverse effects. Otherwise, the overall assessment of benefits and risks will be distorted.

REFERENCES

1. Stadel, BV: Oral contraceptives and cardiovascular disease. New Engl J Med, 305:612, 672, 1981.

2. Ory, HW: The noncontraceptive health benefits from oral contraceptive use. Fam Plan Perspect, 14:182, 1982.

3. Rinehart, W, Piotrow, P: Oral contraceptives-update on usage, safety, and side effects. Popul Rep [A], p 133, 1979.

4. Royal College of General Practitioners: Oral contraceptives and health. London, Pitman Medical, 1970.

5. MacMahon, B, Pugh, TF: Epidemiology: Principles and Methods. Boston, Little, Brown, 1970.

6. Royal College of General Practitioners Oral Contraceptive Study: Oral contraceptives and gallbladder disease. Lancet, 2:957, 1982.

7. WHO Scientific Group: Steroid contraception and the risk of neoplasia. WHO Tech Rep Ser, 619:1, 1978.

8. Kelsey, JL: A review of the epidemiology of human breast cancer. Epidemiol Rev, 1:74, 1979.

9. Baum, JK, Holtz, F, Bookstein, JJ, Klein, EW: Possible association between benign hepatomas and oral contraceptives. Lancet, 2:926, 1973.

10. Rooks, JB, Ory, HW, Ishak, KG, Strauss, LT, Greenspan, JR, Paganini-Hill, A, Tyler, CW: Epidemiology of hepatocellular adenoma: the role of oral contraceptive use. JAMA, 242:644, 1979.

11. Brinton, LA, Williams, RR, Hoover, RN, Stegens, NL, Feinleib, M, Fraumeni, JF: Breast cancer risk factors among screening program participants. J Natl Cancer Inst, 62:37, 1979.

12. Pike, MC, Henderson, BE, Casagrande, JT, Rosario, J, Gray, GE: Oral contraceptive use and early abortion as risk factors for breast cancer in young women. Brit J Cancer, 43:72, 1981.

13. Black, MM, Kwon, CS, Leis, HP, Barday, THC: Family history and oral contraceptives: unique relationship in breast cancer patients. Cancer, 46:2747, 1980.

14. Paffenbarger, RS, Kampert, JB, Chang H-G: Characteristics that predict risk of breast cancer before and after the menopause. Am J Epidemiol, 112:258, 1980.

15. Lees, AW, Burns, PE, Grace, M: Oral contraceptives and breast disease in premenopausal Northern Albertan women. Int J Cancer, 22:700, 1978.

16. The Centers for Disease Control Cancer and Steroid Hormones Study: Long-term oral contraceptive use and the risk of breast cancer. JAMA, 249:1591, 1983.

17. The Centers for Disease Control Cancer and Steroid Hormones Study: Oral contraceptive use and the risk of endometrial cancer. JAMA, 249:1600, 1983.

18. The Centers for Disease Control Cancer and Steroid Hormones Study: Oral contraceptive use and the risk of ovarian cancer. JAMA, 249: 1596, 1983.

19. Hulka, BS: Risk factors for cervical cancer. J Chron Dis, 35:3, 1982.

20. Swan, SH, Brown, WL: Oral contraceptive use, sexual activity, and cervical carcinoma. Am J Obstet Gynecol, 139:52, 1981.

21. Harris, RWC, Brinton, LA, Cowdell, RH, Skegg, DCG, Smith, PG, Vessey, MP, Doll, R: Characteristics of women with dysplasia or carcinoma in situ of the cervix uteri. Br J Cancer, 42:359, 1980.

22. Vessey, MP, Lawless, M, McPherson, K, Yeates, D: Neoplasia of the cervix uteri and contraception: possible adverse effect of the pill. Lancet, 2:930, 1983.

23. Ory, HW, Conger, SB, Naib, Z, Tyler, CW, Hatcher, RA: Preliminary analysis of oral contraceptive use and risk of developing premalignant lesions of the uterine cervix. In Garattini, S, Berendes, HW (Eds): Pharmacology of Steroid Contraceptive Drugs. New York, Raven Press, 1977, p 211.

24. Whitehead, N, Reyner, F, Lindenbaum, J: Megaloblastic changes in the cervical epithelium. JAMA, 226:1421, 1973.

25. Butterworth, CE, Hatch, KD, Gore, H, Mueller, H, Krumdieck, CL: Improvement in cervical dysplasia associated with folic acid therapy in users of oral contraceptives. Am J Clin Nutr, 39:73, 1982.

26. Edmondson, HA, Henderson, B, Benton, B: Liver cell adenomas associated with use of oral contraceptives. New Engl J Med, 294:470, 1976.

27. Beral, V, Ramcharan, S, Faris, R: Malignant melanoma and oral contraceptive use among women in California. Br J Cancer, 36:804, 1977.

28. Kay, CR: Malignant melanoma and oral contraceptives. Brit J Cancer, 44:479, 1981.

29. Holly, EA, Weiss, NS, Liff, JM: Cutaneous melanoma in relation to exogenous hormones and reproductive factors. JNCI, 70:827, 1983.

30. Beral, V, Shaw, H, Evans, S, et al: Malignant melanoma and oral contraceptive use. Final report to the National Institute of Child Health and Human Development. Contract N01-HD-8-2804, 1982.

31. Elashoff, RM, Hunter, JP, Mohilef, E: Epidemiology of melanoma. Final report to the National Institute of Child Health and Human Development, Contract N01-HD-8-2803, 1982.

32. Stevens, RG, Lee, JA, Moolgavkar, SH: No association between oral

contraceptives and malignant melanomas. New Engl J Med, 302:966, 1980.

33. Pituitary Adenoma Study Group: Pituitary adenomas and oral contraceptives: a multicenter case-control study. Fertil Steril, 39:753, 1983.

34. Annegers, JF, Coulam, CB, Abboud, CF, Laws, ER, Kurland, LT: Pituitary adenoma in Olmstead County, Minnesota 1935-1977. A report of an increasing incidence of diagnosis in women of child bearing age. Mayo Clin Proc, 53:641, 1978.

35. Sherman, BM, Harris, CE, Schlechte, J, Duello, TM, Halmi, NS, Van Gilder, S, Chapler, FK, Guenner, DK: Pathogenesis of prolactin-secreting pituitary adenomas. Lancet, 2:1019, 1978.

36. Teperman, L, Futterweit, W, Zappulla, R, Malis, L: Oral contraceptive history as a risk indicator in patients with pituitary tumors with hyperprolactinemia: a case comparison study of twenty patients. Neurosurgery, 7:571, 1980.

37. Committee on Safety of Medicines: Carcinogenicity tests of oral contraceptives: a report by the Committee on Safety of Medicines. London, HMSO, 1972.

38. Vessey, MP: Female hormones and vascular disease: epidemiologic overview. Brit J Fam Plann, Suppl:1, 1980.

39. Sagar, S, Stamatakis, JD, Thomas, DP, Kakkar, VV: Oral contraceptives, antithrombin-III activity, and postoperative deep-vein thrombosis. Lancet, 1:509, 1976.

40. Stamatakis, JD, Lawrence, D, Kakkar, VV: Surgery, venous thrombosis and anti-Xa. Brit J Surg, 64:709, 1977.

41. Alkjaersig, N, Fletcher, A, Burstein, R: Association between oral contraceptive use and thromboembolism: a new approach to its investigation based on plasma fibrinogen chromatography. Am J Obstet Gynecol, 122:199, 1975.

42. Royal College of General Practitioners' Oral Contraception Study: Oral contraceptives, venous thrombosis, and varicose veins. J R Coll Gen Pract, 28:393, 1978.

43. Vessey, MP: Steroid contraception, venous thromboembolism and stroke; data from countries other than the United States. In: Sciarra, JJ, Zatuchni, GI, Speidel, JJ (Eds): Risks, Benefits and Controversies in Fertility Control. Hagerstown, Maryland, Harper and Row, 1978, p 113.

44. Wessler, S, Gitel, SN, Wan, LS, Pasternack, BS: Estrogen-containing oral contraceptive agents: a basis for their thrombogenicity. JAMA, 236:2179, 1976.

45. Sartwell, PE, Masi, AT, Arthes, FG, Greene, G, Smith, HE: Thromboembolism and oral contraceptives; an epidemiologic case-control study, Am J Epidemiol, 90:365, 1969.

46. Boston Collaborative Drug Surveillance Program: Oral contraceptives and venous thromboembolic disease, surgically confirmed gallbladder disease, and breast tumors. Lancet, 1:1399, 1973.

47. Royal College of General Practitioners: Oral contraception and thromboembolic disease. J R Coll Gen Pract, 13:267, 1967.

48. Inman, WHW, Vessey, MP: Investigation of deaths from pulmonary, coronary, and cerebral thrombosis and embolism in women of childbearing age. Brit Med J, 2:193, 1968.

49. Vessey, MP, Doll R: Investigation of relation between use of oral contraceptives and thromboembolic disease. Brit Med J, 2:199, 1968.

50. Vessey, MP, Doll R: Investigation of relation between use of oral contraceptives and thromboemboic disease: a further report. Brit Med J, 2:651, 1969.

51. Vessey, MP, Doll R, Fairbairn, AS, Glober, G: Postoperative thromboembolism and the use of oral contraceptives. Brit Med J, 3:123, 1970.

52. Botiger, LE, Westerholm, B: Oral contraceptives and thromboembolic disease: Swedish experience. Acta Med Scand, 190:455, 1971.

53. Greene, GR, Sartwell, PE: Oral contraceptive use in patients with thromboembolism following surgery, trauma, or infection. Am J Public Health, 62:680, 1972.

54. Stolley, PD, Tonascia, JA, Tockman, MS, Sartwell, PE, Rutledge, AH, Jacobs, MP: Thrombosis with low-estrogen oral contraceptives. Am J Epidemiol, 102:197, 1975.

55. Maguire, MG, Tonascia, J, Sartwell, PE, Stolley, PD, Tockman, MS: Increased risk of thrombosis due to oral contraceptives: a further report. Am J Epidemiol, 110:188, 1979.

56. Petitti, DB, Wingerd, J, Pellegrin, F, Ramcharan, S: Oral contraceptives, smoking, and other factors in relation to risk of venous thromboembolic disease. Am J Epidemiol, 108:480, 1978.

57. Royal College of General Practitioners' Oral Contraception Study: Further analyses of mortality in oral contraceptive users. Lancet, 1:541, 1981.

58. Vessey, MP, McPherson, K, Yeates D: Mortality in oral contraceptive users. Lancet, 1:549, 1981.

59. Inman, WHW, Vessey, MP, Westerholm, B, Engelund, A: Thromboembolic disease and the steroidal content of oral contraceptives: a report to the Committee on Safety of Drugs. Brit Med J, 2:203, 1970.

60. Meade, TW, Greenberg, G, Thompson, SG: Progestogens and cardiovascular reactions associated with oral contraceptives and a comparison of the safety of 50-μg and 30-μg oestrogen preparations. Brit Med J, 280:1157, 1980.

61. Lawson, DH, Davidson, JF, Jick, H: Oral contraceptive use and venous thromboembolism: absence of an effect of smoking. Brit Med J, 2:729, 1977.

62. Jick, H, Slone, D, Westerholm, B, Inman, WHW, Vessey, MP, Shapiro, S, Lewis, GP, Worcester, J: Venous thromboembolic disease and ABO blood type: a cooperative study. Lancet, 1:539, 1969.

63. Irey, NS, Manion, WC, Taylor, HB: Vascular lesions in women taking oral contraceptives. Arch Pathol, 89:1, 1970.

64. Goodrich, SM, Wood, JE: Peripheral venous distensibility and velocity of venous blood flow during pregnancy or during oral contraceptive therapy. Am J Obstet Gynecol, 90:740, 1964.

65. Dugdale, M, Masi, AT: Hormonal contraception and thromboembolic disease: effects of the oral contraceptives on hemostatic mechanisms: a review of the literature. J Chronic Dis, 23:775, 1971.

66. Meade, TW, Brozovic, M, Chakrabarti, R, Howarth, DJ, North, WRS, Stirling, Y: An epidemiological study of the haemostatic and other effects of oral contraceptives. Brit J Haematol, 34:353, 1976.

67. Davies, JA, McNicol, GP: Blood coagulation in pathological thrombus formation and the detection in blood of a thrombotic tendency. Brit Med Bull, 34:113, 1978.

68. Poller, L: Oral contraceptives, blood clotting and thrombosis. Brit Med Bull, 34:151, 1978.

69. Astedt, B: On fibrinolysis in pregnancy, labour, puerperium and during treatment with sex steroids in human ontogenesis and in human organ culture. Acta Obstet Gynecol Scand [Suppl], 18:1, 1972.

70. Arkin, CF, Hartman, AS: The hypercoagulability states. CRC Crit Rev Clin Lab Sci, 10:397, 1979.

71. Petersen, C, Kelly, R, Minard, B, Cawley, LP: Antithrombin III: comparison of functional and immunologic assays. Am J Clin Pathol, 69:500, 1978.

72. Egeberg, O: Inherited antithrombin deficiency causing thrombophilia. Thromb Diath Haemorrh, 13:516, 1965.

73. von Kaulla, E, von Kaulla, KN: Deficiency of antithrombin III activity associated with hereditary thrombosis tendency. J Med, 3:349, 1972.

74. von Kaulla, E, Droegemueller, W, Aoki, N, von Kaulla, KN: Antithrombin III depression and thrombin generation acceleration in women taking oral contraceptives. Am J Obstet Gynecol, 109:868, 1971.

75. Conard, J, Samama, M, Salomon, Y: Antithrombin III and the oestrogen content of combined oestrogen-progestagen contraceptives. Lancet, 2:1148, 1972.

76. Conard J, Samama, M, Horellou, MH, Zorn, JR, Neau, C: Antithrombin III and oral contraception with progestagen-only preparation. Lancet, 2:471, 1979.

77. Fagerhol, MK, Abilgaard, U, Kornstad, L: Antithrombin-III concentration and ABO blood-groups. Lancet, 2:664, 1971.

78. Clayton, JK, Anderson, JA, McNicol, GP: Preoperative prediction of postoperative deep vein thrombosis. Brit Med J, 2:910, 1976.

79. Chakrabarti, R, Hocking, ED, Fearnley, GR, Mann, RD, Attwell, TN, Jackson, D: Fibrinolytic activity and coronary-artery disease. Lancet, 1:987, 1968.

80. Gritsyuk, AI, Schigelsky, VI: Evaluation of blood coagulation and prethrombotic state in patients with coronary atherosclerosis by application of controlled venous blockade. Circulation, 60:220A, 1979.

81. Dreyer, NA, Pizzo, SV: Blood coagulation and idiopathic thromboembolism among fertile women. Contraception, 22:123, 1980.

82. Astedt, B: Low fibrinolytic activity of veins during treatment with ethinyl estradiol. Acta Obstet Gynecol Scand, 50:279, 1971.

83. Astedt, B, Isacson, S, Nilsson, IM, Pandolfi, M: Thrombosis and oral contraceptives: possible predisposition. Brit Med J, 4:631, 1973.

84. Mann, JI, Vessey, MP, Thorogood, M, Doll R: Myocardial infarction in young women with special reference to oral contraceptive practice. Brit Med J, 2:241, 1975.

85. Mann, JI, Doll R, Thorogood, M, Vessey, MP, Waters, WE: Risk factors for myocardial infarction in young women. Brit J Prev Soc Med, 30:94, 1976.

86. Mann, JI, Inman, WHW: Oral contraceptives and death from myocardial infarction. Brit Med J, 2:245, 1975.

87. Mann, JI, Inman, WHW, Thorogood, M. Oral contraceptive use in older women and fatal myocardial infarction. Brit Med J, 2:445, 1976.

88. Slone, D, Shapiro, S, Rosenberg, L, Kaufman, DW, Hartz, SC, Rossi, AC, Stolley, PD, Miettinen, OS: Relation of cigarette smoking to myocardial infarction in young women. New Engl J Med, 298:1273, 1978.

89. Jick, H, Dinan, B, Rothman, KJ: Oral contraceptives and nonfatal myocardial infarction. JAMA, 239:1403, 1978.

90. Shapiro, S, Slone, D, Rosenberg, L, Kaufman, DW, Stolley, PD, Miettinen, OS: Oral contraceptive use in relation to myocardial infarction. Lancet, 1:743, 1979.

91. Rosenberg, L, Hennekens, CH, Rosner, B, Belanger, C, Rothman, KJ, Speizer, FE. Oral contraceptive use in relation to nonfatal myocardial infarction. Am J Epidemiol, 111:59, 1980.

92. Collaborative Group for the Study of Stroke in Young Women: Oral

contraceptives and stroke in young women: associated risk factors. JAMA, 231:718, 1975.

93. Petitti, DB, Wingerd, J: Use of oral contraceptives, cigarette smoking, and risk of subarachnoid haemorrhage. Lancet, 2:234, 1978.

94. Collaborative Group for the Study of Stroke in Young Women: Oral contraception and increased risk of cerebral ischemia or thrombosis. New Engl J Med, 288: 871, 1973.

95. Slone, D, Shapiro, S, Kaufman, DW, Rosenberg, L, Miettinen, OS, Stolley, PD: Risk of myocardial infarction in relation to current and discontinued use of oral contraceptives. New Engl J Med, 305:420, 1981.

96. Jick, H, Porter, J, Rothman, KJ: Oral contraceptives and nonfatal stroke in healthy young women. Ann Intern Med, 89:58, 1978.

97. Inman, WHW: Oral contraceptives and fatal subarachnoid haemorrhage. Brit Med J, 2:1468, 1979.

98. Thorogood, M, Adam, SA, Mann, JI: Fatal subarachnoid hemorrhage in young women: role of oral contraceptives. Brit Med J, 283:762, 1981.

99. Shapiro, S, Slone, D, Neff, ER: Age-specific secular changes in oral contraceptive use. Am J Epidemiol, 114:604, 1981.

100. Vessey, M, Doll, R, Peto, R, Johnson, B, Wiggins, P: A long-term follow-up study of women using different methods of contraception--an interim report. J Biosoc Sci, 8:373, 1976.

101. Zahavi, J, Dreyfuss, F, Kalef, M, Soferman, N: Adenosine diphosphate-induced platelet aggregation in healthy women with and without a combined and a sequential contraceptive pill. Am J Obstet Gynecol, 117:107, 1973.

102. Leff, B, Henriksen, RA, Owen, WG: Effect of oral contraceptive use on platelet prothrombin converting (platelet factor 3) activity. Thromb Res, 15:631, 1979.

103. Royal College of General Practitioners' Oral Contraception Study: Effect on hypertension and benign breast disease of progestagen component in combined oral contraceptives. Lancet, 1:624, 1977.

104. Bradley, DB, Wingerd, J, Petitti, DB, Krauss, RM, Ramcharan, S: Serum high-density-lipoprotein cholesterol in women using oral contraceptives, estrogens and progestins. New Engl J Med, 299:17, 1978.

105. Kannel, WB: Oral contraceptive hypertension and thromboembolism. Int J Gynaecol Obstet, 16:466, 1979.

106. Fisch, IR, Freedman, SH, Hyatt, AV: Oral contraceptives, pregnancy, and blood pressure. In: Ramcharan, S (Ed): The Walnut Creek Contraceptive Drug Study: A Prospective Study of the Side Effects of Oral Contraceptives, Vol. 1. Washington, D.C., Government

Printing Office, 1974, p 105. (DHEW publication no. (NIH)74-562).

107. Ramcharan, S, Pellegrin, FA, Hoag, EJ: The occurrence and course of hypertensive disease in users and nonusers of oral contraceptive drugs. In: Ramcharan, S (Ed): The Walnut Creek Contraceptive Drug Study: A Prospective Study of the Side Effects of Oral Contraceptives, Vol. 2. Washington, D.C., Government Printing Office, 1976, p 1. (DHEW publication no. (NIH) 76-563).

108. Phillips, NR, Duffy, TJ: One hour glucose tolerance in relation to the use of oral contraceptive drugs. In: Ramcharan S (Ed): The Walnut Creek Contraceptive Study: A Prospective Study of the Side Effects of Oral Contraceptives, Vol 1. Washington, D.C., Government Printing Office, 1974, p 169. (DHEW publication no. (NIH) 74-562).

109. Wynn, V, Adams, PW, Godsland, I, Melrose, J, Niththyananthan R, Oakley, NW, Seed, M: Comparison of effects of different combined oral contraceptive formulations on carbohydrate and lipid metabolism. Lancet, 1:1045, 1979.

110. Spellacy, WN, Buhi, WC, Birk, SA: Carbohydrate metabolism with three months of low-estrogen contraceptive use. Am J Obstet Gynecol, 138:151, 1980.

111. Baggett, B, Nash, HA: Effects of contraceptive steroids on serum lipoproteins and cardiovascular disease scrutinized at workshop in Bethesda. Contraception, 21:115, 1980.

112. Ernster, VL: The epidemiology of benign breast disease. Epidemiol Rev, 3:184, 1981.

113. Cole, P, Elwood, JM, Kaplan, SD: Incidence rates and risk factors of benign breast neoplasms. Am J Epidemiol, 108:112, 1978.

114. Brinton, LA, Vessey, MP, Flavel, R, Yeates, D: Risk factors for benign breast disease. Am J Epidemiol, 113:203, 1981.

115. LiVolsi, VA, Stadel, BV, Kelsey, JL, Holford, TR: Fibroadenoma in oral contraceptive users. A histopathologic evaluation of epithelial atypia. New Engl J Med, 44:1778, 1979.

116. LiVolsi, Stadel, BV, Kelsey, JL, Holdford, TR, White, C: Fibrocystic disease in oral contraceptive users. A histopathologic evaluation of epithelial atypia. New Engl J Med, 299:381, 1978.

117. Vessey, MP, Doll, R, Sutton, PM: Oral contraceptives and breast neoplasia: a retrospective study. Brit Med J, 3:719, 1972.

118. Sartwell, PE, Arthes, FG, Tonascia, JA: Epidemiology of benign breast lesions: lack of association with oral contraceptive use. New Engl J Med, 288:551, 1973.

119. Kelsey, JL, Lindfors, KK, White, C: A case-control study of the epidemiology of benign breast disease with reference to oral contraceptive use. Int J Epidemiol, 3:333, 1974.

120. Fasal, E, Paffenbarger, RS: Oral contraceptives as related to cancer

and benign lesions of the breast. J Natl Cancer Inst, 55:767, 1975.

121. Kelsey, JL, Holford, TR, White, C, Mayer, ES, Kilty, SE, Acheson, RM: Oral contraceptives and breast disease: an epidemiological study. Am J Epidemiol, 107:236, 1978.

122. Ravnihar, B, Seigel, DG, Lindtner, J: An epidemiologic study of breast cancer and benign breast neoplasias in relation to oral contraceptive and estrogen use. Eur J Cancer, 15:395, 1979.

123. Ory, H, Cole, P, MacMahon, B, Hoover, R: Oral contraceptives and reduced risk of benign breast diseases. New Engl J Med, 294:419, 1976.

124. Hislop, TG, Elwood, JM: Risk factors for benign breast disease: a 30 year cohort study. Can Med Assoc J, 124:283, 1981.

125. Janerich, DJ, Glebatis, DM, Dugan, JM: Benign breast disease and oral contraceptive use. JAMA, 237:2199, 1977.

126. Hoover, R, Bain, C, Cole, P, MacMahon, B: Oral contraceptive use: association with frequency of hospitalization and chronic disease risk indicators. Am J Public Health, 68:335, 1978.

127. Westoff, CF: Trends in contraceptive practice: 1965-1973. Fam Plan Perspect, 2:54, 1976.

128. Kelsey, JL: A review of the epidemiology of human breast cancer. Epidemiol Rev, 1:74, 1979.

129. Nomura, A, Comstock, GW, Tonascia, JA: Epidemiologic characteristics of benign breast disease. Am J Epidemiol, 105:505, 1977.

130. Ramcharan, S, Pellegrin, FA, Ray, R, Hsu, JP: The Walnut Creek Contraceptive Drug Study: A Prospective Study of the Side Effects of Oral Contraceptives, Vol. 3. Washington, D.C., Government Printing Office, 1981. (DHHS Publication No. (NIH)81-564).

131. Pastides, H, Kelsey, JL, LiVolsi, VA, Holford, TR, Fischer, DB, Goldberg, IS: Oral contraceptive use and fibrocystic breast disease with special reference to its histopathology. J Natl Cancer Inst, 71:5, 1983.

132. Ory, HW, Boston Collaborative Drug Surveillance Program: Functional ovarian cysts and oral contraceptives: negative association confirmed surgically. JAMA, 228:68, 1974.

133. Ory, HW: A review of the association between intrauterine devices and acute pelvic inflammatory disease. J Reprod Med, 20:200, 1978.

134. Senanayake, P, Kramer, DG: Contraception and the etiology of pelvic inflammatory disease: new perspectives. Am J Obstet Gynecol, 138:852, 1980.

135. Rubin, GL, Ory, HW, Lyde, PM: Oral contraceptives and pelvic inflammatory disease. Am J Obstet Gynecol, 144:630, 1982.

136. Burkman, R, The Women's Health Study: Association between intrauterine device and pelvic inflammatory disease. Obstet Gynecol, 57:269, 1981.

137. Royal College of General Practitioners' Oral Contraception Study: Reduction in incidence of rheumatoid arthritis associated with oral contraceptives. Lancet, 1:569, 1978.

138. Linos, A, Worthington, JW, O'Fallon, WM, Kurland, LT: The epidemiology of rheumatoid arthritis in Rochester, Minnesota: a study of incidence, prevalence, and mortality. Am J Epidemiol, 111:87, 1980.

139. Vandenbroucke, JP, Valkenburg, HA, Boersma, JW, Cats, A, Festen JM, Huber-Bruning, O, Raker, JJ: Oral contraceptives and rheumatoid arthritis: further evidence for a preventive effect. Lancet, 2:839, 1982.

140. Linos, A, Worthington, JW, O'Fallon, M, Kurland, LT: Case-control study of rheumatoid arthritis and prior use of oral contraceptives. Lancet, 1:1299, 1983.

141. Silverberg, E: Cancer statistics, 1982. Ca: A Cancer Journal for Clinicians, 32:15, 1982.

142. Weiss, N, Sayvetz, TA: Incidence of endometrial cancer in relation to the use of oral contraceptives. New Engl J Med, 302:551, 1980.

143. Kaufman, DW, Shapiro, S, Slone, D, Rosenberg, L, Miettinen, O, Stolley, P, Knapp, R, Leavitt, T, Watring, W, Rosenstein, N, Lewis, J, Shottenfeld, D, Engle, R: Decreased risk of endometrial cancer among oral contraceptive users. New Engl J Med, 30:1045, 1980.

144. Hulka, BS, Chambless, LE, Kaufman, DG, Fowler, WC, Greenberg, BG: Protection against endometrial carcinoma by combination-product oral contraceptives. JAMA, 247:475, 1982.

145. Weiss, NS, Lyon, JL, Liff, JM, Vollmer, WM, Daling, JR: Incidence of ovarian cancer in relation to the use of oral contraceptives. Int J Cancer, 28:669, 1981.

146. Rosenberg, L, Shapiro, S, Slone, D, Kaufman, DW, Helmrich, SP, Miettinen, OS, Stolley, PD, Rosenshein, NB, Schottenfeld, D, Engle, RL: Epithelial ovarian cancer and combination oral contraceptives. JAMA, 247:3210, 1982.

SECTION 1

COMPARATIVE METABOLISM, PHARMACOKINETICS AND PHARMACOLOGY OF STEROID CONTRACEPTIVES

MODERATOR: EGON DICZFALUSY

INTRODUCTION

Egon Diczfalusy

Reproductive Endocrinology Research Unit
Karolinska Sjukhuset (Swedish Research Medical Council)
Stockholm, Sweden

In September 1976, a group of concerned European pharmacologists met in Sestri Levante and published a report in the European Journal of Clinical Pharmacology entitled "Toward a More Rational Regulation of the Development of New Medicines." I will read a few quotations.

The group was concerned that "undue weight was sometimes attached to results of experiments in animals, when the relevance to man was extremely doubtful. Differences in responses of different species and the limited value of prediction from animal to man were repeatedly noted." And then this committee went on to say, "Current conventional toxicity testing has developed arbitrarily and by casual accretion. The present methods of testing for safety consume time, money and manpower, without a corresponding increase in safety. Some of them originated soon after the tragedy of thalidomide and were the most promising which could be devised at that time. They have since been multiplied in the questionable hope that more extensive testing would achieve still greater safety. They have not been altogether successful in achieving their objective. Toxicity studies cannot be properly planned without knowledge of absorption, blood levels, half-life, excretion routes and plasma binding in the species used."

This is exactly what Dr. Sobel said in his introductory remarks. I am extremely pleased, and looking forward to a challenging three day meeting. Before calling the first speaker, may I also quote another pharmacologist of an earlier generation, Sir Francis Bacon who said in 1625, that, "And he that will not apply new remedies must expect new errors, for time is the greatest innovator." And I suppose this applies also to the testing of the remedies.

THE ROLE OF PHARMACOKINETICS IN PRECLINICAL SAFETY STUDIES OF SYNTHETIC SEX STEROIDS

Michael Humpel, B. Dusterberg, S. Beier,
J. Schuppler, P. Gunzel, and W. Elger

Schering AG
Berlin, West Germany

INTRODUCTION

Having in mind the necessity to contain the world's population and the worldwide influence of U.S. safety requirements for sex steroids, every conference is of great interest in which scientists are given the opportunity to present their data to the regulatory body.

The presentation is in three sections. First, the most relevant pharmacokinetic data of different sex steroids will be given. Thereafter, some results will be presented which were obtained by correlation of kinetics and pharmacology. This will be followed by a retrospective evaluation of toxicity data for some known compounds on the basis of their pharmacokinetics.

The reason why kinetics must be taken into consideration with pharmacology and toxicology, is easy to define. Only pharmacokinetics crosses the borderline of preclinical and clinical investigations offering objective parameters like acute plasma levels, absolute bioavailability, metabolic clearance rates and half-lives for both animal species and humans. However, before presentation of actual data, some general points about the relationship between pharmacokinetics and toxicology will be discussed.

The special interrelationships between kinetics and toxicology stem from the aims of all toxicity studies: to estimate the possible risks to human health caused by drug therapy. Because only a very limited number of animals can be investigated when compared to the total number of possible users, the sensitivity of the test is greatly increased by special conditions like particular animal strains, duration of treatment, increase in dose and frequency of autopsy. Though the animal tests are of limited value for the risk estimation of drugs, all variables of the test should be known as far as possible in order to interpret the animal data meaningfully.

Without discussing the reasons at the moment, we have developed a ranking of pharmacokinetic contributions to toxicology in the case of sex steroids. The most important information is:

- bioavailability as dependent on dose
- rate of metabolism
- half-lives of active principle
- accumulation of active principle

Depending upon the results of these studies and/or specific observations in tolerance studies, additional information may become necessary, such as

- sex differences in pharmacokinetics
- degree of absorption as dependent on dose
- distribution of the active principle
- liver enzyme induction
- site of metabolism
- enterohepatic circulation of the drug
- metabolic pattern
- transplacental passage of drug

Other pharmacokinetic studies will contain less important information for toxicologists, such as:

- rate and routes of elimination of metabolites
- recovery of dose
- concentration of metabolites in tissues
- identification of metabolites

Having listed the contributions that pharmacokinetics can supply in order to reduce the unknown variables in sex steroid toxicity tests, the question arises as to what stage of drug development these data should be available. This is not a formal aspect of research and development divisions in industry but touches on the philosophy of animal toxicity tests. There are two approaches[1]. The idealists would like to carry out long-term toxicity trials, preferably in those animal species which are "closest" to humans with respect to all relevant pharmacokinetic parameters like biotransformation, bioavailability and rate of elimination. Also, the animal species should be close to humans in terms of target tissue sensitivity and the mechanism of endocrine regulation. However, the problem is to define what degree of similarity in any parameter is acceptable and what is unacceptable.

The pragmatists, on the other hand, do not demand studies on metabolism in all laboratory animals prior to long-term tolerance studies but are prepared to include such data, obtained at later stages of drug development, into the final interpretation of the respective animal studies. This procedure may reduce the relevance of the total test and in some cases the test may have to be repeated using another animal species. In order to reduce the probability of such a mishap, we suggest a compromise. In general, data on bioavailability in dose dependency, total or metabolic clearance and terminal half-life of the active principle concentration in plasma should be available on that animal species which is used for 12 week or longer tolerance studies. If there is no common animal species which can fulfill the bioavailability requirement, different routes of administration must be considered for animal testing even for a drug intended for oral use.

To concentrate on the above mentioned parameters is a simplification of the total problem but it has the advantage that those data can usually be generated in a short time and dramatic differences in the rate of metabolism between animal species and humans can be detected.

The results of all other pharmacokinetic studies will have a retrospective character in terms of the evaluation of toxicity tests.

PHARMACOKINETIC PARAMETERS OF SOME SYNTHETIC SEX STEROIDS

At first glance, there are a large number of progestogens on the world's market (Fig. 1). They can be divided into two groups of chemical substances, one line stemming from 19-nortestosterone, the other from progesterone, the so-called C-21 progestogens. The best known compounds of the latter class are medroxyprogesterone acetate, cyproterone (CPA) and chlormadinone acetate. Although there are numerous compounds in the 19-nortestosterone series, the most important compounds are levonorgestrel (LN) its racemate and northisterone (NET), which is the active principle of several other prodrug compounds like lynestrenol, norethynodrel and others.

Although it is known that all 19-nortestosterone derivatives show a partial androgenic effect in humans, worldwide research activities concentrate on this class of chemical structure. The reason for this seems to be a concern about the long-term animal toxicity effects produced by the C-21 steroids such as chlormadinone acetate and medroxyprogesterone acetate. The relevance of these toxic effects in animals was discussed by Benagiano and Fraser on a clinical basis. They found that medroxyprogesterone acetate is not a more toxic drug for humans than 19-nortestosterone progestagens[2].

A detailed discussion of data on the pharmacokinetics of CPA, NET, LN and gestodene[3-9] follows and shows why there are differences in animal tolerance for different sex steroids.

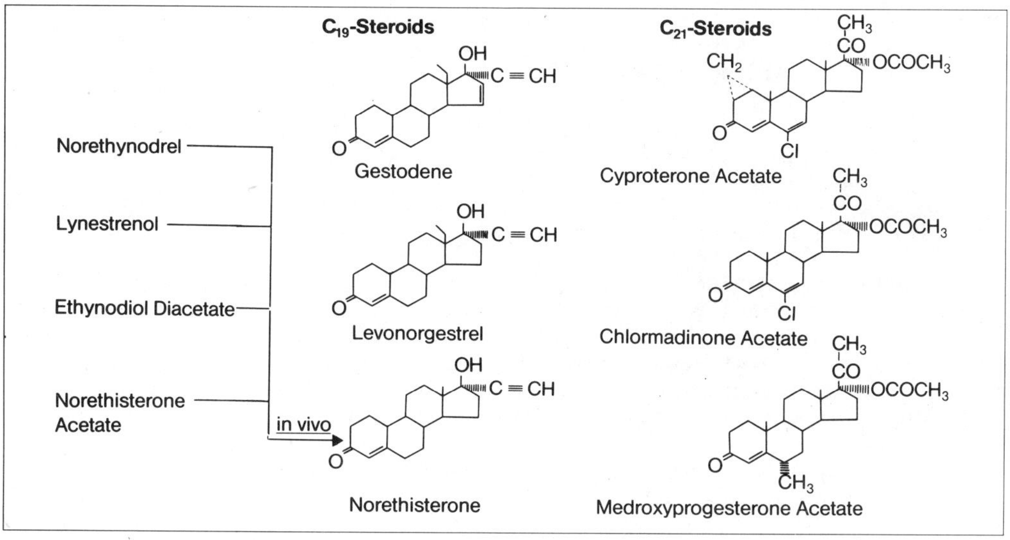

Figure 1. Structural formulas of different progestins.

Table 1. Oral bioavailability of different sex steroids in animals and humans.

Species \ Compound	CPA	LN	NET	GEST	Ethinyl-estradiol
Rat	100 (6.7)	9 (6.7)	31 (6.7)	13 (6.7)	3 (1)
Rabbit	n. d.	n. d.	50 (0.085)	28 (0.25)	<1 (1)
Beagle	75 (0.8)	22 (0.8)	44 (0.8)	36 (0.8)	9 (1)
R. Monkey	91 (1.5)	9 (1.5)	17 (1.5)	9 (1.5)	<1 (1)
Man	100 (0.04)	87 (0.0006)	64 (0.018)	100 (0.002)	40 (0.0016)

n. d. = not determined

Values are given as % of dose.
The dose (mg/kg) for which the parameter was calculated is given in brackets.

Starting with the parameter of absolute bioavailability, the comparison of data clearly demonstrates two results (Table 1). First, the availability for all sex steroids investigated, including ethinyl estradiol, is highest in man. The lowest value was found for the synthetic estrogen, ethinyl estradiol, with about 40 percent of dose, followed by norethisterone with about 64 percent availability of an oral dose. The other three compounds can be regarded as being completely available following oral administration. Comparing the human data with the animal, it must be pointed out that the doses tested in humans were at therapeutic levels whereas animal data were evaluated with much higher doses. Therefore, the bioavailability data may differ even more when evaluated for the same dose in animals and humans. The second result concerns the figures for CPA. This C-21 steroid is the only compound which becomes almost completely available in all animal species and in humans. For the other three C-19 progestogens the values were between 10 percent and 50 percent of oral dose. For ethinyl estradiol the respective values were between 10 percent and less than 1 percent of the oral dose, although this was at 600 times the human dose[9]. The extremely low availability values for ethinyl estradiol are due to conjugation reactions to give sulfates and glucuronides. At least for the rat it was shown that the gut wall contributes to the overall metabolic inactivation of ethinyl estradiol by this route[10].

The same mechanism may be involved in rabbits and rhesus monkeys because oral bioavailability of the estrogen is below 1 percent of the dose. Having reached the systemic circulation, the bioavailable part of the oral dose is distributed throughout and eliminated from the body. Elimination can occur as excretion of unchanged drug or as metabolic inactivation and subsequent excretion of metabolites.

Because sex steroids are highly lipophilic compounds, they cannot be excreted unchanged but must be metabolized to more water soluble derivatives[9,11-13]. Therefore the rate of elimination of active principle from plasma can be taken as an indicator for the rate of drug metabolism. In other words, the plasma clearance rate is equivalent to the metabolic

Table 2. Metabolic clearance rate of different sex steroids in animals and humans. Values are given as ml/min/kg.

Species \ Compound	CPA	LN	NET	GEST	EE_2	Plasma liver flow
Rat	6.8 (6.7)	124 (6.7)	212 (6.7)	168 (6.7)	61* (0.1)	35
Rabbit			35* (0.085)	27* (0.25)	32 (0.1)	26
Beagle	0.59 (0.08)	7.5 (0.08)	9.0 (0.08)	5.2 (0.08)	20* (0.015)	25
R. Monkey	4.7 (0.15)	1.6 (0.15)	9.3 (0.15)	1.4 (0.15)	17* (0.01)	15
Man	1.8 (1.3)	2.2* (0.0006)	6.2* (0.018)	0.63* (0.0013)	4.5* (0.0016)	10

* i.v. dose, all others s.c. or i.m. administration

clearance rate (MCR) (Table 2). There are remarkable differences between compounds in a given animal species and for the same compound between animal species. Values were corrected for body weight. In rats, for example, all three of the 19-nortestosterone derivates show a MCR of above 100 ml/min/kg. In contrast, the MCR of CPA in rats is much lower and accounts for only three percent of the respective NET value.

The clearance rate of NET and gestodene in rabbits is about 15 percent of the respective value in rats. In dogs, the clearance rates of the C-19 steroids are lower than in rabbits and much lower than in rats. However, the respective value for CPA is only 10 percent of the metabolic clearance rate for the C-19 steroids, showing a much slower rate in metabolism of CPA by the dog.

In rhesus monkeys there is no clear difference in this parameter between the two steroid classes. Slow rates of metabolism were found for levonorgestrel and gestodene. The MCR of CPA is about ten times higher than in dogs whereas the respective value for norethisterone is about the same as in dogs.

The metabolic clearance rate of ethinyl estradiol was highest in rats, decreasing successively in rabbit, dog and rhesus monkey. The absolute lowest value was found in humans, accounting for only about 7 percent of the respective figure found in rats.

From the data presented it can be concluded that:

- there are drastic differences in the rate of metabolism of different sex steroids in one animal species
- there are large differences in the rate of metabolic conversion of a given progestin in different animal species
- the dog is a very slow CPA metabolizer

- the rat is an outstandingly fast C-19 steroid metabolizer
- the C-19 steroids were metabolized slowest in man. The rate is not markedly different for CPA.
- NET is the fastest metabolized progestin in all species investigated.
- ethinyl estradiol is metabolized fastest in rats and comparatively slowly by humans.

Because of the extremely high MCR values for all three C-19 progestins and for ethinyl estradiol in the rat, the liver cannot be regarded as the only site of metabolism; other organs and tissues must also contribute to the metabolic rate.

The third pharmacokinetic parameter that can be compared is the half-life of the terminal disposition phase of active ingredient concentration in plasma (Table 3). The data show that half-lives of below one hour exist in the rat for LN and gestodene. Thus the rat eliminates these substances 25-50 times more rapidly than women, although safety studies employ the same dosing interval, namely 24 hours. Calculating six half-lives, during which the concentration will have decreased to almost zero, there is about a 20 hour drug free interval between two consecutive doses in the rat.

Eliminated somewhat slower from plasma are NET in rats, levonorgestrel and gestodene in rhesus monkeys and gestodene in dogs. In rabbits and dogs NET is eliminated at a rate which is similar to that found in humans.

Only the dog eliminates CPA more slowly. In this case, a marked accumulation of drug will occur in the dog during daily administration. Compared to the half-lives found for the C-19 progestogens in rats and rhesus monkeys, the respective values for CPA again demonstrates the outstanding pharmacokinetic position of this substance. This is also demonstrated by steady state plasma levels of CPA, NET and LN after a 14 day oral treatment with 3 mg/kg in a beagle (Fig. 2). While almost undetectable or very low levels were found with LN and NET, respectively,

Table 3. Terminal half-lives of different sex steroids in animals and humans.

Compound / Species	CPA	LN	NET	GEST	Ethinyl-estradiol
Rat	26 (24 – 72)	0.5 (0.17 – 7)	3.7 (2 – 12)	0.4 (0.1 – 4)	1.1 (1 – 8)
Rabbit			7.4 (6 – 24)	2.2 (2 – 8)	1.2 (1 – 10)
Beagle	109 (5 – 96)	1.2 (3 – 9)	6.3 (5 – 12)	4.6 (7 – 24)	2.9 (3 – 10)
R. Monkey	25 (12 – 72)	4.4 (2 – 30)	1.9 (2 – 12)	4.0 (2 – 30)	0.7 (1 – 8)
Man	48 (24 – 120)	26 (24 – 120)	7 – 10 (6 – 24)	10 (4 – 48)	25 (10 – 48)

Values are given as hours.
The time period during which the parameter was calculated is given in brackets (hours).

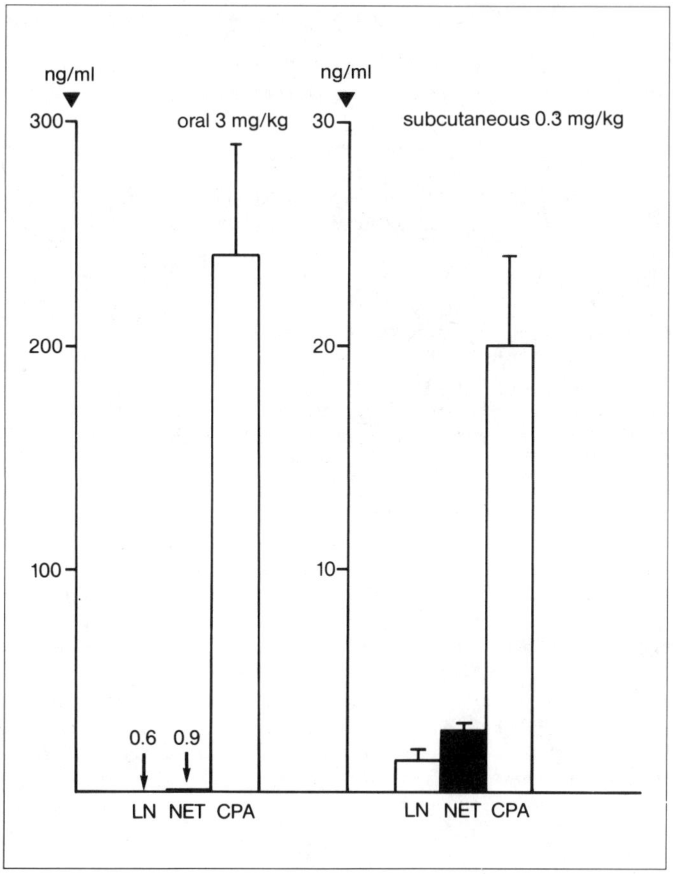

Figure 2. Active ingredient steady state plasma levels of levonorgestrel (LN), norethisterone (NET) and cyproterone acetate (CPA) after daily oral or subcutaneous administration to three beagle dogs.

the high bioavailability and slow elimination produced very high steady state levels of CPA[14]. When given subcutaneously, the differences in plasma levels are less dramatic although clearly visible. The differences in steady state levels can be explained by the comparatively low CPA clearance in the dog leading to a high accumulation during daily treatment[14]. Biotransformation is the subject of a subsequent lecture but general conclusions are as follows:

- The principal routes of biotransformation in animals and humans are known for sex steroids. They do not differ qualitatively.
- C-19 progestins, C-21 progestins and ethinyl estradiol are metabolized with different rates by all enzyme systems involved. This results in quantitative differences in metabolic pattern.
- Most of the highly hydroxylated sex steroid metabolites have not been identified.
- There are no signs that sex steroids develop toxic metabolites.

The following conclusion may be drawn for the data presented on sex steroids:

- Risk estimations for potential hazards to humans on the basis of short or long-term tolerance studies in animal species are useless for synthetic sex steroids without knowing the pharmacokinetics of each drug for each species.
- It is recommended to employ doses in tolerance studies that result in multiples of human bioavailable doses or of human acute plasma levels.
- For some widely marketed or developed C-19 progestins, animal tolerance studies should have been carried out using the parenteral route of administration instead of increasing the oral dose.
- It can be anticipated that a parenteral tolerance testing of C-19 steroids would show that there are no marked differences between the toxicity of C-19 and C-21 progestins if multiples of human plasma levels of respective active principle were compared. In addition it can be suggested that the results of those studies would drastically lower the "safety factors."
- "Clean" long-term oral tolerance studies (for instance those for norethisterone, d,l-norgestrel and levonorgestrel) show the low toxicity of all metabolites.
- Because of its human-like pharmacokinetics in rats and rhesus monkeys, toxicity tests of CPA are adequate for risk estimation. Although detailed information on pharmacokinetics of the other C-21 progestins are not available, findings should be very similar for chlormadinone acetate and medroxyprogesterone acetate.
- Due to extremely low bioavailabilities and short half-lives, the oral tolerance testing of ethinyl estradiol in animal species is obsolete from the pharmacokinetic point of view. Rather low "no effect dose levels" (which will be mentioned later) clearly demonstrate for ethinyl estradiol that kinetics is only one part of the total story of those toxic effects originated from an endocrine pharmacological "overeffect."

PHARMACOKINETICS AND PHARMACOLOGY

Although we are far from knowing the effective threshold plasma levels of different progestins in different animal species and of target tissue threshold concentrations, there is a growing understanding about the influence of species specific pharmacokinetic properties of a given compound on its pharmacology. The pharmacological effect of a sex steroid is achieved by at least two factors, the affinity for receptors, called intrinsic activity, and the product of time and concentration of the active principle at the receptor site.

Plasma levels are regarded as a fairly good indicator of the latter factor, although it should be borne in mind that target tissues may represent deep compartments with the consequence that its drug exchange with plasma cannot be monitored properly. The product of concentration of a drug in plasma and time is called AUC, the area under the plasma level versus time curve. As pointed out before, the magnitude of the area may differ for different routes of administration and when bioavailability is not optimal.

In addition, the shape of the area may change with the route of administration or by dose splitting and administration interval shortening.

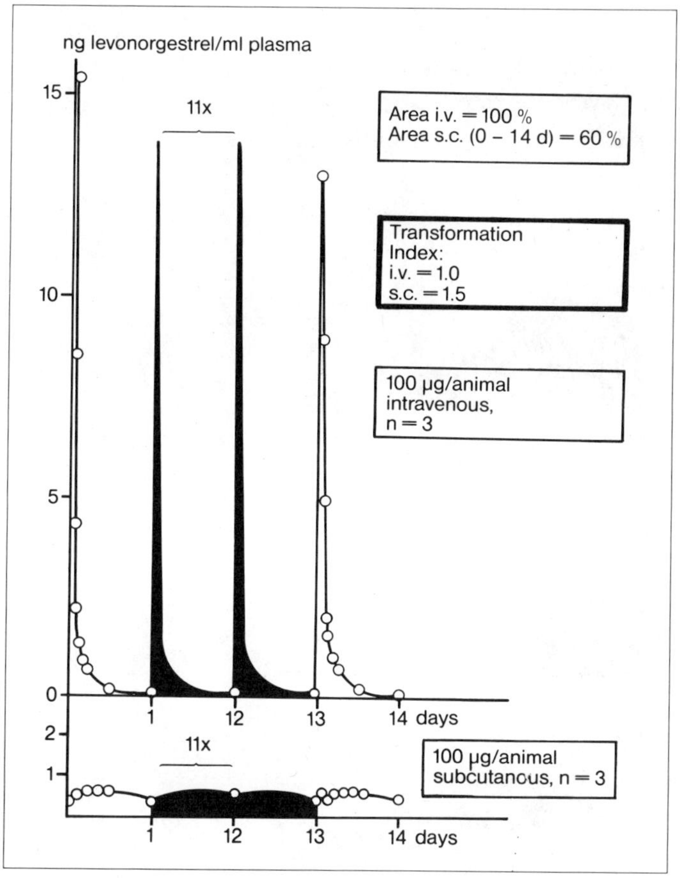

Figure 3. Plasma levonorgestrel levels during the quantitative gestagen bioassay in each 3 female beagles (cross over design); o = measured values, ■ = simulated time course.

Both parameters of the area, the size and the shape, will influence the overall pharmacological effect and a knowledge of both is necessary to understand experimental results.

This can be demonstrated with different progestins in the beagle dog, a model which has been extensively studied[14]. The influence of the shape of the area was investigated in our laboratories using levonorgestrel in the quantitative canine progestogen bioassay[9].

In this assay the progestogenic activity of a given compound is quantified by the transformatory state of the estrogen-primed endometrium of ovariectomized beagles. In a cross-over study with three animals, 100 µg of levonorgestrel was administered either intravenously (I.V.) or subcutaneously (S.C.) daily for 14 days (Fig. 3). Although the maximum concentration of LN in plasma was 20-30 times higher in the I.V. group for a short time each day and although only 60 percent of the total dose in the S.C. group was liberated by the time of analysis, the transformatory effect on the endometrium was identical to that of an effective threshold dose (index 1.5) whereas in the I.V. group only a marginal effect was

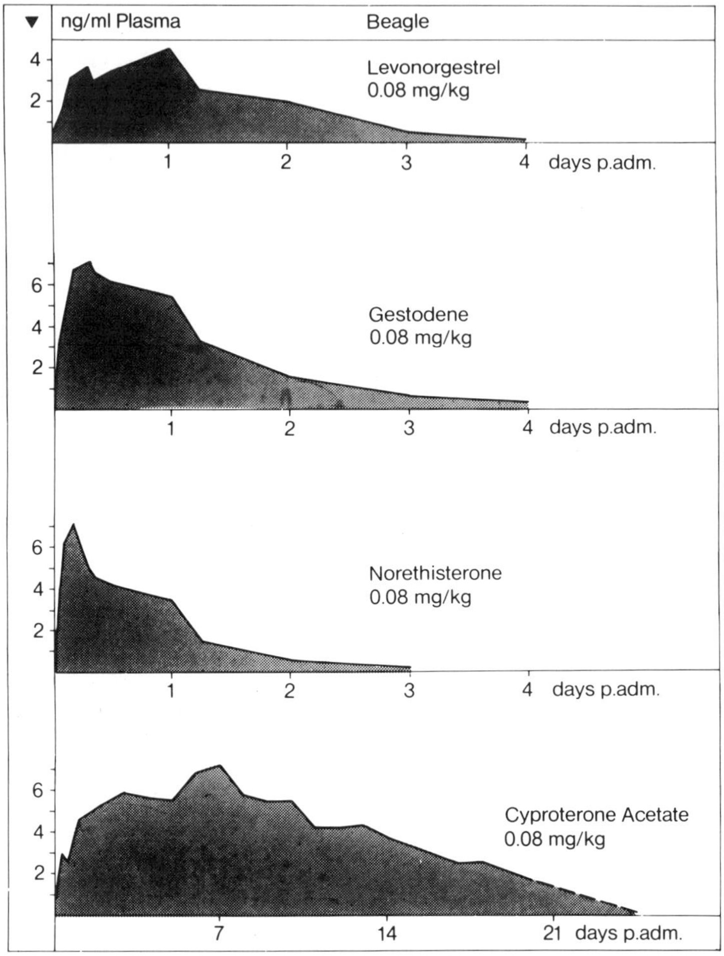

Figure 4. Plasma levels of active ingredient following single subcutaneous injection of different progestins into dogs. Compounds were dissolved in oil.

seen (index 1.0). From these data it can be concluded that constant plasma levels of active ingredient are much more effective than highly fluctuating ones. The threshold plasma level of levonorgestrel in this animal model was 0.5-1 ng/ml.

As was shown earlier, the size of the area cannot be predicted by the oral dose of a progestin because of different degrees of first-pass metabolism. Therefore, different progestins were tested in the above bioassay using both the oral and subcutaneous route of administration. In contrast to the oral treatment, where half-lives of drug elimination from plasma determine the degree of accumulation during repeated administration, after subcutaneous administrations the release rate from the depot is mainly responsible for accumulation. As could be shown for all three C-19 sex steroids and CPA[9], the release rates were different, reflecting differences in lipophilicity and metabolic clearance rates

Table 4. Effective threshold active ingredient plasma levels of levonorgestrel, norethisterone and cyproterone acetate in the beagle.

Effective dose and active ingredient levels of three progestines in the quantitative canine bioassay as measured by endometrial transformation						
Compound	LN		NET			CPA
Route of administr.	s.c.	p.o.	s.c.	p.o.	s.c.	p.o.
Effective threshold dose (mg/d)	0.1–0.3	~1.0	~1.0	≧30	~0.3	~0.1
Effective threshold plasma level (ng/ml)	0.5–1.5	0.23*	5.9	6.0*	20	9.1*
* minimum concentrations (24 hours values)						

(Fig. 4). For NET, LN and gestodene, half-lives of release of 13-20 hours were calculated whereas for CPA the half-life was 180 h (7.5 d). As a result, high levels of CPA were found in steady state conditions of the bioassay when compared to equal doses of NET and LN (Table 4). The threshold dose levels and the threshold steady state plasma levels for CPA, LN and NET in the quantitative canine bioassay show drastic differences in effective oral dose but not in effective plasma levels, which were independent of the route of administration. As a consequence, the effective threshold active ingredient plasma levels are about 1 ng/ml for levonorgestrel, 6 ng/ml for norethisterone and about 15 ng/ml for cyproterone acetate[14].

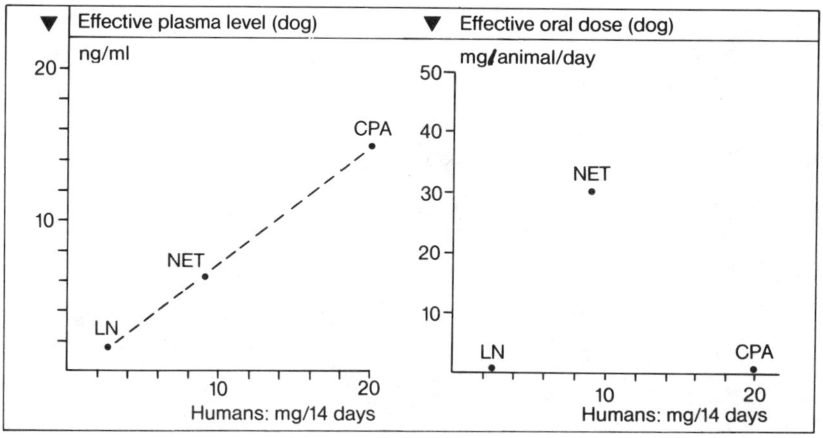

Figure 5. Correlation of effective threshold dose and plasma levels of three progestins in the beagle dog with the transformation dose in humans (Kaufmann test). The effective oral dose for norethisterone in humans represents the bioavailable part of the dose (60 percent of 13 mg per 14 d).

Comparison of these animal values with human data taken from the endometrial transformation test, the so-called "Kaufmann test," shows a good correlation for different intrinsic activities of the compounds as a slope (Fig. 5). The transformation dose in animals, on the other hand, does not correlate at all with the respective human values. This would have led to the misconception of rather different intrinsic activities of the progestins in both species. We believe this is a good example of how pharmacokinetics can link animal and human data and how advantageous it may be to use such data.

PHARMACOKINETICS AND TOXICOLOGY

The long-term safety studies of ethinyl estradiol in animal species indicate that the no-effect levels are rather low (Table 5). The no-effect dose level appears to be 5 µg/kg in rats and 10 µg/kg in dogs. The monkey tolerated up to 50 µg/kg without toxic effects showing only less body weight gain. Correction of the nominally administered dose for the bioavailable reveals two interesting facts. First, the absolute dose levels tested in rhesus monkeys were below or just equal to the bioavailable dose in humans of 400 ng/kg. Second, bioavailable dose levels tolerated by rats were lower than the human ones, whereas in dogs a two- to six-fold human dose became bioavailable and was tolerated.

The fact that rat and rhesus monkey cannot be burdened with ethinyl estradiol on a high bioavailable dose level without showing estrogen related toxic effects again demonstrates the limitations of the test for human risk estimation. We wonder which conclusions can be drawn from these studies in terms of the safe use of ethinyl estradiol in man.

A similar situation exists with long-term toxicity studies of progestins (Fig. 6). A recent paper by Fitzgerald et al[15] reported on a 10-year toxicity study of NET-Ac in rhesus monkeys. They stated that, "The

Table 5. Toxicity of ethinyl estradiol (EE_2) in animal species.

Species	EE_2-Dose µg/kg	Treatment schedule	Toxic effects	Estimated bioavailable dose (ng/kg)	Ratio to women* (BV)
Rat M+F	8	2 yr chr.	above limit of tolerance	240	0.6
Rat M+F	50	2 yr chr.	clearly toxic	1500	3.8
Dog	10	2 yr chr.	limit of tolerance	900	2.3
Dog	25	7 yr cycl.	endometrial inflammations, no other toxic damages	2250	5.6
R. Monkey	2	8 yr cycl.	no effect	20	0.05
	10		decrease of body weight gain	100	0.25
	50			500	1.3

* The bioavailable EE_2-dose in oral contraceptives using women is 400 ng/kg (50 µg EE_2 containing pills)
1) Evaluated from an internal report of Schering

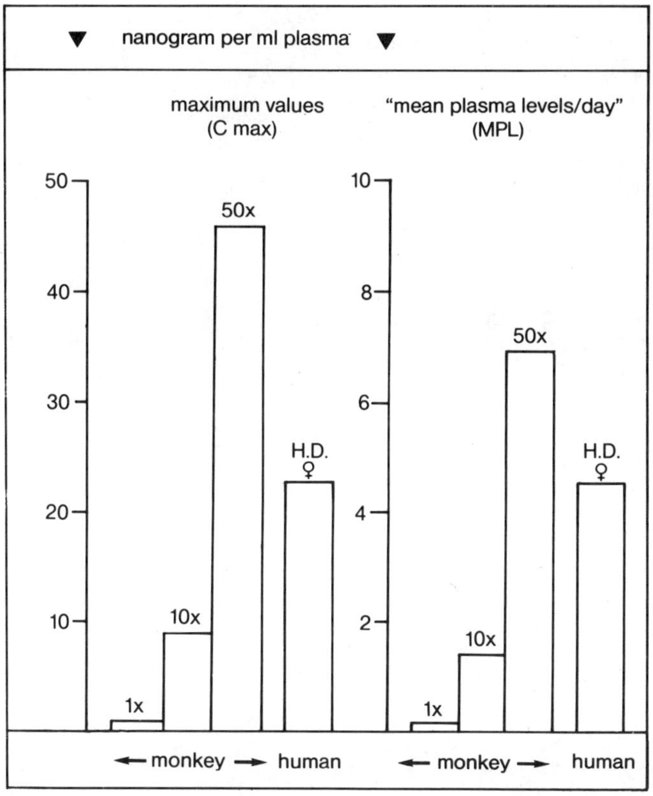

Figure 6. Maximum daily NET plasma levels and calculated "mean plasma levels" during 10 years tolerance study in female rhesus monkeys treated with 1, 10 and 50 times the human dose (H.D. = 0.05 mg/kg).

results of this study indicate that Norlestrin had no significant toxic manifestations or tumorigenic potential when administered on a cyclic regimen to female rhesus monkeys at levels up to 50 times the human dose for ten years."

However, what was really tested? For the different animal groups, maximum plasma NET levels of 0.9, 9 and 46 ng/ml can be calculated. Because these concentrations are maintained for much shorter periods than in humans, it seems to be more appropriate to compare the "mean daily plasma levels" which can be calculated to be 0.14, 1.4 and 6.9 ng/ml, respectively. The respective values for women using 2.5 mg NET-Ac containing pills are 22 ng/ml as the maximum concentration and 4.5 ng/ml as the mean "daily" plasma level[5]. On the basis of this comparison, only the highest dose animals were burdened greater (by a factor of 1.5) than normal OC users. Compared to somewhat higher dose oral contraceptives on the market, there is no difference in absolute NET plasma levels between the highest dose animal group and users. Therefore this study demonstrated nothing more than the safety of Norlestrin for rhesus monkeys at the effective oral contraceptive dose level for humans.

Focusing on the 7-year beagle study and the 10-year monkey study with

Table 6. Dose levels and calculated daily maximum plasma levels (C_{max}) and daily "mean plasma levels" (MPL) of active principle in long-term toxicity studies with levonorgestrel and d, l-norgestrel.

Study N° (IRDC)	Species (time)	Compound	Dose (μg/kg/d)	C_{max} ng/ml	MPL ng/ml	MPL Animal (% of human)
238 – 008	Dog 7 yr	d,l NG chron.	3	0.09	0.03	2
			15	0.46	0.15	12
			37.5	1.15	0.37	29
238 – 016	Dog 7 yr	LNG cycl.	10	0.62	0.2	15
			50	3.1	0.99	76
			125	7.8	2.5	192
238 – 008			500	31	9.9	762
238 – 004	Monkey 10 yr	d,l NG chron.	3	0.08	0.06	5
			15	0.38	0.31	25
			75	1.9	1.55	119
	Monkey	LNG cycl.	1000	50	41	3150
	Human	LNG cycl.	3	3.2	1.3	100

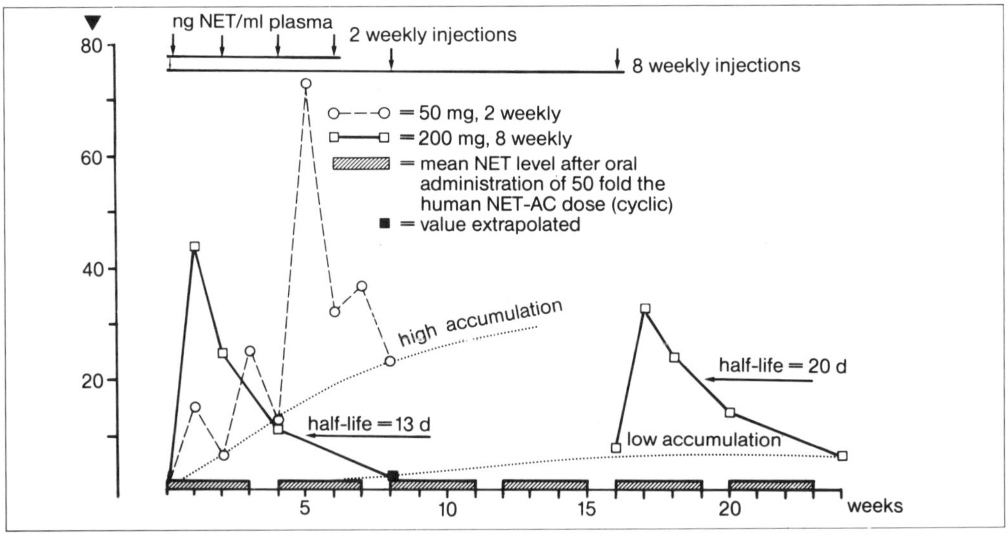

Figure 7. Norethisterone (NET) plasma levels following repeated subcutaneous injection of 200 mg NET-enanthate/kg into female rats 8 weekly or 50 mg/kg fortnightly; from: ongoing study under NIH-contract.

d, l-norgestrel, the situation is even of greater concern (Table 6). The highest oral dose was 37.5 μg/kg/d in dogs and 75 μg/kg in rhesus monkeys. Using the same parameters for comparison with humans as described previous-

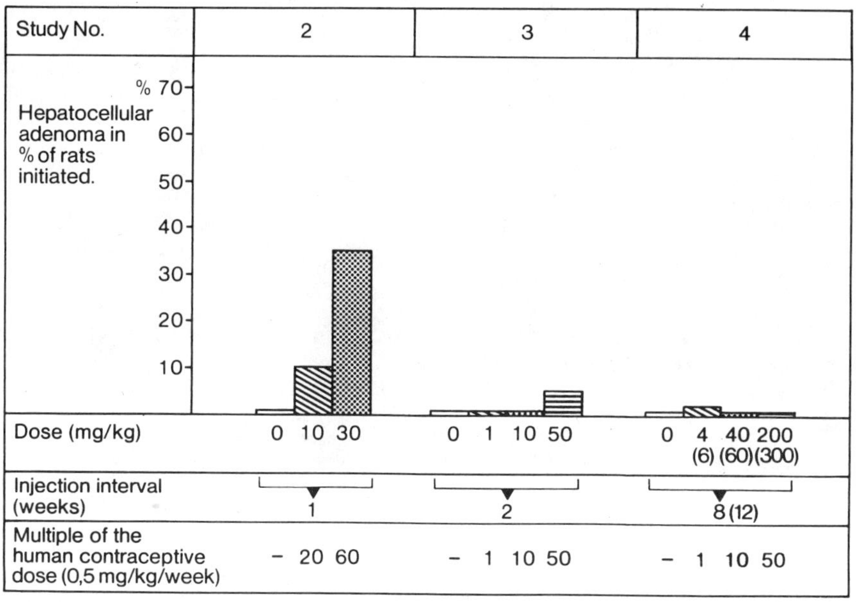

Figure 8. Incidence of hepatocellular adenoma in female rats given norethisterone enanthate by i.m. injection for up to 2 years.

ly, several conclusions emerge. The dogs were burdened with levonorgestrel to only 30 percent of the mean daily plasma level when compared to the respective values in women using 150 μg levonorgestrel. In the highest dose rhesus monkeys, roughly the same levels were reached as in women. In newer long term studies with levonorgestrel, the highest doses were drastically increased to a maximum of 0.5 mg/kg dog and 1 mg/kg monkey corresponding to a 170-fold and 330-fold human dose of 3 μg/kg. Mean plasma levels were estimated to be seven times higher in dogs and 30 times higher in rhesus monkeys than in women. Therefore only in these dose groups was a higher burden with active ingredient achieved than is normally present with low dose oral contraceptives in women.

Compared to oral tolerance studies with progestins the parenteral route of administration ensures a much higher body burden with the drug by circumventing first-pass metabolism (Fig. 7). In contrast to orally administered compounds given daily, the dosing interval of a parenterally administered depot progestogen in animals should be based on pharmacokinetic observations. If this point is neglected a sizable overdosing may result by accumulation[16]. For instance, a single subcutaneous injection of 200 mg of NET-EN/kg in rats (50 times the human dose) leads to a mean plasma NET level of about 15 ng/ml for eight weeks. The corresponding value for humans can be calculated as 5 ng/ml. Therefore the rats are burdened with a 3-fold "mean plasma level."

A marked increase in NET plasma level can be generated in rats by accumulation if the treatment schedule is changed to 50 mg/kg every two weeks, a period which was thought to simulate the number of ovarian cycles in the rat to the number of menstrual cycles in the women per injection interval. Although the "mean plasma level" of NET is only dependent on dose and not on injection intervals, the behavior over time of active ingredient levels is totally different during the two treatment schedules. While animals treated every eight weeks are exposed to rather highly fluctuating levels, the fortnightly injection group is exposed to medium levels for the whole time, which is different from the situation in humans and which should increase the toxicity related to the endocrine pharmacological effect. Exactly this was seen in long-term toxicity studies with NET-enanthate in rats (Fig. 8). The drastic influence of the injection interval can best be demonstrated by the incidence of hepatocellular adenomas.

In summation, we believe that the examples given show the necessity of:

- reappraising "old" animal tolerance studies to ensure its relevance to estimate the risks in humans
- planning future studies on the basis of pharmacokinetic data in animal and humans
- interpreting the toxicity of a given sex steroid under the aspect of active principle bioavailability and direct comparison of plasma levels in humans and animal species.

It is our belief that on this basis we should eliminate the high multiples of human dose which may not have a biological foundation. In addition, it can be anticipated that toxicity[17] of parenterally given sex steroids will not be higher than orally administered compounds.

REFERENCES

1. Glocklin, VC: General considerations for studies of the metabolism of drugs and other chemicals. 65th Annual FASEB Meeting, Atlanta, April 16, 1981.

2. Benagiano, G, Fraser, I: The Depo-Provera debate. Commentary on the article "Depo-Provera, a critical analysis." Contraception, 24:493, 1981.

3. Dusterberg, B, Humpel, M, Speck, U: Terminal halflives in plasma and bioavailability of norethisterone, levonorgestrel, cyproterone acetate and gestodene in rats, beagles and rhesus monkeys. Contraception, 24:673, 1981.

4. Back, DJ, Breckenridge, AM, Crawford, FE, Orme, ML'E, Rowe, PH, Smith, E: First-pass effect of norethindrone in rabbits and rats. J Pharmacol Exp Ther, 207:555, 1978.

5. Back, DJ, Breckenridge, AM, Crawford, FE, McIver, M, Orme, ML'E, Rowe, PH, Smith, E: Kinetics of norethindrone in women. II. Single-dose kinetics. Clin Pharmacol Ther, 24:448, 1978.

6. Becker, H, Dusterberg, B, Klosterhalfen, H: Bioverfugbarkeit von Cyproteronacetat nach oraler und intramuskularer applikation von Androcur™ bei mannern. Urologia Internationalis, 35:381, 1980.

7. Humpel, M, Wendt, H, Pommerenke, G, Weiss, C, Speck, U: Investigations of pharmacokinetics of levonorgestrel to specific consideration of a possible first-pass effect in women. Contraception, 17:207, 1978.

8. Humpel, M, Nieuweboer, B, Wendt, H, Speck, U: Investigations of pharmacokinetics of ethinyloestradiol to specific consideration of a possible first-pass effect. Contraception, 19:421, 1979.

9. Humpel, M: Unpublished results.

10. Back, DJ, Bates, MW, Breckenridge, AM, Crawford, FE, Orme, ML'E, Rowe, PH, Smiles, G, Smith, E: The metabolism of norethisterone and ethinyloestradiol by rat gut wall. J Steroid Biochem, 9:823, 1978.

11. Humpel, M: Pharmacokinetics and biotransformation of norethisterone in animals. A Review. Contraception, 26:83, 1982.

12. Sisenwine, SF, Kimmel, HB, Liu, AL, Ruelius, HW: The metabolic disposition of norgestrel in female rhesus monkeys. Drug Metab Disposition, 7:1, 1979.

13. Helton, ED, Goldzieher, JW: The pharmacokinetics of ethynyl estrogens. A review. Contraception, 15:255, 1977.

14. Beier, S, Haase, F, Kosub, B, Dusterberg, B, Elger, W: The progestational activity of different gestagens used for human contraception in the beagle bitch. Contraception, 20:533, 1979.

15. Fitzgerald, J, de la Iglesia, F, Goldenthal, EI: Ten-year oral toxicity study with Norlestrin in rhesus monkeys. J Toxicol Environ Health, 10:879, 1982.

16. Humpel, M, Dusterberg, B: The role of pharmacokinetics in the development and use of long-acting progestogens. In: Benagiano, G, Zulli, E, Diczfalusy, E (Eds.): Progestogens in Therapy, New York, Raven Press, in press.

17. Grahame-Smith, DG: Preclinical toxicological testing and safeguards in clinical trials. Eur J Clin Pharmacol, 22:1, 1982.

DISCUSSION

PROFESSOR VON EICKSTEDT: I question why you considered the distribution of the steroid and its metabolite of low importance, since the distribution, should be discussed in detail.

DR. HUMPEL: We have also considered the time axis during drug development. The most important information needed at a rather early point of development is active principle bioavailability, half-life and metabolic clearance rate in order to get an impression of the drug's pharmacokinetics. I did not say that we would not carry out these studies, but we would include these data at a later stage of development. The results of these studies are not a prerequisite for starting the tolerance studies but may serve for its interpretation.

DR. WESSLER: This may be a somewhat naive question, but I wasn't clear when you used the word "toxic" whether you were referring to toxic levels. Could you clarify that, or did I possibly miss something in your presentation?

DR. HUMPEL: I think that this question should be answered by my colleague Dr. Schuppler.

DR. SCHUPPLER: It is very difficult to differentiate toxic levels with sex steroids, i.e., is it an exaggerated pharmacological effect or is it a frank toxic effect? By toxic effect, we have generally observed some slight decrease in, say, body weight for a threshold or endocrinological parameters. With estradiol, a toxic effect would be a depression of erythropoiesis. Does that answer your question?

DR. WESSLER: I see, but in the literature the degree of the depression or augmentation was identified, so that this risk is defined someplace. I didn't see it in the presentation. Am I correct to say that it is available in the literature?

DR. SCHUPPLER: That is correct.

DR. LIPSETT: I appreciated your very thoughtful presentation of pharmacokinetics. Can you define oral bioavailability and how you get it?

DR. HUMPEL: Oral bioavailability is defined as the quotient of the area under the concentration versus time curve measured after oral administration and after either I.V., S.C. or I.M. injection (in any case parenteral) times one hundred.

DR. LIPSETT: Is that area determined until the material disappears from the plasma?

DR. HUMPEL: That is correct.

DR. LIPSETT: I assume from your data there are wide variations among species with respect to plasma binding. So you wouldn't take that into account?

DR. HUMPEL: No. We always measured total plasma concentration of the active ingredient.

DR. LIPSETT: Do you know what happens to C-19 androgens in the rat? They are clearly being metabolized and the rate of clearance is higher than the cardiac output. So something must be happening in the blood. Do you have any information about that?

DR. HUMPEL: No, but extrahepatic metabolism can be suggested.

DR. EDGREN: Two questions, one very specific one. Is cyproterone acetate (CPA) associated with an increased incidence of breast nodules in dogs?

DR. HUMPEL: Yes.

DR. EDGREN: The other one is far more philosophical. Is the mean plasma level with daily administration of these materials a meaningful concept in view of the broad excursions which we see, at least in humans, depending on dose. Is just taking a mean a really meaningful parameter to work with?

DR. HUMPEL: That is a good question. I thought about it during the preparation of the presentation, but I didn't find any better parameter. It is just a calculated number, that stands for the total area.

DR. FOTHERBY: Could I raise a philosophical question also resulting from one of your slides. You stated that the toxicity of the metabolites is low but how do we know anything about toxicity of the metabolites if we don't know what the metabolites are?

DR. HUMPEL: This is a conclusion from the long-term studies. We know that the drugs in question are well absorbed, although bioavailability may be very low. In animals the total dose reaches the systemic circulation mostly in form of steroid metabolites. When the animals are burdened with a high amount of metabolites for ten years and nothing happens, I would conclude they are not toxic.

DR. EDGREN: There are a number of reasonably well defined metabolites for NET, norgestrel, etc. and at various times in the past I have tried to run down their biological effects in very massive doses. We have always found them to be biologically of a very low order of potency and I can't remember having killed animals this way. So I think acute toxicity is unlikely.

DR. HUMPEL: Thank you very much.

PHARMACOKINETICS OF CONTRACEPTIVE STEROIDS IN HUMANS

Uwe Goebelsmann*

Department of Obstetrics and Gynecology
UCLA College of Medicine
Los Angeles, California

INTRODUCTION

In contrast to our longstanding and enormous clinical experience with contraceptive steroids, most of our knowledge about the pharmacokinetics of these drugs in man has been obtained only in recent years, appears limited and, in many aspects, is quite inadequate. A major obstacle used to be the lack of reliable radioimmunoassays (RIAs) to determine the minute concentrations of contraceptive steroids in serum or plasma. This problem has been solved to a certain degree in recent years. Yet, a number of methodological problems and inadequacies remain, not only with regard to RIAs but also with regard to subject selection, dosing, sampling, conditions of study as well as data analysis. Meaningful pharmacokinetic studies of contraceptive steroids in humans are laborious and costly. However, such studies are essential for the selection and timing of drug doses, for evaluating the pharmacokinetic action and particularly for the selection of appropriate animal models and the design of animal toxicity studies. If the pharmacokinetics of a certain contraceptive steroid in a given animal model differ significantly from the human pharmacokinetics of this drug, then the particular animal model is unsuitable for pharmacokinetic and toxicologic studies of this contraceptive steroid.

TERMINOLOGY OF PHARMACOKINETICS

Before reviewing the pharmacokinetics of specific contraceptive steroids following various routes of administration, I wish to introduce a number of pharmacokinetic terms in a very brief introductory discourse on pharmacokinetics in general.

Taken from an excellent two-part introduction to this subject by Greenblatt and Koch-Weser[1,2], Figure 1 describes the patterns of serum concentrations of a drug after intravenous or oral administration, after both complete and incomplete as well as rapid and slow absorption following oral administration. The intravenous administration delivers the entire dose of the drug into the bloodstream while oral administration may result in either complete or incomplete absorption. The latter, independent of

* Deceased

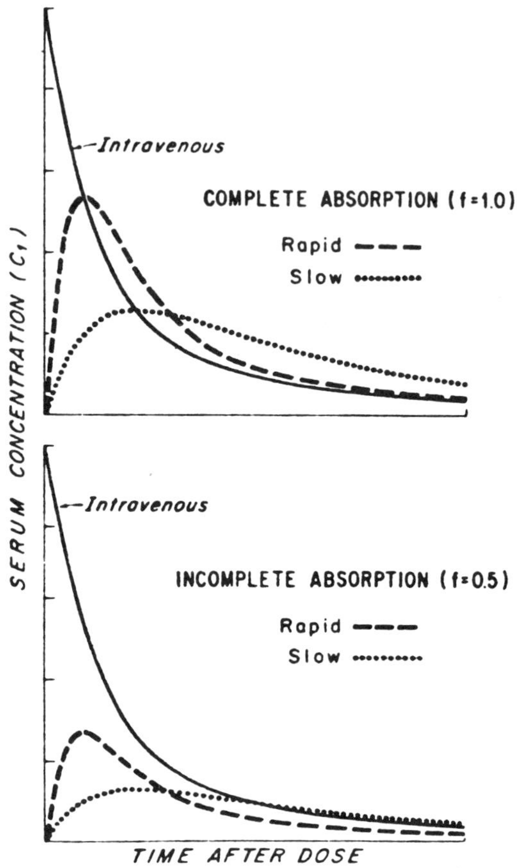

Figure 1. Serum concentrations of drugs following intravenous and oral administration: Effects of completeness and rate of absorption. From Greenblatt and Koch-Weser (2).

its rate, may be either rapid or slow. The rate of absorption is not related to the completeness of this process. The extent of absorption (completeness) is reflected by the area under the serum drug concentration versus time curve or, in brief, the "area under the curve" abbreviated as AUC. If the AUC of a drug after oral administration (AUC_o) equals the AUC after intravenous injection (AUC_{iv}), then absorption of this drug after oral administration is termed complete. The ratio of AUC_o to AUC_{iv} is termed F ratio (equation 1).

$$\frac{AUC_o}{AUC_{iv}} = F \qquad \text{equation 1}$$

If, however, for a certain drug the ratio of AUC_o to AUC_{iv} is only 0.5 (F = 0.5), then only 50 percent of the oral dose of the drug is absorbed into the circulation. The F ratio is also known as systemic bioavailability.

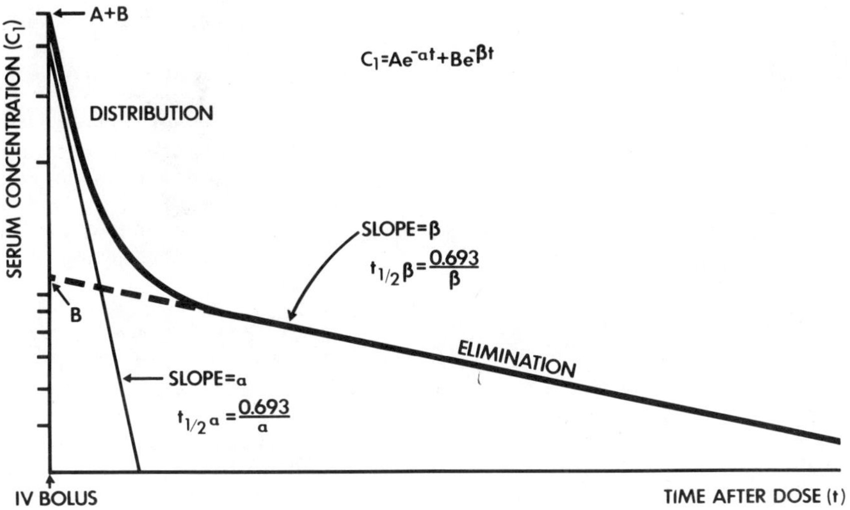

Figure 2. Pharmacokinetics of an intravenously administered drug as predicted by a two-compartment open model. Redrawn from Greenblatt and Koch-Weser (1).

The rate of absorption of a drug (rapid versus slow) is indicated by the slope of the ascending portion of the serum concentration curve of the drug.

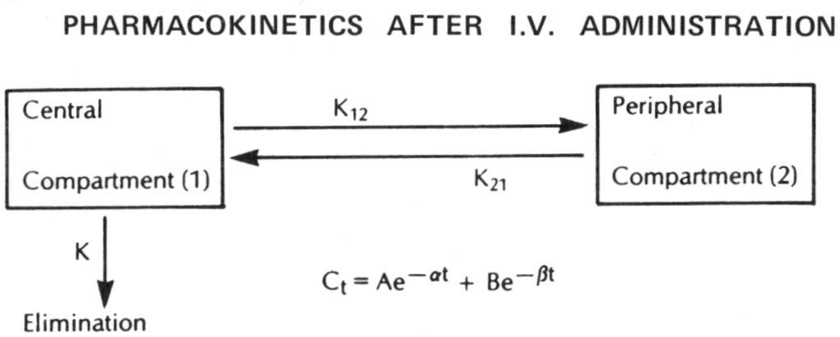

C_t = plasma concentration at time t.

A = plasma concentration at time zero for rapid disposition curve.

B = plasma concentration at time zero for slow disposition curve.

α = first order rate constant for disposition from the central compartment to the peripheral compartment.

β = apparent elimination rate constant.

K_{12} & K_{21} = first order distribution constants between the central and peripheral compartments.

K = overall elimination rate constant.

Figure 3. Pharmacokinetics after intravenous administration. From Goldzieher et al (3).

In the majority of instances, the pharmacokinetics of a contraceptive steroid are best described by a two-compartment open model. Figure 2 introduces the pharmacokinetics of such a two-compartment open model for the more simple intravenous administration. The serum drug curve in this semilogarithmic plot is approximated by two lines describing the initial distribution phase (α) with rapidly declining serum concentrations of the drug and the subsequent elimination phase (β) during which drug levels decrease in a more protracted fashion. The so-called method of residuals is employed for separating the drug concentration curve into its various exponential components: in this simplified case there are only two such components.

The half-life ($t_{1/2}$) of the distribution and elimination phase is obtained by dividing the natural logarithm of 2 by the slope of the line depicting the declining drug concentration during each phase. The y intercepts of these lines (A and B) represent serum drug concentrations at the beginning of the distribution and elimination phase, respectively. Their sum (A + B) equals the serum drug concentration at the time the intravenous bolus was injected. The drug concentration in serum for time t is then calculated according to the equation listed in Figure 3.

Figure 3 introduces the first order distribution constants k_{12} and k_{21} which represent the rate of transfer of the drug from the first or central compartment to the second or peripheral compartment (k_{12}) and the rate of transfer in the opposite direction (k_{21}) as well as the overall elimination rate constant k which represents elimination of the drug which takes place exclusively from the central (first) compartment.

PHARMACOKINETICS AFTER ORAL ADMINISTRATION

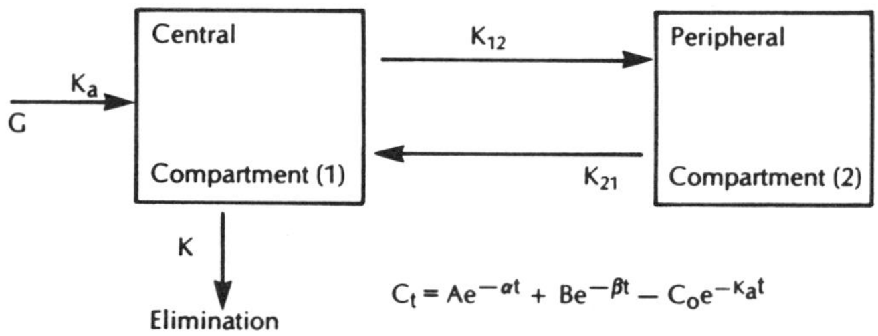

$$C_t = Ae^{-\alpha t} + Be^{-\beta t} - C_o e^{-K_a t}$$

$$t_{1/2\alpha} = \frac{0.693}{\alpha} \qquad K_{12} = \alpha + \beta - K_{21} - K$$

$$t_{1/2\beta} = \frac{0.693}{\beta} \qquad \int_0^\infty AUC = \frac{A}{\alpha} + \frac{B}{\beta} - \frac{C_o}{K_a}$$

$$t_{1/2}K_a = \frac{0.693}{K_a} \qquad V_d = \frac{dose}{\beta \cdot AUC}$$

$$K_{21} = \frac{A\beta + B\alpha}{A + B} \qquad f = \frac{\beta}{K}$$

$$K = \frac{\alpha\beta}{K_{21}}$$

Figure 4. Pharmacokinetics in a two-compartment open model for oral drug administration. From Goldzieher et al (3).

Figure 4 represents the two-compartment open model for oral administration which is generally used in pharmacokinetic studies of oral contraceptives. This figure introduces another rate constant, k_a, which describes the rate of absorption of a drug, i.e., absorption from the gastrointestinal tract as well as passage through the portal system and the liver. These rate constants k_a, K_{12}, k_{21} and k will appear in a number of the following figures and tables which present pharmacokinetic parameters for various contraceptive steroids. The absorption phase half-life $t_{1/2}k_a$ as well as the other rate constants are readily calculated as described in Figure 4. V_d represents the apparent volume of distribution. Time does not permit me to discuss the calculation of serum (plasma) drug levels at various times (C_t) according to the equation listed in Figure 4 or according to equation 2, nor to elaborate on various pharmacokinetic parameters for oral drug administration which are pertinent to oral contraceptive steroids and are based upon a two-compartment open model. Instead, reference is made to papers by Goldzieher et al[3], Stanczyk et al[4] and the textbook on pharmacokinetics by Gibaldi and Perrier[5].

$$C_p = \frac{k_a FD}{V_1} \cdot \left[\frac{(k_{21} - \alpha) \cdot e^{-\alpha t}}{(k_a - \alpha) \cdot (\beta - \alpha)} + \frac{(k_{21} - \beta) \cdot e^{-\beta t}}{(k_a - \beta) \cdot (\alpha - \beta)} + \frac{(k_{21} - k_a) \cdot e^{-k_a t}}{(\alpha - k_a) \cdot (\beta - k_a)} \right] \qquad \text{Equation 2}$$

C_p = Plasma Concentration

FD = Fraction of Dose (D) Entering Systemic Circulation

k_a = Absorption Constant

k_{21} = Intercompartment Transfer Rate (Peripheral to Central)

α = Distribution Rate Constant

β = Elimination Rate Constant

V_1 = Apparent Volume of Distribution (Central Compartment)

From Stanczyk et al[4]

PHARMACOKINETICS OF SPECIFIC CONTRACEPTIVE STEROIDS FOR VARIOUS ROUTES OF ADMINISTRATION

Following this introduction, I would like to review the pharmacokinetics of specific contraceptive steroids in man in the following order: first, I would like to address the pharmacokinetics of 1) ethinylestradiol (EE), 2) norethindrone (NET), 3) levonorgestrel (LNG) following oral administration and 4) conditions affecting the pharmacokinetics of oral EE, NET and LNG, then those of intramuscular medroxyprogesterone acetate (MPA) and norethindrone enanthate (NET-EN), and finally those of subdermal LNG implants, intravaginal steroid-containing rings and vaginal EE suppositories.

Oral Administration

Ethinylestradiol (EE)

Using a celite column chromatographic separation procedure in conjunction with a specific antibody against EE[6,7], we measured plasma EE in 24 women in a bioequivalency study of a single oral dose of 120 μg EE plus 1.0 mg NET contained in two tablets or dissolved in a weak alcoholic solution[4]. The resulting mean plasma EE concentrations achieved following intake of the solution and tablets are shown in Figure 5 which demonstrates bioequivalency of the two formulations used based upon 1) essentially identical drug levels at all times at which measurements were made, 2) virtually identical areas under the curve and 3) virtually identical maximum drug levels in plasma (C_{max}) which were reached at 1.54 and 1.52 hours following administration of the EE solution and tablets, respectively.

The mean plasma EE levels found in our study (Figure 5) are in close agreement with those reported by Goldzieher et al[3] in a group of 10 women

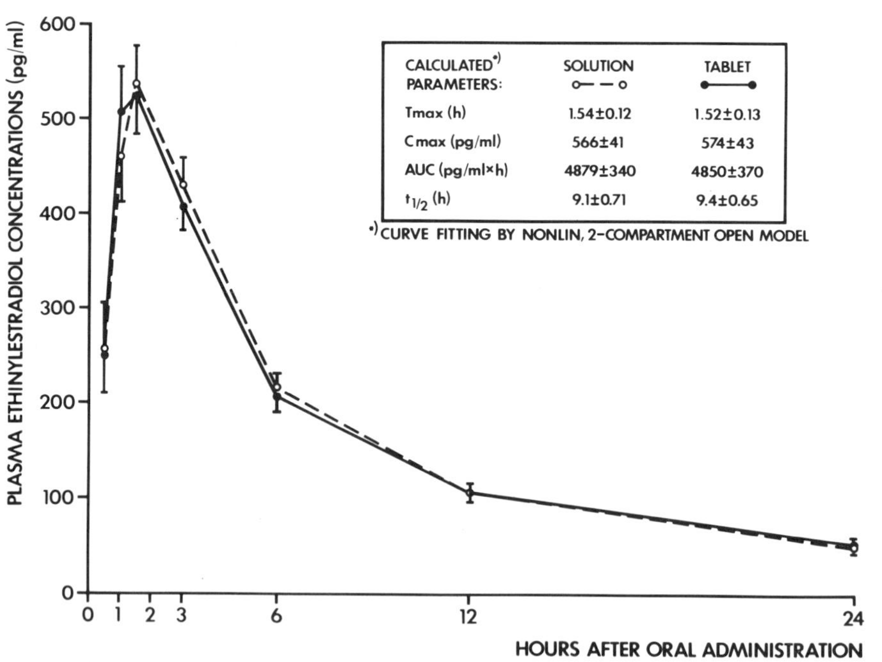

Figure 5. Mean (± SEM) plasma ethinylestradiol (EE) levels in 24 women ingesting a weak alcoholic solution or two tablets containing 120 μg of EE plus 1.0 mg of norethindrone in a bioequivalence study. Drawn from data by Stanczyk et al[4].

from Tucson who received 100 μg of EE in a double-crossover study when the levels reported by the latter authors, published as pg/ml/m^2, are converted into pg/ml using the body surface figures provided by these authors[3] (Figure 6).

The data reported by Goldzieher et al[3], those of a WHO collaborative study[8] and those obtained in our recent study[4] revealed marked subject to subject variations in plasma or serum EE concentrations. This observation mandates that a sufficiently large number of subjects be studied if meaningful pharmacokinetic data are to be obtained. Furthermore, both the study of Goldzieher et al[3] and the WHO collaborative study[8] reveal differences in the pharmacokinetics of EE between various populations studied in different locations around the world. Table 1 presents an overview of the pharmacokinetic parameters obtained or calculated from the data published in the above three studies[3,4,8]. The pharmacokinetic parameters for oral EE calculated in our study[4] with the aid of a NONLIN computer program using a two compartment open model[9] are in good agreement with those reported by Goldzieher et al[3] for their Tucson and Palo Alto populations. This agreement lends credence to the validity of these pharmacokinetic parameters for the oral administration of EE to women. A summary of the information presented in Table 1 indicates that EE is rapidly absorbed with an approximate $t_{1/2}k_a$ of 20 minutes, has a rapid distribution phase with a half-life ($t_{1/2}\alpha$) of one to two hours and an elimination half-life ($t_{1/2}\beta$) of six to 15 hours. The apparent volume of distribution ranged from 198 to 235 l[3]. Only 17.8 to 44.3 percent of the administered oral doses of EE entered the central compartment.

Of considerable importance is the finding of Goldzieher et al[3] that the mean peak plasma EE concentrations are closely related to the mean AUC

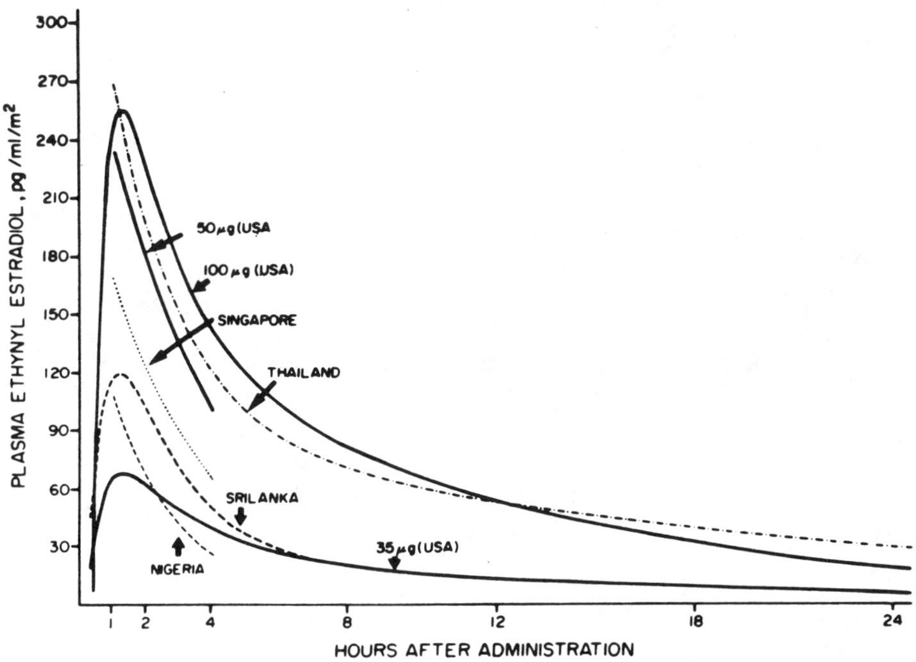

Figure 6. Mean plasma ethinylestradiol (EE) concentrations at various times following a single oral dose of various amounts of EE to women of different countries. From Goldzieher (3).

Table 1. Pharmacokinetic parameters of orally administered ethinylestradiol (EE).

EE DOSE (μg)		120	100	80	50	50	35
k_a	(h^{-1})	2.3		2.4	2.9	1.837	1.972
α	(h^{-1})	0.58	0.565	0.662	0.42	0.568	0.476
β	(h^{-1})	0.064	0.086	0.109	0.05	0.055	0.069
k_{21}	(h^{-1})	0.190	0.250	0.245	0.11	0.101	0.170
k_{12}	(h^{-1})	0.259	0.207	0.231	0.17	0.212	0.182
k	(h^{-1})	0.195	0.194	0.294		0.309	0.193
$t_{1/2}k_a$	(h)	0.30		0.28	0.29	0.37	0.35
$t_{1/2}\alpha$	(h)	1.19	1.22	1.03	1.8	1.22	1.46
$t_{1/2}\beta$	(h)	10.8	8.07	6.35	15.3	12.6	10.0
f		0.328	0.443	0.371	0.30	0.178	0.358
LOCATION OF SUBJECTS		Palo Alto	Tucson	Sri Lanka	4	Sri Lanka	Palo Alto
NO. OF SUBJECTS		20	10 x 2*	10	82	8	30 x 2*
AUTHORS		1	2	2	3	2	2

1) Stanczyk et al. (4); 2) Goldzieher et al. (3); 3) WHO study (8); 4) 14 cities around the world; *) Double crossover study

irrespective of locality and dose (r = 0.95) as shown in Figure 7. As the AUC is an important parameter of bioavailability, the most important EE plasma levels to obtain in any study are therefore peak plasma EE levels and plasma EE levels obtained closely before and soon after the peak. This observation is of importance in the design of pharmacokinetic studies because appropriately timed sampling may mean less frequent sampling without loss of essential information. This would be helpful in reducing the high expenses of such studies without losing critical information.

The systemic bioavailability (F) for EE has been determined in crossover studies in which subjects received a given dose of EE by oral and intravenous administration. According to the studies of Back et al[10,11] and Humpel et al[12], the overall systemic bioavailability of oral EE amounts to only 40 percent (Table 2). Without or with concomitant ingestion of norethindrone acetate, the F ratio ranged from 0.36 to 0.45 for EE doses ranging from 30 to 100 µg, i.e., approximately 60 percent of oral EE does not enter the central compartment.

Much less is known about the pharmacokinetics of mestranol (MEE). Upon ingestion, MEE is converted to the pharmacologically active EE. Peak plasma EE levels occur about four hours after MEE ingestion[13]. Helton and Goldzieher et al[14] reported that peak EE levels after MEE administration are lower but broader than those observed after EE intake. According to Bird and Clark[15], the metabolic clearance rate (MCR) determined by the

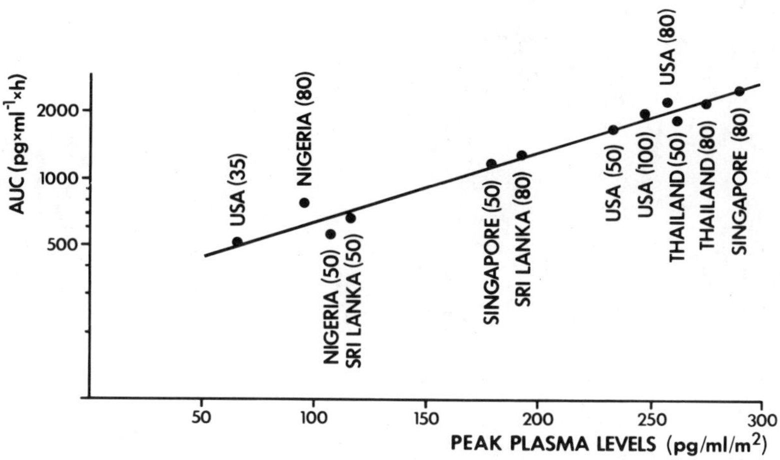

Figure 7. Correlation of mean peak plasma ethinylestradiol levels with mean area under curve (AUC) by locality and dose. Redrawn from Goldzieher et al (3).

Table 2. Systemic bioavailability of ethinylestradiol (EE): An approximately 60% first-pass effect.

EE DOSE	SYSTEMIC BIOAVAILABILITY (F)*	AUTHORS
30 μg	0.45 ± 0.09 (n = 5)	BACK et al., (11)
50 μg**	0.42 (n = 6)	BACK et al., (10)
100 μg	0.36 (n = 3)	HŬMPEL et al., (12)

*MEAN ± SEM, F = AUC_o/AUC_{iv}. **ALONE AND WITH NORETHINDRONE ACETATE

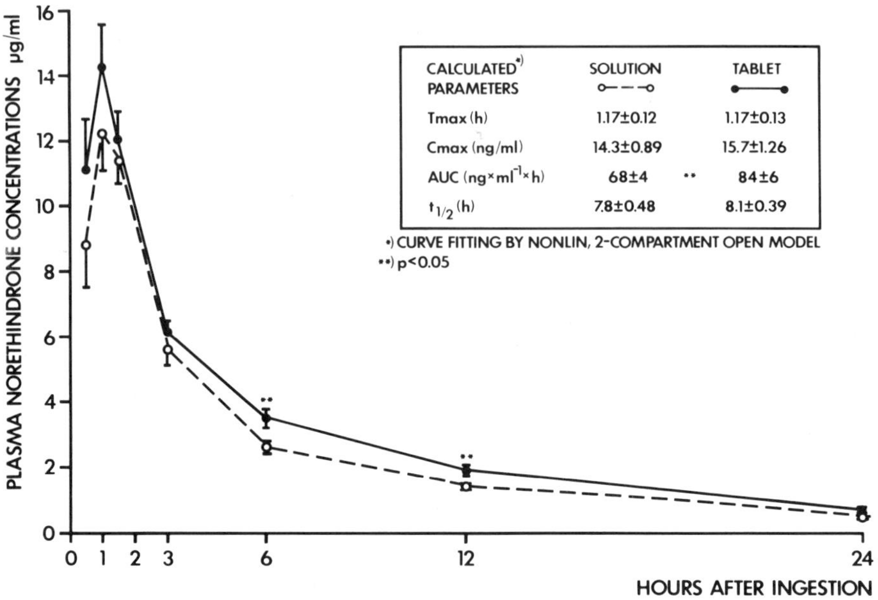

Figure 8. Mean (± SEM) plasma norethindrone (NET) levels in 24 women ingesting a weak alcoholic solution or two tablets containing 1.0 mg NET plus 120 µg of ethinylestradiol in a bioequivalence study. Drawn from data by Stanczyk et al (4).

classical constant infusion technique using labeled MEE and EE is greater for MEE (1741 l/24h) than for EE (1345 l/24h). The principal circulating metabolite of both EE and MEE is ethinylestradiol sulfate (EE-S): the mean conversion ratio of MEE to EE-S was found to be 3.369 and that of EE to EE-S was determined to be 6.476[15]. Mills et al[16] using the single injection technique found a mean MCR for MEE of 1247 l/day.

Norethindrone (NET)

The pharmacokinetics of orally administered NET using data obtained in our recent study[4] will be reviewed next. In this bioequivalence study, 1.0 mg of NET was given to 24 women in combination with 120 µg of EE contained either in a weak alcoholic solution or in two tablets and given in a crossover fashion. The mean plasma NET levels obtained following intake of solution and tablets are shown in Figure 8.

The data presented in Figure 8 indicate rapid absorption of the drug after oral administration followed by a relatively short distribution and prolonged elimination phase. Maximum plasma levels achieved 1.17 hours after intake of both the solution and the tablets. No significant difference was observed between the means of the maximum plasma concentration (C_{max}) or the overall elimination half-life ($t_{1/2}$) as calculated by a NONLIN computer program using a two compartment open model[9]. However, the AUC was significantly greater after intake of the tablet than following ingestion of the solution. This astonishing result indicating greater bioavailability following the tablets than the solution cannot be explained. However, this finding suggests that it may not be correct to presume that absorption of oral contraceptive steroids contained in tablet, capsules or any other form is best compared with that of a contraceptive steroid dissolved in a weak alcoholic solution. Is it generally presumed that the highest bioavailability is reached with a weak alcoholic solutIon as the vehicle. The latter serves as the standard formulation for bioavailability and bioequivalence studies. However, our data[4] suggest that it may not always be appropriate to use absorption from a weak alcoholic contraceptive steroid solution as the standard against which other vehicles for other contraceptive steroids are compared.

Our absolute plasma NET concentrations are higher than those reported by Fotherby et al[17] in his comprehensive WHO collaborative study. Similarly, the mean AUC obtained after ingestion of 1.0 mg NET in our study[4] was larger than that reported by Back et al[18] as listed in Table 3. This discrepancy may be due, in part, to differences in NET RIA methodology. On the other hand, the distribution (α) and elimination phase (β) half-life estimated by Back et al[18] are in agreement with those observed in our study[4] as depicted in Table 3. Our data indicate a rapid absorption phase with a mean $t_{1/2}k_a$ of only 0.21 hours[4]. As mentioned above, these data are derived by computerized curve fitting for a two-compartment open model according to the NONLIN program[4,9]. Back et al[18] estimated the plasma clearance rate for NET as 576 and 521 1/24 hours. These figures are in excellent agreement with the MCR of 551 1/24 hours determined by Mills et al[19] who employed the single isotope (^{3}H-NET) injection technique.

Back et al[18] measured the systemic bioavailability (F) for oral NET and NET acetate (NET-AC) by determining the AUC for plasma NET after intravenous and oral administration of NET and NET-AC in conjunction with

Table 3. Pharmacokinetics of oral norethindrone (NET) and NET acetate (NET-AC).

DOSE (mg)	1.0 NET-AC	1.05 NET	1.0 NET
k_a (h^{-1})			3.3
k_{21} (h^{-1})			0.24
k_{12} (h^{-1})			0.56
k (h^{-1})			0.38
$t_{1/2}k_a$ (h)			0.21
$t_{1/2}\alpha$ (h)	1.03	1.03	0.63
$t_{1/2}\beta$ (h)	7.0	7.14	8.35
AUC (ng x ml^{-1} x h)	30.9	29.9	84
CLEARANCE* (l/24h)	576	521	
NO. OF SUBJECTS	6	6	20
AUTHORS	BACK et al. (18)		STANCZYK et al. (4)

*I.V. NET: 511 1/24h; Mills et al. (19): MCR = 551/24h

Table 4. Systemic bioavailability of oral norethindrone (NET) and NET acetate (NET-AC): apparent 40% first-pass effect.

DOSE (mg)*		SYSTEMIC BIOAVAILABILITY (F)**
1.0	NET–AC	0.64 ± 0.04 (n = 6)
1.05	NET	0.64 ± 0.08 (n = 6)
3.0	NET–AC	0.52 ± 0.06 (n = 6)

Back et al. (18). *Plus 50 μg ethinylestradiol. **Mean ± SEM, F = AUC_o/AUC_{iv}

50 g of EE (Table 4). The F ratio (AUC_o/AUC_{iv}) averaged 0.6 and was the same for NET and NET-AC. These data indicate that only 60 percent of orally administered NET becomes systemically bioavailable. It should be pointed out that the variation in the F ratio between study subjects is much smaller than the inter-subject variation of plasma (serum) oral contraceptive levels or absolute AUC values. Thus, a relatively small number of subjects appears to suffice to obtain accurate systemic bioavailability data (F ratios), whereas a considerably larger number of study subjects is needed to obtain statistically meaningful results for other pharmacokinetic parameters. The findings of Fotherby et al[17] in their 14-center WHO collaborative study are quite remarkable in this regard. These authors compared the pharmacokinetics of orally administered NET in subjects studied in 14 different centers around the world and found that the intercenter differences were of the same order of magnitude as the intracenter differences in the rate of metabolism.

Levonorgestrel (LNG)

Levonorgestrel (LNG) is the biologically active enantiomer of the two forms (d and l) of norgestrel. It should be mentioned that the former d-norgestrel is now LNG. Only LNG plasma (serum) concentrations and pharmacokinetics will be mentioned in this review.

The pharmacokinetics of LNG have been studied by Humpel et al[20,21], Back et al[11] and many others. Figure 9, which has been drawn from data reported by Humpel et al[21], shows mean (± SEM) serum LNG concentrations following ingestion of 150 g of LNG in combination with 30 g of EE by 6 women. The serum LNG concentration curve shown in Figure 9 depicts a rapid absorption phase of 0.29 hours, a rapid first disposition phase (comparable to the distribution or -phase) and a quite protracted second disposition phase (also called elimination or -phase). The second disposition or elimination ( ) phase of LNG is actually more protracted than that of EE or NET. It is conceivable that the disappearance curve of LNG from serum (plasma) may be broken down into a first, second and third disposition phase. The fact that, according to Humpel et al[21], a significant serum LNG concentration (0.36 ± 0.007 ng/ml, x̄ ± SEM) remains 24 hours after ingestion of 150 g of LNG plus 30 g

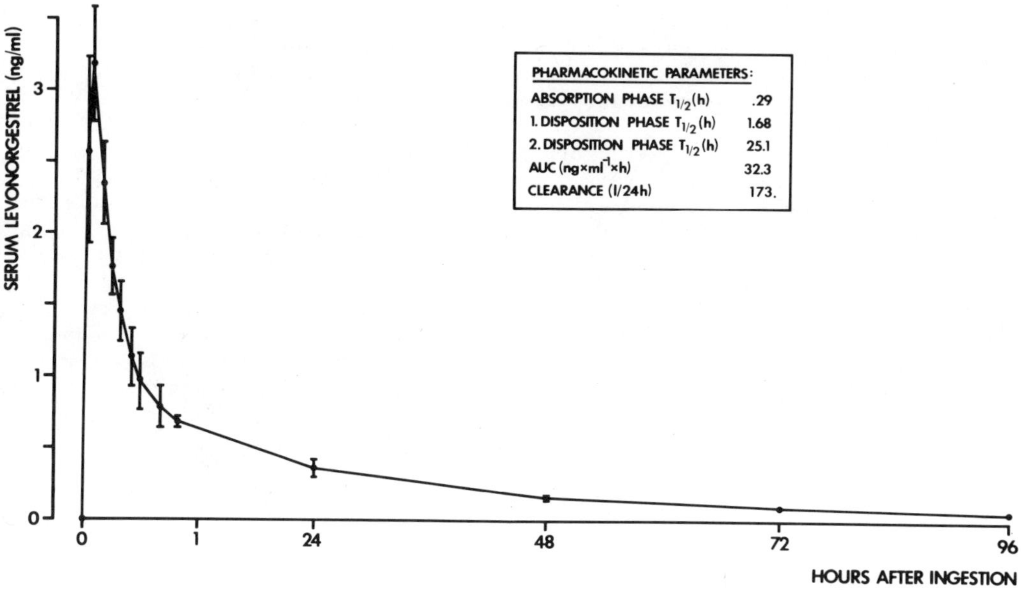

Figure 9. Mean (± SEM) serum levonorgestrel (LNG) concentrations in 6 women following a single oral dose of 150 µg LNG in combination with 30 µg of ethinylestradiol. Drawn from data published by Humpel et al (21).

of EE suggests that one should expect a considerable rise in serum (plasma) LNG levels when this dose of LNG plus EE is ingested on a continuous daily basis.

Table 5. Pharmacokinetics of oral levonorgestrel (LNG) in women (mean ± SD).

PARAMETERS	LNG/ETHINYLESTRADIOL DOSE (µg) 250/50	150/30	250/50	150/30
T_{max} (h)	2.2 ± 1.3	~2	< 2	< 2
C_{max} (ng/ml)	7.1 ± 2.0	3.2 ± 1.0	5.0 ± 1.6	3.6 ± 1.1
$t_{½}$ D_1 (h)	3.0 ± 0.6	1.6 ± 0.3	0.9 ± 0.4*	1.0 ± 0.4*
$t_{½}$ D_2 (h)	26 ± 7.2	27 ± 4.6	8.8 ± 2.9**	11 ± 2.9**
AUC_0 (ng/ml x h)		32 ± 10	33 ± 7.6	20 ± 6.7
CLEARANCE (l/24 h)		173	163	152
VOL. DISTR. (l/kg)			1.6 ± 0.7	1.9 ± 0.7
NO. OF SUBJECTS	6	6	5	5
AUTHORS	HÜMPEL et al. (20)	HÜMPEL et al. (21)	BACK et al. (11)	

*Distribution and **elimination phase half-lives instead of first and second disposition phase half-lives of Hümpel et al. (20) and (21)

Table 5 summarizes the pharmacokinetic parameters for LNG. Peak serum (plasma) LNG levels are achieved at about two hours following its ingestion and the means of the maximum serum (plasma) LNG concentrations of the two groups of investigators are in close agreement despite a limited number of subjects in each study group. The distribution phase is rapid with a mean half-life of approximately one hour according to Back et al[11] whereas the elimination phase half-life averages 8.8 and 11 hours for the 250 and 150 µg dose of LNG, respectively. The protracted elimination of circulating LNG as described by Back et al[11] is in agreement with the long $t_{1/2}$ of the second distribution phase (D_2) of Humpel et al[20,21] as listed in Table 5. The halflives of D_1 and D_2 by Humpel et al[20,21] have been calculated differently than the distribution and elimination phase half-lives by Back et al[11]. Hence, the absolute values listed in Table 5 cannot be compared directly, however, they lead to the same conclusion: oral LNG is rapidly absorbed and readily distributed but it is eliminated more slowly than NET or EE. The same LNG clearance rates calculated by both groups of authors are smaller than that of NET and the apparent volume of distribution of LNG appears to be smaller than that of NET. The possible reasons for these differences will be discussed below.

In contrast to EE and NET, LNG is not subject to any appreciable firstpass effect (Table 6). Two groups of investigators[11,21] determined the systemic bioavailability (F) of orally administered LNG for doses of 30, 150 and 250 µg, respectively. The F ratio (AUC_o/AUC_{iv}) ranged from 0.87 to 0.99, indicating that essentially all the LNG ingested becomes systemically bioavailable. This apparent lack of a first-pass effect for LNG differs markedly from the average 60 and 40 percent first-pass effects described for orally administered EE and NET, respectively (see Table 7).

Table 7 represents a brief side by side comparison of a number of pharmacokinetic parameters reported for orally administered EE, NET and LNG. All three compounds are rapidly absorbed and distributed but LNG is eliminated more slowly than NET as is evident from the parallel comparison by Humpel et al[20]. Our direct comparison of NET and EE pharmacokinetics[4] indicates that both the $t_{1/2}\ \alpha$ and the $t_{1/2}\ \beta$ are shorter for NET than for EE and the apparent volume of distribution of NET also appears to be

Table 6. Oral levonorgestrel (LNG): apparent lack of first-pass effect.

LNG DOSE	SYSTEMIC BIOAVAILABILITY (F)*	AUTHORS
30 µg	0.87 ± 0.05 (n = 3)	HÜMPEL et al. (21)
150 µg (+ 30 µg EE)	0.89 ± 0.06 (n = 5)	BACK et al. (11)
250 µg (+ 50 µg EE)	0.99 ± 0.09 (n = 3)	BACK et al. (11)

*MEAN ± SEM, F = AUC_o/AUC_{iv}.

Table 7. Comparison of average values reported for a number of pharmacokinetic parameters for orally administered ethinylestradiol (EE), norethindrone (NET) and levonorgestrel (LNG).

PARAMETERS		EE	NET	LNG
ABSORPTION $t_{1/2}k_a$	(h)	0.28 — 0.37	0.21	0.29
DISTRIBUTION $t_{1/2}\alpha$	(h)	1.03 — 1.46	0.63 — 1.03	0.9 — 1.0
ELIMINATION $t_{1/2}\beta$	(h)	6.35 — 12.6	7.0 — 8.35	8.8 — 11.
T_{max}	(h)	1.5	1.2	2 — 2.2
BIOAVAILABILITY F		0.36 — 0.45	0.52 — 0.64	0.87 — 0.99
SHBG-BOUND	(%)		63	80
VOLUME DISTRIBUTION	(l/kg)	3.8	3.6 — 4.3	1.6 — 1.9
CLEARANCE RATE	(l/24h)		511 — 576*	152 — 176

MCR by constant infusion technique: *551 l/24h

smaller than that of EE. The difference in the apparent volume of distribution between NET and LNG as well as their clearance rates is thought to be due to the fact that more LNG than NET is bound to sex hormone binding globulin (SHBG).

Conditions Affecting the Pharmacokinetics of Oral EE, NET and LNG

Pharmacokinetic studies on oral contraceptive steroids are usually performed under highly idealized conditions. Subjects chosen for such studies must not have been pregnant for two or three months and must not have taken any contraceptive steroids for a certain period of time. The studies are started in the morning after overnight fasting and are followed by a washout period of one to four weeks, and usually only a single dose is administered. In real life, however, women take birth control pills daily, sometimes every morning, sometimes every evening, and they start four to six weeks after a term pregnancy and often immediately after a first trimester abortion. The possible effects of these various conditions of oral contraceptive intake on the pharmacokinetics of oral contraceptive steroids have been studied by a number of investigators.

Kiriwat and Fotherby[22] addressed the question whether the pharmacokinetics of oral contraceptive steroids would be altered if they were administered at different times of the day. These investigators determined serum EE (Figure 10) and NET levels (Figure 11) in a group of women who were given oral doses of 50 μg EE plus 1.0 mg NET either in the morning or at night. Various pharmacokinetic parameters of the morning and the evening administrations were determined and compared; no significant difference was found. These results, although obtained in a limited number of subjects, suggest that the time of day at which oral contraceptives are taken does not significantly affect the pharmacokinetics of these agents in women.

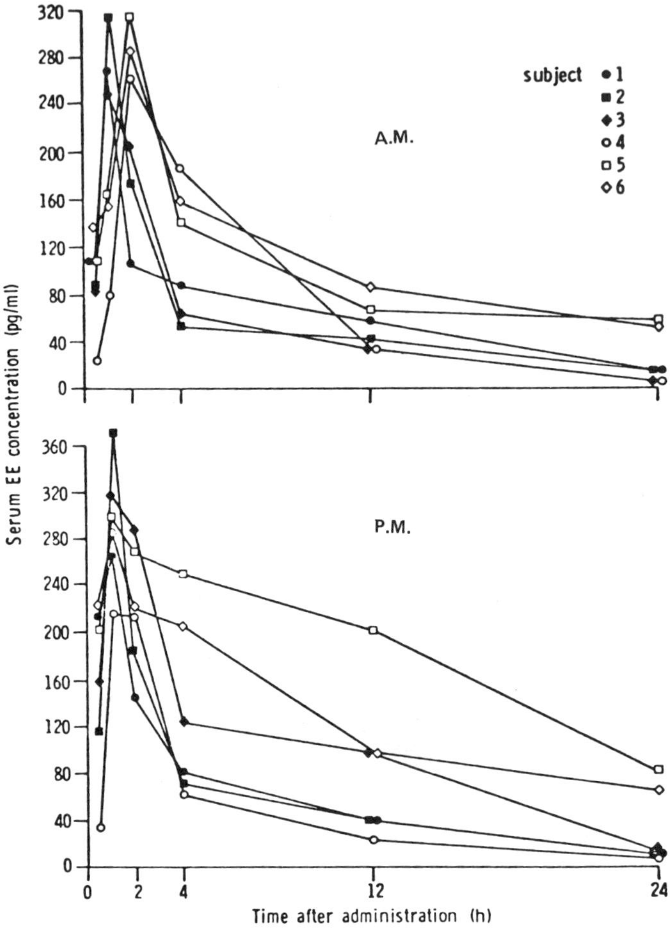

Figure 10. Serum ethinylestradiol (EE) levels after morning or evening ingestion of 50 μg EE plus 1 mg norethindrone: no significant difference in pharmacokinetics. From Kiriwat and Fotherby (22).

Multiple dosing, on the other hand, affects the pharmacokinetics of oral contraceptives as was shown by Brenner et al[23]. Figure 12 depicts a progressive rise of serum LNG concentrations prior to as well as three hours after the daily ingestion of 500 μg of dl-norgestrel (dl-NG) in combination with 50 μg EE (Ovral), of 300 μg dl-NG plus 30 μg EE (Lo/Ovral) and of 75 μg dl-NG (Ovrette). A similar rise of plasma LNG has been described by Weiner et al[24] in women taking 150 μg LNG plus 30 μg EE or 250 μg LNG plus 50 μg EE but not in those ingesting only 30 μg of LNG per day.

The data depicted in Figure 13 indicate that the progressive rise of serum LNG levels measured three hours after the daily ingestion of 500 μg of dl-NG plus 50 μg of EE (Ovral) continues for approximately seven days and plateaus thereafter. During the second cycle of Ovral use, however, there appears to be a higher serum LNG level already on the first day of pill intake than was observed on day 1 of the first pill cycle and only a minor rise thereafter for the next few days[23].

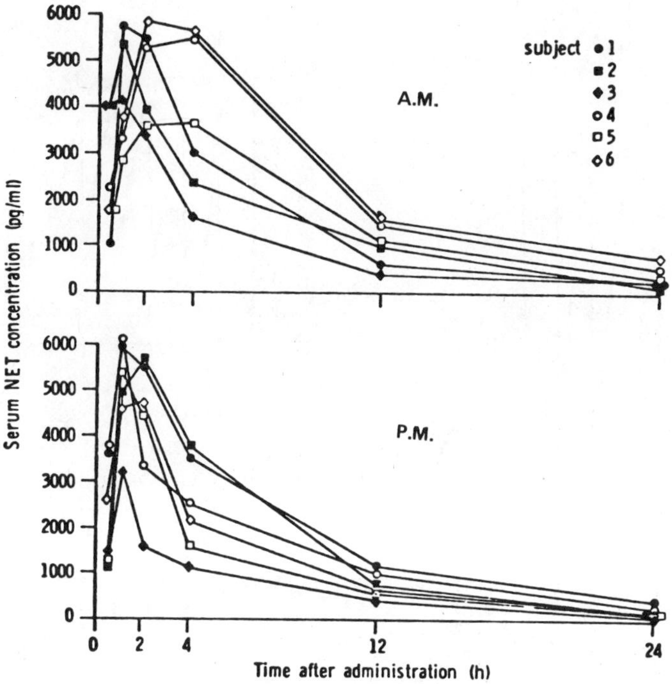

Figure 11. Serum norethindrone (NET) levels after morning or evening ingestion of 1 mg NET plus 50 μg ethinylestradiol: no significant difference in pharmacokinetics. From Kiriwat and Fotherby (22).

The same phenomenon has been observed by Back et al[25] as shown in Figure 14. Plasma NET levels rose progressively in four women during their first 20-day cycle of daily ingestion of 1 mg of NET-AC plus 50 μg of EE. However, during the subsequent cycle, the plasma NET level measured 12 hours after the first dose was about twice as high as that 12 hours after the first tablet given in the first cycle and subsequent plasma NET levels rose much more slowly during the second cycle. Back et al[25] found that the plasma half-life of NET during long-term therapy with contraceptive steroids did not differ from the halflife observed after a single dose. However, these authors found a correlation between plasma NET concentrations and sex hormone binding globulin-binding capacity (SHBG-BC) and postulated that the increase in SHBG-BC resulted in a reduction in the apparent volume of distribution of NET and thus in an elevation of circulating NET levels.

These findings are well explained by the results of the study of Odlind et al[26] as shown in Figure 15. Victor et al[27] in 1976 originally described the binding of LNG (then "d-NG") to SHBG. The binding of the contraceptive steroids LNG and NET to human plasma proteins was further investigated by Jenkins and Fotherby[28] among various other investigators. The study by Odlind et al[26] clearly demonstrates that the rise in total plasma NET is due to an increase in SHBG-bound but not in non-SHBG bound nor unbound plasma NET. The rise in total and SHBG-bound plasma NET levels parallels that of SHBG-BC in plasma.

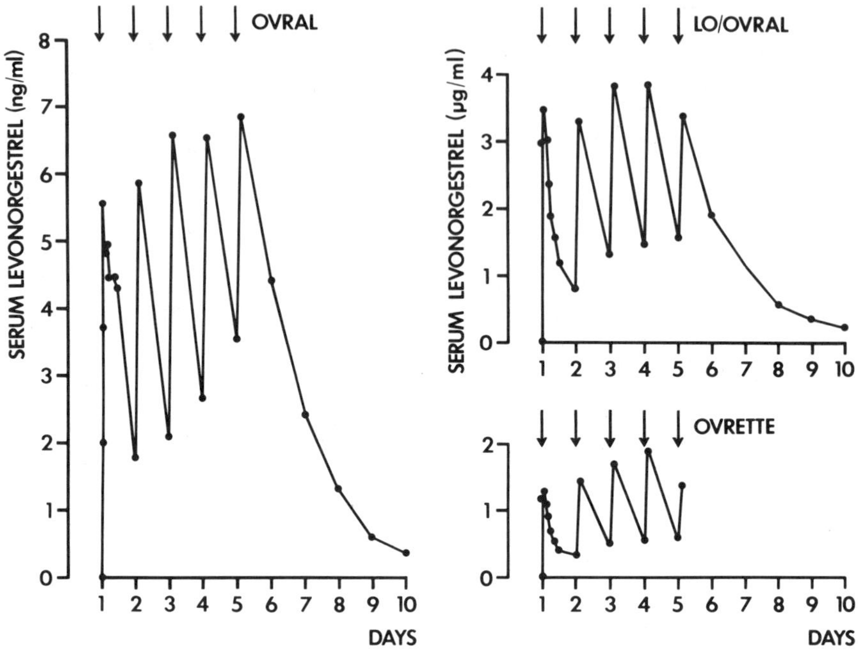

Figure 12. Mean serum levonorgestrel concentrations in three groups of 3 women, each prior to and following ingestion (↓) of 500 µg dl-Norgestrel (dl-NG) plus 50 µg of ethinylestradiol (EE) (Ovral), of 300 µg dl-NG plus 30 µg EE (Lo/Ovral) or of 75 µg dl-NG (Ovrette). Drawn from data by Brenner et al (23).

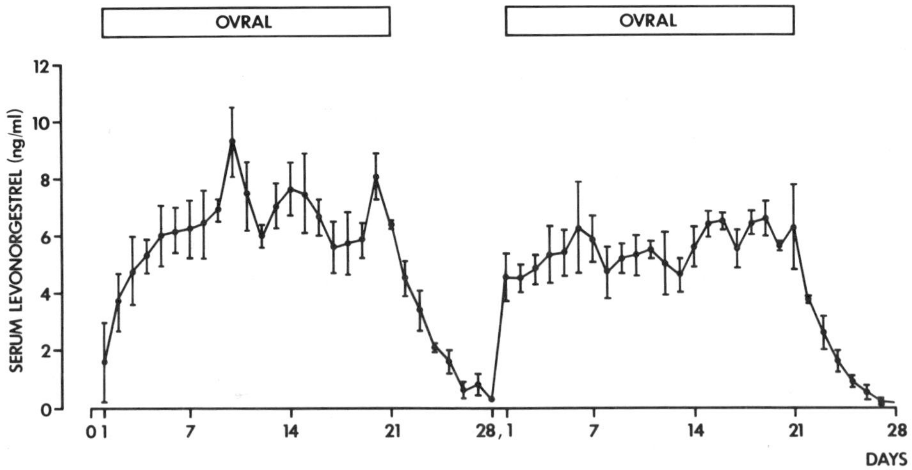

Figure 13. Serum levonorgestrel (d-NG) concentrations (mean ± SEM) in 3 women 3 hours after daily ingestion of 500 µg dl-NG and 50 µg ethinylestradiol (EE) in tablets (Ovral) for 2 consecurive weeks. Drawn from data by Brenner et al (23).

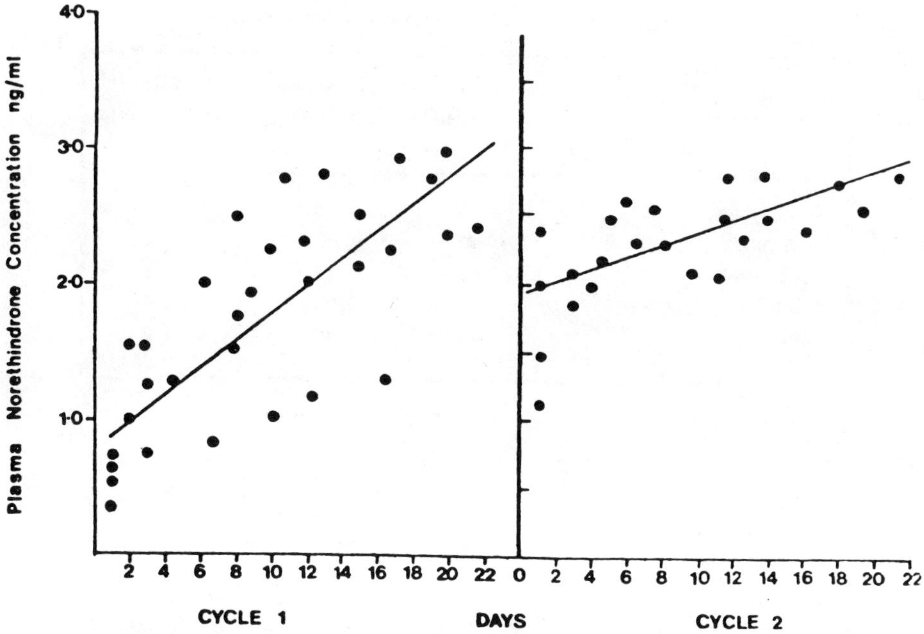

Figure 14. Plasma norethindrone (NET) levels 12 hours after ingestion of 1 mg NET acetate and 50 μg ethinylestradiol by 4 subjects for two cycles. From Back et al (25).

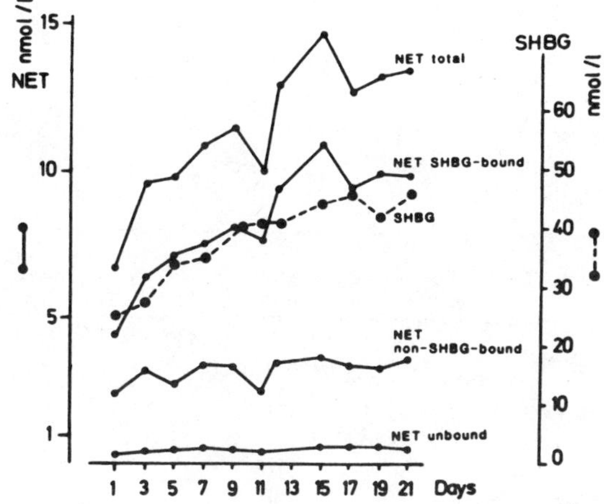

Figure 15. Mean plasma total, SHBG-bound and unbound norethindrone (NET) and SHBG in 5 women ingesting 3 mg NET acetate plus 50 μg ethinylestradiol daily for one cycle. From Odlind et al (26).

Table 8. Hormone binding to plasma proteins.

HORMONE	SHBG-BOUND %	ALBUMIN-BOUND %	FREE DIALYZABLE %
TESTOSTERONE*	60	40	2
DIHYDROTESTOSTERONE*	80	20	2
LEVONORGESTREL**	80	14	
NORETHINDRONE***	63	33	4
ESTRADIOL*	40	60	2

*Pardridge (29); **Jenkins & Fotherby (28);
***Odlind et al. (26)

Binding of LNG and NET to SHBG thus modifies their pharmacokinetics. The binding of these progestins to SHBG and albumin is compared with that of testosterone, dihydrotestosterone and estradiol in Table 8, which contains data by Pardridge[29], Jenkins and Fotherby[28] as well as Odlind et al[26]. The data shown in Table 8 indicate that a larger portion of circulating LNG than of NET is bound to SHBG as has already been stated above. Noteworthy is that the "binding" of these steroids to albumin is a low affinity binding. Therefore, it appears appropriate to distinguish between a "SHBG-bound" and a "non-SHBG bound" fraction of plasma (serum) steroids whereby the latter fraction may be subdivided into an "albumin-bound" or "albumin-associated" with an "unbound" (i.e., freely dialyzable) portion. Plasma EE is not bound to SHBG, but EE-S the principal EE metabolite[14,15], is extensively bound to albumin with affinities of $1 \times 10^6\ M^{-1}$ and $1.8 \times 10^4\ M^{-1}$ [30]. Jenkins and Fotherby[31], when studying the binding of NET and LNG to SHBG and albumin in various species, found

Table 9. Sex hormone binding globulin (SHBG) in various states. Data represent means ± SEM of SHBG-binding capacity. From Pardridge (29).

PATIENT CATEGORY & NO.		SHBG (nM)
PREGNANCY	(9)	323 ± 28
ORAL CONTRACEPTIVES	(8)	126 ± 16
THIN POSTMENOPAUSAL	(9)	74 ± 9
NORMAL PREMENOPAUSAL	(9)	65 ± 9
OBESE POSTMENOPAUSAL	(9)	43 ± 4
NORMAL MALE	(8)	28 ± 3
HIRSUTE FEMALE	(5)	17 ± 2

significant differences. In the human, baboon and rhesus monkey, binding of LNG and NET occurred mainly to SHBG with a greater affinity for LNG than for NET and to lesser extent to albumin. Although some binding of these progestins to SHBG was found in the dog and rabbit, this was much less than in the primates studied, and a larger portion of the progestins was bound to albumin. In the guinea pig and rat, binding was limited to albumin[31]. In his review on the transport of protein-bound hormones into tissues, Pardridge[29] discussed the factors and mechanisms which determine the extent to which protein-bound steroids reach their tissue receptors. From this review, it becomes evident that plasma protein binding is an important determinant of hormone action and that total plasma (serum) steroid levels without additional information on protein binding do not adequately describe the extent to which a contraceptive steroid may become truly bioavailable. Furthermore, it is obvious that animals whose plasma protein binding of contraceptive steroid hormones differs significantly from that in the human may constitute unsuitable models for pharmacologic and toxicologic studies of contraceptive steroids used in man. Based upon the work of Jenkins and Fotherby[31], baboon and rhesus monkey but none of the other species tested (including the dog) appear to be useful models with regard to contraceptive steroid hormone binding to plasma proteins.

As outlined in Table 9, considerable differences are encountered in SHBG-BC among individuals. It is highest in pregnant women followed by

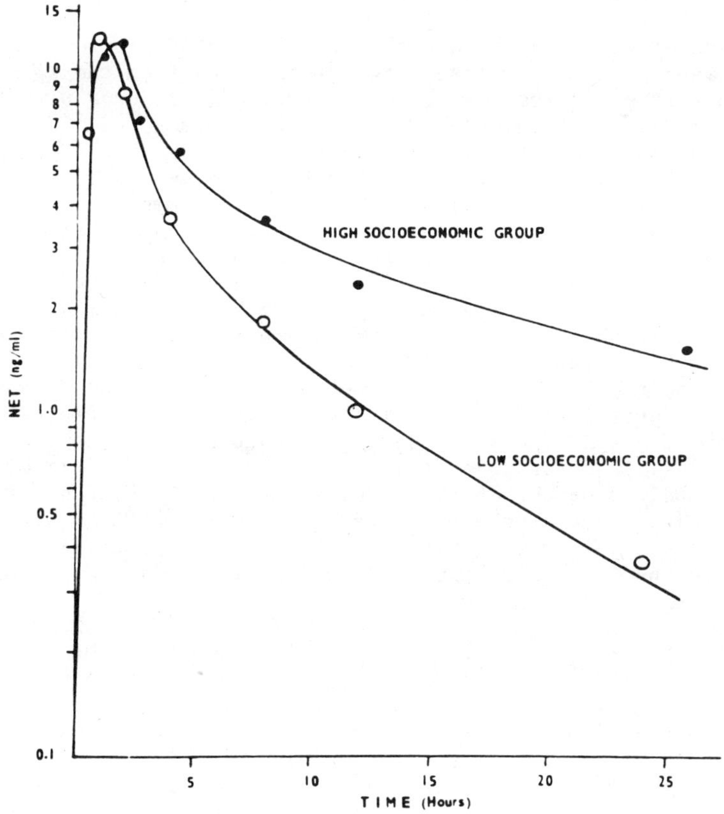

Figure 16. Mean serum norethindrone levels in 5 women of a high and 11 women of a low socioeconomic group. From Prasad et al (32).

women who are taking EE or MEE containing contraceptive steroids. SHBG-BC is higher in thin than obese women and low in men and hirsute women. The information contained in Table 9 emphasizes the importance of subject selection for pharmacokinetic studies of contraceptive steroids. Assessment of a prospective study subject's SHBG-BC, therefore, appears to be as important as ascertaining that her liver function tests are within normal limits before she is enrolled in a pharmacokinetic study of contraceptive steroids if the latter are known or suspected to bind to SHBG.

The effect on SHBG-BC as outlined in Table 9 may be only one of several factors by which body weight affects the pharmacokinetics of contraceptive steroids. As shown in Figure 16, Prasad et al[32] found a significant difference between the half-life of plasma NET in women of a low socioeconomic group with poor nutritional status ($t_{1/2}$ = 5.9 hours) and that of well-nourished women belonging to a high socio-economic group ($t_{1/2}$ = 13.4 hours). Thus, it is important to include anthropometric indices in the results of pharmacokinetic studies of contraceptive steroids.

Long-Term Injectable Contraceptive Steroids

Medroxyprogesterone Acetate (MPA)

Microcrystalline medroxyprogesterone acetate (MPA) under the trade name Depo-Provera (DMPA) was the first long-term injectable contraceptive steroid used. It is well established that intramuscular doses of 150 mg of DMPA given once every three months are associated with excellent contraceptive efficacy but also with a delayed return of fertility[3]. The latter is due to a slow absorption of the drug from the injection site or the DMPA microcrystals. Ovarian cyclicity returns with the eventual decrease in circulating MPA concentrations[33-35]. In contrast, serum MPA levels rise rapidly and thereafter fall progressively following oral MPA administration with pharmacokinetics similar to those described for NET and LNG[36]. However, values for the most common pharmacokinetic parameters (bioavailability, absorption, distribution and elimination phase half-lives, rate constants, etc.) have not been established for orally administered MPA. These data would be useful for the interpretation of intramuscularly administered DMPA. Figure 17 depicts mean serum MPA concentrations in three women following a single intramuscular injection of 150 mg of DMPA. Our serum MPA levels shown in Figure 17 are lower than those reported by Kirton and Cornette[33], Jeppsson and Johansson[34] as well as Fotherby et al[37], most likely due to RIA specificity based upon our use of a specific antibody in conjunction with the 3-O-carboximino-^{125}I-iodohistamine derivative of MPA as radioligand[36]. However, regardless of the absolute values, the pattern of declining serum MPA levels following a single intramuscular dose of DMPA is quite similar in most studies. In our investigation (Figure 17), serum MPA levels were detectable for up to nine months[36]. Immediately following DMPA injection, they ranged from 1.5 to 3 ng/ml.

In our study, subjects resumed ovulation when serum MPA levels had fallen below 0.1 ng/ml, i.e., positive LH feedback in response to rising serum estradiol levels was suppressed above that MPA level. On the other hand, serum estradiol levels rose to preovulatory levels when serum MPA concentrations fell below 0.5 to 0.25 ng/ml. As shown in Figure 17, about 25 percent of the MPA that became bioavailable within 30 weeks following DMPA injection did so within the first four weeks, about 50 percent

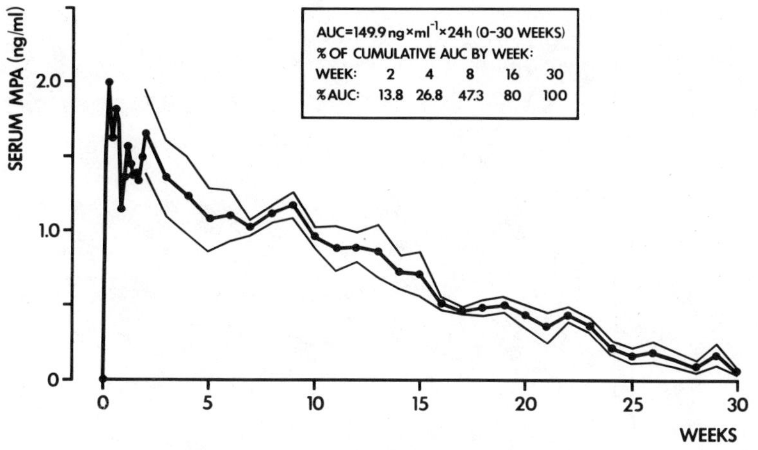

Figure 17. Serum medroxyprogesterone acetate (MPA) concentrations (means ± SE) in 3 women following a single intramuscular injection of 150 mg depo-Provera. Drawn from data by Ortiz et al (35).

within the first eight and 80 percent within the first 16 weeks after injection. If repeated injections of DMPA are given every three months, there will be a rise in circulating MPA levels due to an accumulation of MPA microcrystals at the injection sites. This will not prolong the time interval between the last DMPA injection and the final disappearance of MPA from the circulation.

In a larger study, Fotherby et al[37] investigated the pharmacokinetics of intramuscular DMPA following different doses (20, 50, 100 and 150 mg, respectively). The resulting mean serum DMPA levels are shown in Figure 18. The fact that only one of the five subjects who received 150 mg of DMPA had detectable serum MPA levels after 100 days following injection is in contrast to previous reports[33,35]. However, this study[37] was conducted in Thailand. It is conceivable that population and/or activity differences may be responsible for this discrepancy in DMPA pharmacokinetics.

Norethindrone Enanthate (NET-EN)

One of the earliest pharmacokinetic studies of norethindrone enanthate (NET-EN) is the one by Gerhards et al[38]. Figure 19 taken from the latter study[38], depicts plasma levels of total unconjugated ^{3}H-labeled material, of ^{3}H-NET-EN and ^{3}H-NET following a single intramuscular injection of ^{3}H-NET-EN into two postmenopausal women. It is emphasized that approximately 90 percent of the circulating unconjugated ^{3}H-labeled material is not ^{3}H-NET. Thus, if plasma or serum NET is determined following NET-EN injection, only some 10 percent of the circulating NET-EN derived steroids are being measured as NET. This fact must raise certain concerns, but the remaining 90 percent, as Dr. Humpel has mentioned and Dr. Edgren has alluded to in

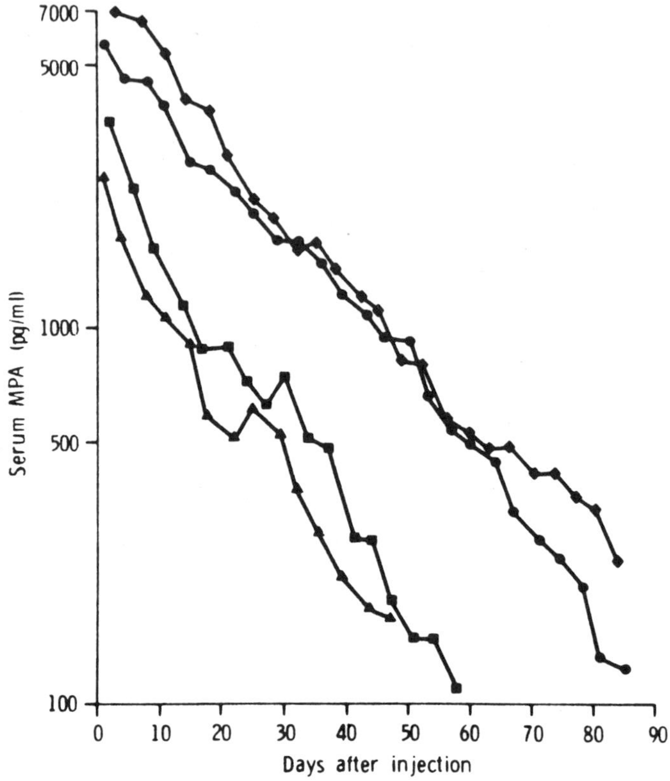

Figure 18. Mean serum medroxyprogesterone acetate (MPA) levels following intramuscular injection of 150, 100, 50 and 25 mg of depo-MPA to groups of 5 women each. From Fotherby et al (37).

the preceding discussion, probably represents substances which do not possess any acute toxicity. Dr. Gerhard's study[38] also showed that the levels of circulating NET, except during the very first days after injection, exceeded those of the parent compound NET-EN. This finding may be the result of NET binding to SHBG.

Saxena et al[39] developed a RIA for NET-EN and substantiated the findings of Gerhards et al[38] that, following intramuscular NET-EN injection, serum NET levels exceeded serum NET-EN concentrations. In a more recent study by Dr. Fotherby's group, Sang et al[40] showed similar results in nine subjects who received a single intramuscular injection of NET-EN (Figure 20). The latter authors[40] studied the pharmacokinetics of intramuscularly administered NET-EN and compared the elimination of circulating NET-EN with that of NET (see Table 10).

Plasma or serum levels of NET following intramuscular injection of NET-EN have been measured and reported by several groups of investigators[41-45]. The effects of circulating NET upon serum gonadotropins, estradiol and/or progesterone levels have also been described[41,44-46].

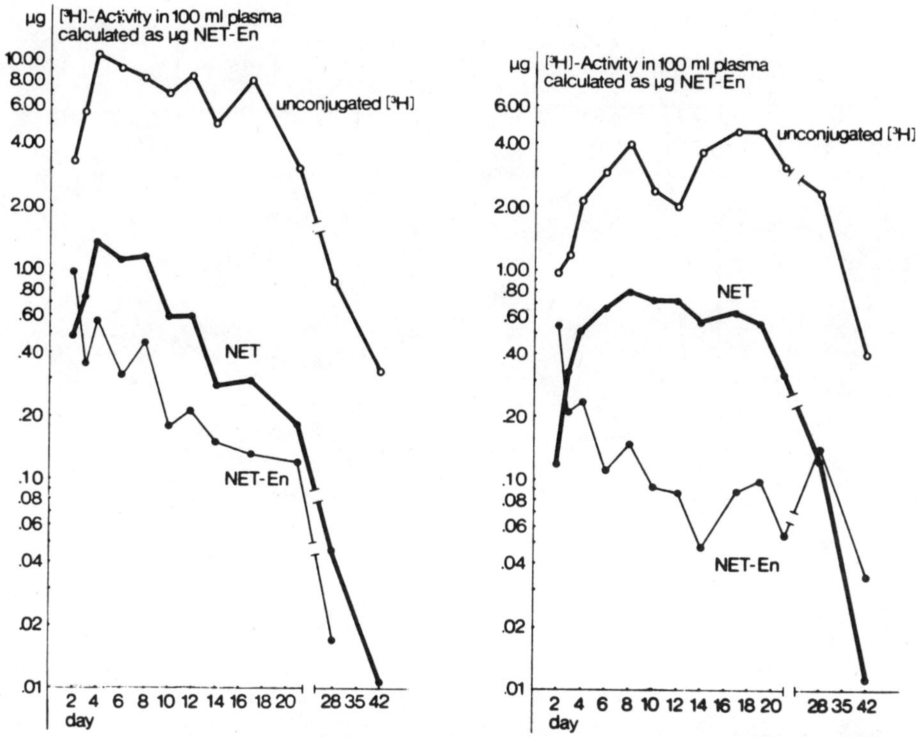

Figure 19. Plasma norethindrone (NET) and NET enanthate (NET-EN) concentrations following a single intramuscular injection of 200 mg ^{3}H-NET-EN to 2 postmenopausal women. From Gerhards et al (38).

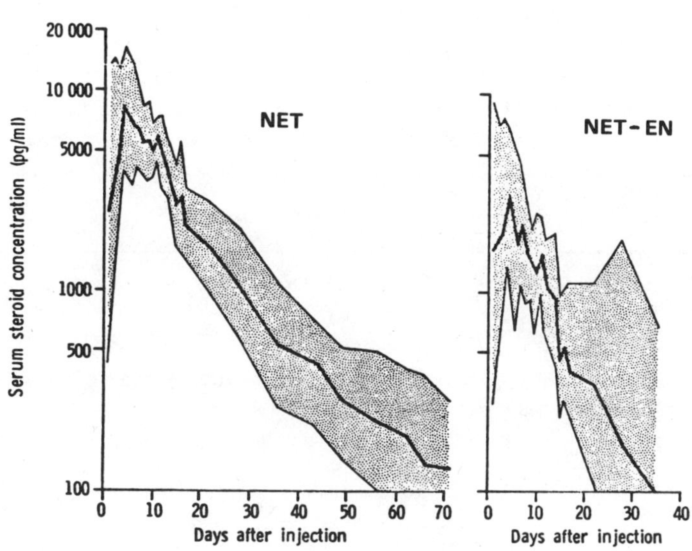

Figure 20. Serum norethindrone (NET) and NET enanthate (NET-EN) concentrations following intramuscular injection of 200 mg of NET-EN in 9 subjects. From Sang et al (40).

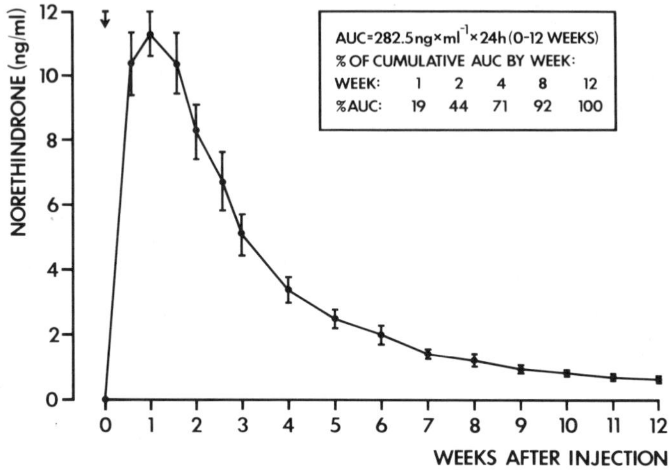

Figure 21. Mean (± SE) serum norethindrone (NET) concentrations in 15 women following intramuscular injection of 200 mg NET enanthate marked by arrow. From Goebelsmann et al (44).

Figure 21 depicts mean (± SEM) serum NET levels in 15 women following a single intramuscular injection of 200 mg of NET-EN. Ten of the 15 women were included in a previous report[44] and the remaining five subjects were studied soon after completion of the original investigation. The mean serum NET levels found in our study[44], as shown in Figure 21, are in

Table 10. Pharmacokinetics of norethindrone enanthate (NET-EN) following a 200 mg intramuscular injection (means ± SEM).

	NET-EN	NET	NET
PEAK LEVELS (ng/ml)	5.2 ± 1.5	11.1 ± 2.5	12.4 ± 3.6
DAYS TO PEAK LEVELS	4.5	4.3	6.5 ± 0.9
AUC (ng/ml x 24h)	50.2	143.5	282.4
CLEARANCE (l/24h)	560 ± 144	1080 ± 100	
ABSORPTION $t_{1/2}$ (24h)	13.2 ± 2.2		
ELIMINATION $t_{1/2}$ (24h)	8.1 ± 1.2	11.6 ± 1.5	
NUMBER OF SUBJECTS	9	9	15
AUTHORS	SANG et al. (40)		GOEBELSMANN et al. (44)

agreement with those reported by Weiner and Johansson[41] and by Sang et al[40]. Our data revealed a positive correlation between the AUC and the peak serum NET concentrations measured as previously described by Goldzieher et al[3] for orally administered EE (compare Figure 7). However, the AUC is also related to the rate of decline of serum NET concentrations. The latter was found to differ significantly between subjects in our study[44] as well as in other reports[40-42]. The observation that the rate of decline of serum NET levels differs considerably from subject to subject is of great importance with regard to dose frequency and contraceptive efficacy because suppression of ovarian follicle maturation and positive feedback inhibition of the preovulatory LH surge are related to serum NET concentrations. In our study[44], positive feedback inhibition occurred at serum NET levels ranging from 0.1 to 1.8 ng/ml and return of ovulation was observed after a mean time interval of 98 days after NET-EN injection.

The data shown in Figure 21 also indicate that about 70 percent of the NET-EN dose, which is absorbed and converted to circulating NET, reaches the central compartment within the first four weeks following intramuscular injection and less than 10 percent becomes bioavailable after eight weeks. This finding is in good agreement with that of Sang et al[40] who reported that less than five percent of the biovailable NET was released after 60 days. There appears to be a considerable variation of absorption rates between subjects which, in part, may be explained by anthropometric as well as activity differences. Although the bulk of NET which becomes bioavailable following intramuscular NET-EN injection does so within the first eight weeks, NET remains detectable in serum for up to 12 months[44]. Hence, serum NET concentrations rise in women who receive multiple injections of NET-EN at 10 or 12 week intervals[43].

Table 10 summarizes the pharmacokinetics of intramuscular NET-EN. Peak serum NET levels averaging 11 to 12 ng/ml are obtained after an intramuscular dose of 200 mg of NET-EN about four to seven days following injection. Peak circulating NET-EN are lower than peak NET concentrations. The absorption half-life for intramuscular NET-EN averages 13.2 days and the mean elimination half-life of NET-EN is 8.1 days as compared to 11.6 days for NET. The AUC for NET reported by Sang et al[40] was only half that observed in our study[44]. The low AUC of Sang et al[40] may be explained, in part, by the relative rapid clearance which is twice as high as that reported by Back et al[18] and by Mills et al[19].

Equation 3 represents an attempt of approximating the bioavailability of NET following the injection of 200 mg of NET-EN based upon the data shown in Figure 21. The sum of the daily serum production rates (PRs) calculated for the first 12 weeks is calculated by adding the individual daily PRs calculated for days 1-4, 5-7 and so on until days 78-84. The latter ones were calculated as the product of the MCR for serum NET and the mean serum NET concentration measured for each time interval. The MCR for NET was determined by Back et al[18] as 521 l/day. The mean cumulative PR for circulating NET according to equation 3 was found to be 144 mg in 84 days. This indicates that essentially all the NET-EN injected (200 mg of NET-EN corresponds to 145 mg of NET) reached the circulation as NET. It should be added, however, that the MCR calculated for NET by Back et al[18] pertains to a single dose administration and may not necessarily be applicable for a long-term administration of NET via intramuscular NET-EN that is absorbed and hydrolyzed to NET.

$$\sum_{d\ 0-84} PR = PR_{d\ 1-4} + PR_{d\ 5-7} \bullet\bullet\bullet\bullet\bullet + PR_{d\ 78-84}$$

$$PR = MCR \times C$$

$$MCR = 511\ l/day\ \text{(Back et al, 18)}$$

$$= 144\ mg/84\ days$$

Equation 3

Intramuscularly injected NET-EN is absorbed from the site of injection and appears to enter the fat tissue where it may be stored temporarily. Hydrolysis of the ester does occur in liver and extrahepatic tissues in man but not in rabbits. This has been shown by Back et al[14] in a study on the enzymatic cleavage of NET-EN in man, dog, goat, guinea pig, rat and rabbit (Figure 22). Particularly in rabbits, but to a certain extent also in other animals, NET-EN is hydrolyzed in muscle and blood. It is obvious that such species differences in the sites of NET-EN metabolism will cause differences in the pharmacokinetics of NET-EN between various species. The rabbit appears to be a poor model for human NET-EN pharmacokinetics[47] and other animals may have similar drawbacks.

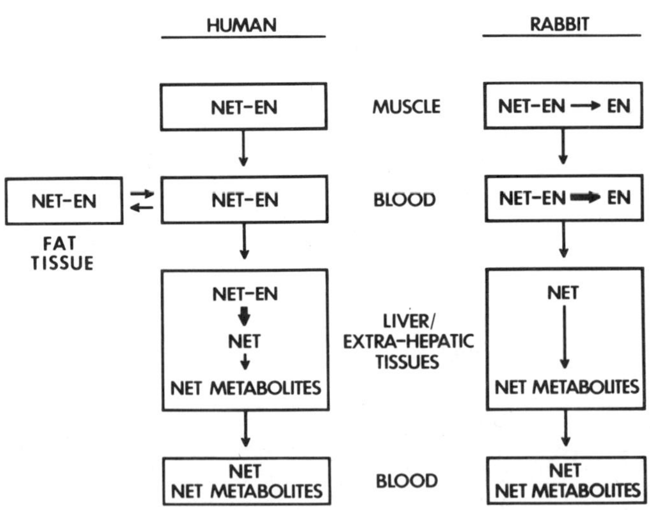

Figure 22. Postulated scheme for hydrolysis of norethindrone enanthate (NET-EN) in humans and rabbits after intramuscular injection. From Back et al (47).

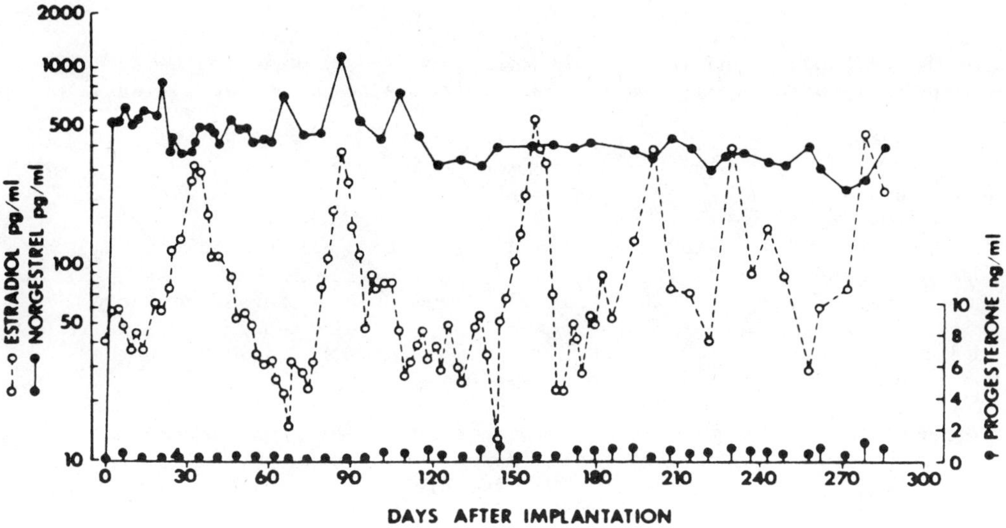

Figure 23. Serum levonorgestrel (LNG) concentrations in a woman with six silastic capsules, each containing 34 mg of LNG. From Moore et al (49).

Other Nonparenteral Routes of Contraceptive Steroid Administration

Subdermal Implants

Plasma or serum LNG concentrations have been measured in women who carried subdermal LNG implants[48-51]. These implants usually consist of six silastic (polydimethylsiloxane) capsules which contain approximately 30 mg of LNG each.

Table 11. Sustained zero order release of levonorgestrel (LNG) from six silastic subdermal implants containing a total of 204 mg of LNG. Values represent mean ± SEM plasma LNG levels.

YEAR FROM IMPLANT	LNG CONCENTRATIONS GROUP 1*		REPORTED BY GROUP 2**	
	ng/ml	n	ng/ml	n
1			0.35 ± 0.03	27
2	0.44 ± 0.03	9	0.31 ± 0.02	23
3	0.44 ± 0.03	36	0.34 ± 0.02	30
4	0.42 ± 0.03	38	0.32 ± 0.03	8
5	0.39 ± 0.05	17	0.29 ± 0.02	42
6	0.43 ± 0.05	16		

*ALVAREZ et al. (51); **CROXATTO et al. (50)

Figure 23 depicts serum LNG concentrations in a woman with six silastic LNG capsules and a combined content of 204 mg LNG. The serum LNG levels remained virtually constant over a period of nine months during which serum estradiol levels rose periodically to preovulatory levels but serum progesterone levels remained in the preovulatory range, indicating presence of follicle maturation but positive feedback inhibition (i.e., no midcycle LH peak and hence no ovulation). Similar results were reported by Weiner and Johansson[48].

Croxatto et al[50] and Alvarez and associates [51] measured plasma LNG concentrations in women with subdermal LNG implants for up to six years. Their results, summarized in Table 11, document a sustained zero order release of LNG in large groups of women who had six subdermal silastic implants totaling 204 mg of LNG. The mean plasma LNG levels reported by these investigators[50,51] are in agreement.

Near zero order release rates were observed by Laumas et al[52] for NET-AC in women with a single silastic implant consisting of a silastic tubing filled with 40 mg of crystalline NET-AC which released an average of 180 to 200 µg of NET-AC each day as determined from the remaining amount of steroid following removal of the implants. However, the steroid release from these NET-AC implants decreased noticeably; serum NET levels fell from an average level of 1 ng/ml during the first and 0.5 ng/ml or less during the sixth month after implantation.

Only the release rates were determined <u>in vitro</u> and <u>in vivo</u>, the latter by measuring steroid content prior to insertion and following removal of these subdermal implants, and the plasma or serum steroid levels were measured, but no pharmacokinetic parameters have been reported for this route of contraceptive steroid administration that is characterized by a sustained zero order drug release rate.

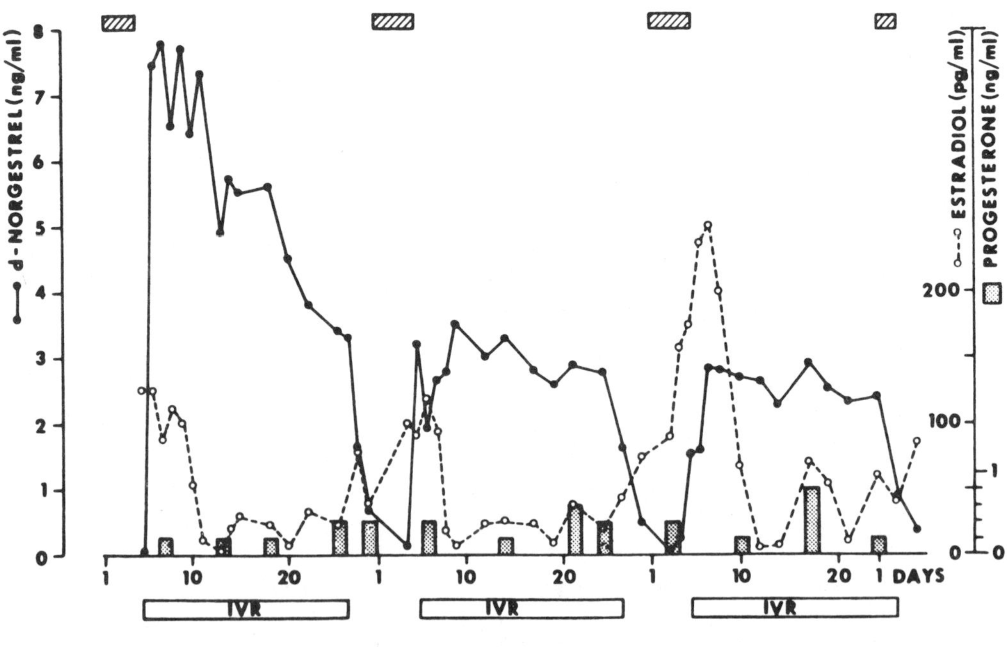

Figure 24. Serum levonorgestrel, estradiol and progesterone levels in a woman using an intravaginal ring (IVR) impregnated with 100 mg of dl-Norgestrel. From Stanczyk et al (54).

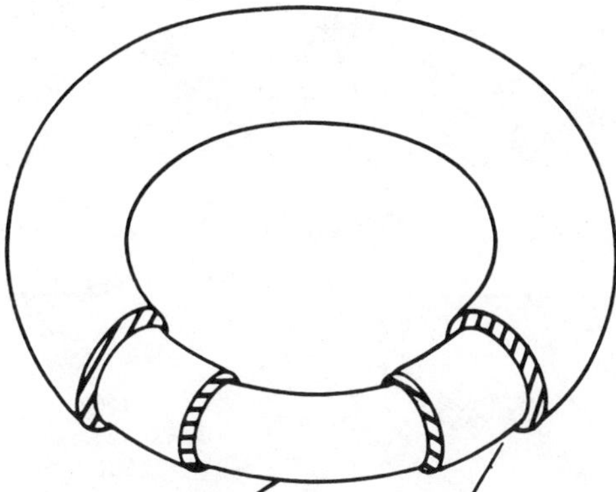

Figure 25. Sectional view of the "shell" ring with zero order steroid release rates. From Jackanicz (56).

Intravaginal Rings

Early studies employed polysiloxane intravaginal rings (IVRs) which were homogeneously impregnated with NET of dl-NG[53]. Serum levels of LNG in a woman wearing an IVR impregnated with 100 mg of dl-NG are depicted in Figure 24. Our data of Figure 24[54] reveal relatively high serum LNG concentrations immediately following the first IVR insertion which decline gradually to less than 50 percent of the initial peak levels by the 21st and last day of the first IVR cycle. During all subsequent IVR cycles, serum LNG levels were constant throughout the entire cycle. When the IVRs were removed, serum LNG levels fell precipitously as one would expect according to oral LNG pharmacokinetics. Essentially identical data were reported by Victor et al[55]. These results indicated that the initial release of dl-NG occurred in a burst-like fashion. This was followed by a subsequent sustained near zero order release rate.

The initial burst-like release of steroids from the silastic IVR was essentially abolished with the new "shell" design as outlined by Jackanicz[56]. As shown in Figure 25, the "shell" IVR consists of an inert inner core which is covered by a 0.15 mm thick steroid-containing layer and a 0.25 mm outer "metering" layer.

Landgren et al[57] in a very careful study found only a very short burst-like release of LNG within the first 24 hours after IVR insertion with a similar shell-type LNG-releasing IVR[58] as shown in Table 12. The mean plasma LNG levels observed in women wearing these devices were relatively constant over a three month period over which they declined by about 20 percent of the initial concentrations, indicating a near zero order release rate of LNG (Figure 26). The *in vitro* determination of the nominal release rate as described by Burton *et al*[58], apparently a problem in this study, measures release of the steroid into an isotonic saline solution. It is quite conceivable that the conditions for steroid release within the vagina are different from those in the isotonic perfusion chamber.

Table 12. Initial absorption of levonorgestrel from intravaginal rings (n = 7) expressed as percent of subsequent plateau levels (geometric means and 95% confidence limits, C.L.). From Landgren et al (57).

HOURS AFTER INSERTION	MEAN LEVEL (%)	95% C.L.
0.5	96	70 – 131
1	164	122 – 219
2	208	159 – 270
4	216	145 – 322
8	201	136 – 297
16	176	120 – 258
24	156	119 – 205

Landgren et al[59] were able to document complete absence of any initial burst-like release of steroid from NET-containing IVRs of the "shell" design[58] as is documented by the data in Table 13. These authors found essentially zero order release rates from these NET-releasing IVRs when they measured serum NET levels in two groups of women who used IVRs which released 200 and 50 μg NET per 24 hours, respectively (see Figure 27).

The study by Landgren et al[59] shows a gradual rise of plasma NET concentrations during the initial postinsertion period to a plateau which is reached at 24 hours. From thereon, during the 90 days of the study, plasma NET levels remained constant and decreased only very slowly with an average daily decrease of 0.1 to 0.2 percent.

By comparison, the subdermal silastic implants release contraceptive

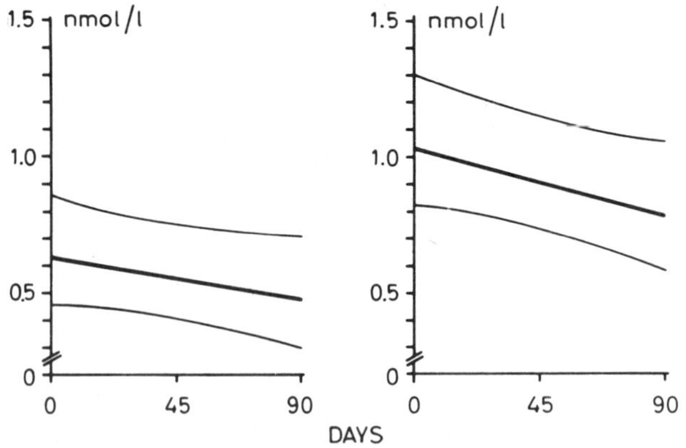

Figure 26. Geometric mean plasma levonorgestrel (LNG) levels (with 95% C.L.) in women using intravaginal rings which release LNG at the nominal rate of 20 (left) and 10 μg/24 hours (right) in 10 and 7 subjects, respectively. From Landgren et al (57).

Table 13. Initial absorption of norethindrone from intravaginal rings (n = 8) expressed as percent of subsequent plateau level (geometric means and 95% confidence limits, C.L.). From Landgren et al (59).

HOURS AFTER INSERTION	MEAN LEVEL (%)	95% C.L.
0.5	19	14 — 25
1	32	26 — 39
2	51	45 — 58
4	62	55 — 71
8	82	76 — 88
16	94	85 — 105
24	106	98 — 116

steroids at a very constant zero order rate for many years whereas the shelltype IVRs release contraceptive steroids at a nearly zero order rate for a more limited period of time. The release rate by the latter devices appears to decrease by about 0.1 to 0.2 percent per day. Unfortunately, time does not permit me to expand on the interesting pharmacodynamics of these modes of contraceptive steroid administration[57,59].

Vaginal Ethinylestradiol Suppositories

In 1977, Rigg et al[60] presented evidence that intravaginal adminis-

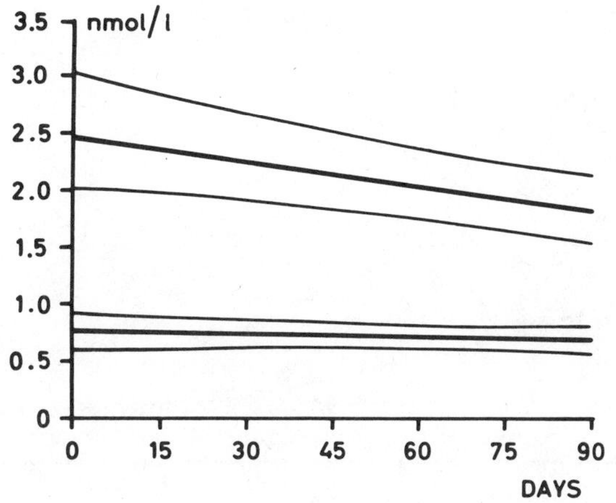

Figure 27. Geometric mean plasma norethindrone (NET) levels (with 95% C.L.) in two groups of 15 women, each using intravaginal rings which release NET at 200 and 50 μg/24 hours, respectively. From Landgren et al (59).

tration of estradiol (E_2) circumvented the high conversion of E_2 to estrone (E_1) thought to occur on its first pass through the liver following ingestion of micronized E_2 and absorption from the intestinal tract[61]. Thus, it was envisioned that parenteral routes of administration of EE might likewise result in a diminution of the hepatic effects of EE[62] which is subject to a very pronounced first pass effect[10-12]. In order to test whether vaginal administration of EE would selectively reduce its pronounced hepatic effect, we prepared polyethylene glycol (PEG) suppositories containing 120 μg of EE[63]. The mean serum EE levels obtained with this regimen were significantly lower than those obtained following ingestion of a single dose of 120 μg of EE (Figure 28). Peak serum EE levels after vaginal administration averaged 25 percent of those observed after oral administration and were achieved between three and six hours after EE suppository insertion. The AUC for the initial 24 hours for vaginal EE amounted to only 30 percent of the AUC obtained for the first 24 hours after ingestion of the same dose of EE (120 μg). The decline of the serum EE concentration curve after peak EE levels had been reached was much more protracted than its counterpart following oral administration (Figure 28).

These data indicate that 1) vaginal absorption of EE administered as a PEG suppository is much more protracted than absorption following oral administration and 2) a smaller portion of the vaginal than of the oral dose becomes bioavailable. Incidentally, vaginal administration of EE did not

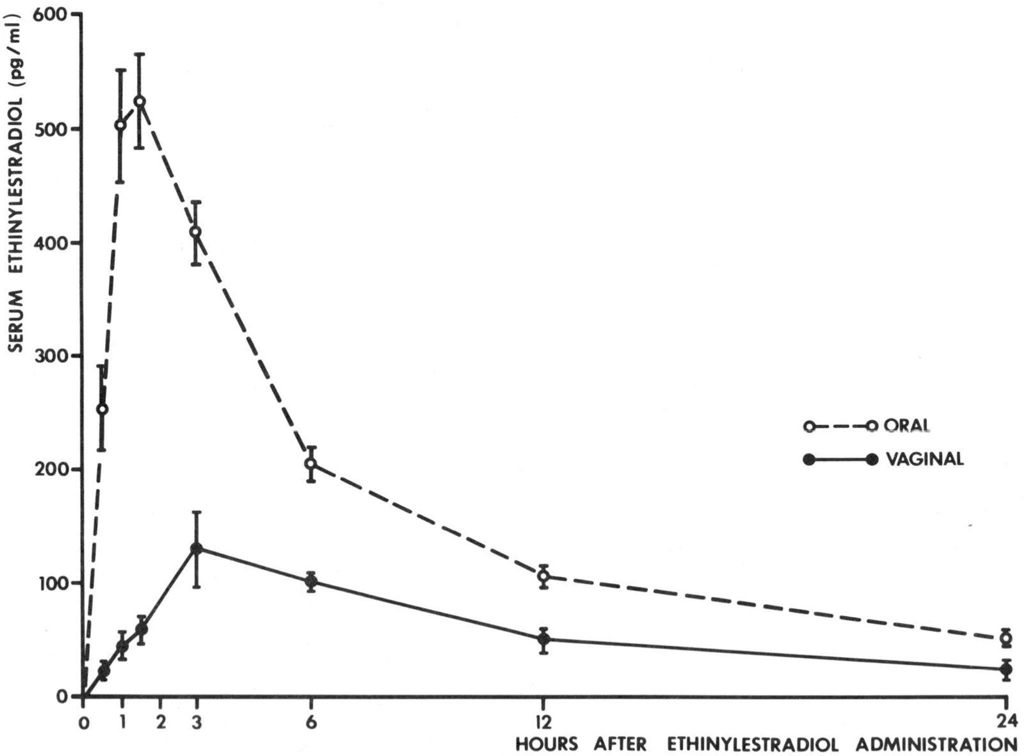

Figure 28. Mean ($\pm$ SE) serum ethinylestradiol concentrations following oral and vaginal (EE) administration to 24 and 5 healthy women, respectively. From Mashchak et al (63).

result in a selective reduction of the pronounced hepatic effects of EE[63] known to occur after oral administration[62,64]. This conclusion is consistent with the findings of Schwartz et al[65] and by us[63] and may be due to the fact that Schwartz et al inserted EE tablets while we administered PEG suppositories of EE. The PEG mixture which loses its solid state at body temperature may actually compete with the vaginal mucosa for the EE and thus retain a portion of the EE causing protracted and decreased absorption through the vaginal mucosa.

This concludes my brief review of the pharmacokinetics of contraceptive steroids in humans. This summary of pertinent publications and ongoing research is far from complete. In addition to presenting factual information on the subject, I have tried to point out some of the shortcomings of past and present pharmacokinetic studies on contraceptive steroids in man as well as of their interpretation. Bioavailability, as defined in pharmacokinetic terms, cannot always be equated with the presence or magnitude of an effect at the cellular site of drug action because the former considers total contraceptive steroid hormone levels while the latter is modified by 1) the affinity to and rate of dissociation from their binding proteins and 2) the capillary transit time for the target tissue in question[29]. Thus, we may safely conclude that it is necessary that the pharmacokinetics of a contraceptive steroid in a given animal model match those found in humans. However, the latter condition does not suffice to accept the animal in question as a suitable model for pharmacologic and toxicologic studies from which one may safely extrapolate to humans.

ACKNOWLEDGEMENT

The author is indebted to Miss Antje Goebelsmann for drawing all the figures which have been contributed by the author.

REFERENCES

1. Greenblatt, DJ, Koch-Weser, J: Drug Therapy. Clinical pharmacokinetics. (First of two parts). N Engl J Med, 293:702, 1975.

2. Greenblatt, DJ, Koch-Weser, J: Drug Therapy. Clinical pharmacokinetics. (Second of two parts). N Engl J Med, 293:964, 1975.

3. Goldzieher, JW, Dozier, TS, de la Pena, A: Plasma levels and pharmacokinetics of ethynyl estrogens in various populations. I. Ethynylestradiol. Contraception, 21:1, 1980.

4. Stanczyk, FZ, Mroszczaka, EJ, Ling, T, Runkel, R, Henzl, M, Miyakawa, I, Goebelsmann, U: Plasma levels and pharmacokinetics of norethindrone and ethinylestradiol administered in solution and as tablets to women. Contraception, in press.

5. Gibaldi, M, Perrier, D: Pharmacokinetics. New York and Basel, Marcel Dekker, Inc. 1982.

6. Stanczyk, FZ, Gale, JA, Goebelsmann, U, Nerenberg, C, Matin, S: Radioimmunoassay of plasma ethinylestradiol in the presence of circulating norethindrone. Contraception, 22:457, 1980.

7. Cook CE, Tallent, CR, Christensen, HD: Antigens from synthetic and natural estrogens: formation by conjugation with protein through a thiopropionic acid line. Life Sci, 14:1075, 1974.

8. Fotherby, K et al. (WHO Collaborative Study). Pharmacokinetics of ethinyloestradiol in women from different populations. Contraception, 23:487, 1981.

9. Metzler, CM, Elfring, GL, McEwen, JM: A user's manual for NONLIN and associated program. Research Biostatistics. The Upjohn Company, Kalamazoo, Michigan, April 20, 1974.

10. Back, DJ, Breckenridge, AM, Crawford, FE, MacIver, M, Orme, ML'E, Rowe, PH, Watts, MJ: An investigation of the pharmacokinetics of ethynylestradiol in women using radioimmunoassay. Contraception, 20:263, 1979.

11. Back, DJ, Bates, M, Breckenridge, AM, Hall, JM, MacIver, M, Orme, ML'E, Park, BK, Rowe, PH: The pharmacokinetics of levonorgestrel and ethinylestradiol in women - studies with Ovran and Ovranette. Contraception, 23:229, 1981.

12. Humpel, M, Nieuweboer, B, Wendt, H, Speck, U: Investigations of Pharmacokinetics of ethinyloestradiol to specific consideration of a possible first-pass effect in women. Contraception, 19:421, 1979.

13. Warren, RJ, Fotherby, K: Plasma levels of ethynyloestradiol after administration of ethynyloestradiol or mestranol to human subjects. J Endocrinol, 59:369, 1973.

14. Helton, ED, Goldzieher, JW: The pharmacokinetics of ethynyl estrogens. A review. Contraception, 15:255, 1977.

15. Bird, CE, Clark, AF: Metabolic clearance rates and metabolism of mestranol and ethynylestradiol in normal young women. J Clin Endocrinol Metab, 36:296, 1973.

16. Mills, TM, Lin, TJ, Hernandez-Ayup, S, Greenblatt, RB, Ellegood, JO, Mahesh, VB: The metabolic clearance rate and urinary excretion of oral contraceptive drugs. II. Mestranol. Am J Obstet Gynecol, 120:773, 1974.

17. Fotherby, K, et al: (WHO Collaborative Study). Rate of metabolism of norethisterone in women from different populations. Contraception, 19:39, 1979.

18. Back, DJ, Breckenridge, AM, Crawford, FE, McIver, M, Orme, ML'E, Rowe, PH, Smith, E: Kinetics of norethindrone in women. II. Single-dose kinetics. Clin Pharmacol Ther, 24:448, 1978.

19. Mills, TM, Lin, TJ, Hernandez-Ayup, S, Greenblatt, RB, Ellegood, JO, Mahesh, VB: The metabolic clearance rate and urinary excretion of oral contraceptive drugs. I. Norethindrone. Am J Obstet Gynecol, 120:764, 1974.

20. Humpel, M, Wendt, H, Dogs, G, Weiss, Chr, Rietz, S, Speck, U: Intraindividual comparison of pharmacokinetic parameters of d-norges-

trel, lynestrenol and cyproterone acetate in 6 women. Contraception, 16:199, 1977.

21. Humpel, M, Wendt, H, Pommerenke, G, Weiss, Chr, Speck, U: Investigations of pharmacokinetics of levonorgestrel to specific consideration of a possible first-pass effect in women. Contraception, 17:207, 1978.

22. Kiriwat, O, Fotherby, K: Pharmacokinetics of oral contraceptive steroids after morning and evening administration. Contraception, 27:153, 1983.

23. Brenner, PF, Mishell, DR, Jr, Stanczyk, FZ, Goebelsmann, U: Serum levels of d-norgestrel, luteinizing hormone, follicle-stimulating hormone, estradiol and progesterone in women during and following ingestion of combination oral contraceptives containing dl-norgestrel. Am J Obstet Gynecol, 129:133, 1977.

24. Weiner, E, Victor, A, Johansson, EDB: Plasma levels of d-norgestrel after oral administration. Contraception, 14:563, 1976.

25. Back, DJ, Breckenridge, AM, Crawford, FE, McIver, M, Orme, ML'E, Park, BK, Rowe, PH, Smith, E: Kinetics of norethindrone in women. I. Radioimmunoassay and concentrations during multiple dosing. Clin Pharmacol Ther, 24:439, 1978.

26. Odlind, V, Victor, A, Johansson, EDB: Plasma protein binding of norethisterone. Contraception, 25:457, 1982.

27. Victor, A, Weiner, E, Johansson, EDB: Sex hormone binding globulin: the carrier protein for d-norgestrel. J Clin Endocrinol Metab, 43: 244, 1976.

28. Jenkins, N, Fotherby, K: Binding of the contraceptive steroids norgestrel and norethisterone in human plasma. J Steroid Biochem, 13:521, 1980.

29. Pardridge, WM: Transport of protein-bound hormones into tissues in vivo. Endocrine Reviews, 2:103, 1981.

30. Reed, MJ, Fotherby, K: Interaction of ethynyloestradiol sulphate with plasma proteins. J Steroid Biochem, 13:495, 1980.

31. Jenkins, N, Fotherby, K: Binding of the gestagens norethisterone and levonorgestrel in blood of various species. J Steroid Biochem, 14:1055, 1981.

32. Prasad, KVS, Narasinga Rao, BS, Sivakumar, B, Prema, K: Pharmacokinetics of norethindrone in Indian women. Contraception, 20:77, 1979.

33. Kirton, KT, Cornette, JC: Return of ovulatory cyclicity following an intramuscular injection of medroxyprogesterone acetate (Provera™). Contraception, 10:39, 1974.

34. Jeppsson, S, Johansson, EDB: Medroxyprogesterone acetate, estradiol, FSH and LH in peripheral blood after intramuscular administration of

DepoProvera to women. Contraception, 14:461, 1976.

35. Ortiz, A, Hiroi, M, Stanczyk, FZ, Goebelsmann, U, Mishell, DR, Jr: Serum medroxyprogesterone acetate (MPA) concentrations and ovarian function following intramuscular injection of depo-MPA. J Clin Endocrinol Metab, 44:32, 1977.

36. Hiroi, M, Stanczyk, FZ, Goebelsmann, U, Brenner, PF, Lumkin, ME, Mishell, DR, Jr: Radioimmunoassay of serum medroxyprogesterone acetate (Provera™) in women following oral and intravaginal administration. Steroids, 26:373, 1975.

37. Fotherby, K, Koetsawang, S, Mathrubutham, M: Pharmacokinetic study of different doses of Depo-Provera. Contraception, 22:527, 1980.

38. Gerhards, E, Hecker, W, Bellmann, O: Studies on the kinetics and metabolism of 17β-heptanoyl-17α-ethinyl-4-oestren-3-one-7^{3}H norethisterone enanthate in humans following intramuscular injection. Arzneim-Forsch (Drug Res), 26:1611, 1976.

39. Saxena, BN, Shrimanker, K, Fotherby, K: Radioimmunoassay of serum norethisterone oenanthate levels in women after intramuscular administration. J Steroid Biochem, 8:1117, 1977.

40. Sang, GW, Fotherby, F, Howard, G, Elder, M, Bye, PG: Pharmacokinetics of norethisterone oenanthate in humans. Contraception, 24:15, 1981.

41. Weiner, E, Johansson, EDB: Plasma levels of norethindrone after I.M. injection of 200 mg of norethindrone enanthate. Contraception, 11: 419, 1975.

42. Howard, G, Warren, RJ, Fotherby, K: Plasma levels of norethisterone in women receiving norethisterone oenanthate intramuscularly. Contraception, 12:45, 1975.

43. Fotherby, K, Howard, G, Shrimanker, K, Elder, M, Bye, PG: Plasma levels of norethisterone after single and multiple injections of norethisterone oenanthate. Contraception, 18:1, 1978.

44. Goebelsmann, U, Stanczyk, FZ, Brenner, PF, Goebelsmann, AE, Gentzschein, EK, Mishell, DR, Jr: Serum norethindrone (NET) concentrations following intramuscular NET enanthate injection. Effect upon serum LH, FSH, estradiol and progesterone. Contraception, 19:283, 1979.

45. Prasad, KVS, Madhavan Nair, K, Sivakumar, B, Prema, K, Narasinga Rao, BS: Plasma levels of norethindrone in Indian women receiving norethindrone enanthate (20 mg) injectable. Contraception, 23:497, 1981.

46. Fotherby, K, Howard, G, Shrimanker, K, Elder, M, Bye, PG: Effect of norethisterone oenanthate on serum gonadotropin levels. Contraception, 16:591, 1977.

47. Back, DJ, Breckenridge, AM, Chapman, CR, Crawford, FE, Elsen, KA, Orme, ML'E, Rowe, PH: Studies on the enzymatic cleavage of norethisterone oenanthate. Contraception, 23:125, 1981.

48. Weiner, E, Johansson, EDB: Plasma levels of d-norgestrel, estradiol

and progesterone during treatment with silastic implants containing d-norgestrel. Contraception, 14:81, 1976.

49. Moore, DE, Roy, S, Stanfzyk, FZ, Mishell, DR, Jr: Bleeding and serum d-norgestrel subdermal polysiloxane capsules for contraception. Contraception, 23:197, 1981.

50. Croxatto, HB, Diaz, S, Miranda, P, Elamsson, K, Johansson, EDB: Plasma levels of levonorgestrel in women during long term use of norplant. Contraception, 23:197, 1981.

51. Alvarez, F, Brache, V, Faundes, A, Johansson, EDB, Odlind, V, Nash, H: Levonorgestrel plasma levels during continuous administration with different models of subdermal implants. Contraception, 27:123, 1983.

52. Laumas, V, Jain, AK, Jha, P, Rahman, SA, Jumar, D, Malik, BK, Sarkar, NN, Takkar, D, Hingorani, V, Laumas, KR: Correlation between the serum norethindrone (NET) levels attained after insertion of a silastic implant releasing norethindrone acetate and the endogenous hormones particularly progesterone. Contraception, 23:211, 1981.

53. Mishell, DR, Jr, Lumkin, ME, Jackanicz, T: Initial clinical studies of intravaginal rings containing norethindrone and norgestrel. Contraception, 12:253, 1975.

54. Stanczyk, FZ, Hiroi, M, Goebelsmann, U, Brenner, PF, Lumkin, ME, Mishell, DR, Jr: Radioimmunoassay of serum d-norgestrel in women following oral and intravaginal administration. Contraception, 12: 279, 1975.

55. Victor, A, Edqvist, LE, Lindberg, P, Elamsson, K, Johansson, EDB: Peripheral plasma levels of d-norgestrel in women after oral administration of d-norgestrel and when using intravaginal rings implanted with dl-norgestrel. Contraception, 12:261, 1975.

56. Jackanicz, TM: Levonorgestrel and estradiol release from an improved contraceptive vaginal ring. Contraception, 24:323, 1981.

57. Landgren, B-M, Johannisson, E, Masironi, B, Diczfalusy, E: Pharmacokinetic and pharmacodynamic investigations with vaginal devices releasing levonorgestrel at a constant, near zero order rate. Contraception, 26:567, 1982.

58. Burton, FG, Skiens, WE, Gordon, NR, Veal, JT, Kalkwarf, DR, Duncan, GW: Fabrication and testing of vaginal contraceptive devices designed for release of prespecified dose levels of steroids. Contraception, 17:221 1978.

59. Landgren, B-M, Oriowo, MA, Diczfalusy, E: Pharmacokinetic and pharmacodynamic studies with vaginal devices releasing norethisterone at a constant near zero order. Contraception, 24:29, 1981.

60. Rigg, LA, Milanes, B, Villanueva, B, Yen, SSC: Efficacy of intravaginal and intranasal administration of micronized estradiol-17β. J Clinical Endocrinol Metab, 45:1261, 1977.

61. Yen, SSC, Martin, PL, Burnier, AM, Czekala, NM, Greaney, MO, Jr,

Callantine, M: Circulating estradiol, estrone and gonadotropin levels following the administration of orally active 17β-estradiol in postmenopausal women. J Clin Endocrinol Metab, 40:518, 1975.

62. Mandel, FP, Geola, FL, Lu, JKH, Eggena, P, Sambhi, MP, Hershman, JM, Judd, HL: Biologic effects of various doses of ethinyl estradiol in postmenopausal women. Obstet Gynecol, 59:673, 1982.

63. Mashchak, CA, Mishell, DR, Jr, Goebelsmann, U: Comparison of hepatic alterations produced by oral and vaginal administration of ethinylestradiol. J Clin Endocrinol Metab, in press.

64. Mashchak, CA, Lobo, RA, Dozona-Takano, R, Eggena, P, Nakamura, RM, Brenner, PF, Mishell, DR, Jr: Comparison of pharmacodynamic properties of various estrogen formulations. Am J Obstet Gynecol, 144:511, 1982.

65. Schwartz, U, Schneller, E, Moltz, L, Hammerstein, J: Vaginal administration of ethinylestradiol: effects on ovulation and hepatic transcortin synthesis. Contraception, 25:253, 1982.

DISCUSSION

DR. BLYE: Dr. Goebelsmann, in your "weak alcoholic solution" dosing, how weak was the alcoholic solution? Was the steroid completely dissolved?

DR. GOEBELSMANN: The steroid was completely dissolved in the following manner. The steroid is first dissolved in 95 percent ethanol (USP), and then distilled water is added to achieve 23 percent alcohol by volume. The steroids remain in solution. Studies were undertaken to determine the stability of the drug in this solution, for the completeness of solution and for the drug concentration. There was no doubt that this "weak alcoholic solution" delivered the correct dose, particularly in the view of our unexpected findings.

DR. HUMPEL: I would like to comment on the volume of distribution for levonorgestrel. This is a number calculated from the total concentration in plasma and I think it should be stated that at the maximum, perhaps one or two percent of total dose is in plasma. That means 99 or 98 percent of the dose is in the tissues, the volume of distribution of levonorgestrel should not be very different from that of norethisterone.

DR. GOEBELSMANN: I agree with you that these volume of distribution values are great approximations derived from calculations which have many assumptions, some of which may be wrong. However, I would say that they have a relative meaning. On a relative basis, the volume of distribution for levonorgestrel appears smaller than that for norethindrone. Again, if one would have a direct assessment for the volume of distribution, this would be much more valuable than the calculated values. Limitations in time did not permit me to go into the details of such calculations which can be derived from pharmacology texts.

DR. GOLDZIEHER: I think one of the things that deserves mention is the importance of the stomach as the place of absorption, and in that sense, I think gastric content has much greater influence than we might expect. We have been doing some studies on oral slow release formulations and find that if we delay release until estrogen gets into the duodenum, then sulfation of the compound and its bioavailability becomes increasingly important to the point where you defeat the purpose of the slow release. I think one of the interesting phenomena in your alcoholic solution versus your tablet might be explained by the volume of alcoholic solution plus whatever water you took afterward compared to the amount of water you gave with the tablet. If you gave a large volume of water with the tablet, you essentially might have been comparing an aqueous solution with an aqueous alcoholic solution, and the absorption of both is so rapid that you can't really see any difference.

DR. GOEBELSMANN: This is true. We have learned this while conducting these studies. In ongoing pharmacokinetic studies we actually normalize the fluid intake and gastric content. We request that subjects do not eat or drink anything the night prior to the study. I think your comment is absolutely important. Overnight fasting, then drinking just the steroid solution, followed by a small standard volume of water, and for the first four hours thereafter nothing else constitutes our routine for pharmacokinetic studies.

DR. KATZENELLENBOGEN: You showed a study indicating quite large differences in the clearance time for SHBG among different socioeconomic groups. How important a variable do you think this is among women in general in terms of clearance rates, and what do you think that is related to? Is it diet associated? How much SHBG is hormone associated? What about liver function?

DR. GOEBELSMANN: I think that SHBG binding capacity is very important for norethindrone and levonorgestrel clearance when measuring total plasma levels and basing all calculations and conclusions on total plasma levels.

What causes the differences in SHBG binding capacity or SHBG concentration (if you measure SHBG as a protein by radioassay) remains largely unknown. Differences may be nutrition related. We only know that, in general, obese women do have smaller and lean women have higher levels of SHBG. In addition, the androgen as well as their estrogen levels in these women may be important. Their liver function may also be important. Numerous factors affect hepatic SHBG synthesis and, unfortunately, too little is known.

Thus, it might be useful to circumvene all these questions of what does affect hepatic SHBG synthesis and SHBG binding capacity by testing subjects for SHBG binding capacity or SHBG before enrolling them in a pharmacokinetic study and thus evaluate and perhaps normalize the study population.

DR. DICZFALUSY: Just a comment on this last point. In the WHO studies, there are a number of those differences which seem to suggest that there are population differences. It may well be that women in Thailand are given, for example, too much Depo-Provera, because original binding study data were derived from investigations conducted in the western part of the world.

DR. BARDIN: In the experiments, where there was a difference between the metabolic clearance rate determined by the constant infusion technique and the other technique that you mentioned, were you trying to compare an orally administered drug versus the constant infusion technique, or was that i.v. a single injection versus constant infusion?

DR. GOEBELSMANN: It was done by i.v. versus oral or just by oral administration. Actually, the clearance rate can be determined or approximated by using mathematical formulas. In this particular instance, the calculated clearance rates have not been checked simultaneously in the same patients with a classical technique, as developed by Tate and others.

Dr. Goldzieher's study has shown how to determine the clearance rate if one has an accurate assessment of the volume of distribution, knows the dose, and has determined the bioavailability constant. The volume of distribution is very, very difficult to assess. It is a very tenuous figure. If we use one uncertain value to calculate the clearance rate, then we cannot place much credence into the clearance rate determinations based on pharmacokinetic parameters unless they are corroborated by the classical technique.

DR. BARDIN: I want to make a point. The issue here is to try to establish a few reliable pharmacokinetic parameters. There will be no difference in the metabolic clearance rate when measured by a single injection or a constant infusion, provided you don't try to select the number of compartments in advance and provided you sample long enough. I think enough questions have been raised about the volume of distribution here to indicate that it is really not a reliable parameter. Erlio Gurpide's book relates how you can alter the the estimation by 100 percent just selecting different time points when you take blood samples.

One of the concerns we can dicuss and we have a lot of authorities here in the room, is to what are kinetic parameters that can be reliably measured. I think Dr. Humpel may have alluded to it. He used the metabolic clearance rate and the terminal phase elimination time. Can we agree that those are parameters that can be accurately measured and are not so dependent upon different experimental designs. Dr. Fotherby's point is really well taken, a lot of these measurements can vary depending on time of blood sampling or experimental design. I believe a little discussion may be in order about what would be accurate or useful to measure, because we can measure ten things, but they are not all useful.

DR. AKSEL: In view of the purpose of this meeting, which is the animal testing requirements, based on the human data which animal model or models would you select to duplicate your data?

DR. GOEBELSMANN: With regard to ethinylestradiol, Dr. Goldzieher's study has reported that the baboon probably is the animal model closest to the human. These studies have been done by the same investigator who did the human studies using the same criteria. We have used the same approach in our laboratory and find that the results obtained in these two species are closely related.

With regard to norethindrone and levonorgestrel, I cannot make such a firm statement.

DR. VON EICKSTEDT: Dr. Bardin questioned which data are really relevant. I would like to ask Dr. Goebelsmann to discuss the sulfates of steroids and what really should be measured, the actual, the normal, the long-term measured blood levels, sex steroid hormone binding globulins, the hormones bound to a protein or, as you mentioned, the conjugates?

Since these steroids undergo enterohaptic circulation, the conjugates (sulfates or glucuronides) become important and should be taken into account when considering availability of the receptor.

Do conjugates have to be measured and enterohepatic circulation taken into account, or can you rely on the pharmacodynamic data we have had for more than ten years?

DR. GOEBELSMANN: We can not rely solely on those pharmacokinetic data. I think they are inadequate. The question remains as to what extent we must expand on these data. As long as there is the possibility that we regenerate biologically active steroids from any conjugate, the conjugate, whether in the general circulation or in the enterohepatic circulation, will have to be measured. We definitely should take into account the question of how much is SHBG-bound. This could be accomplished very simply by dividing between SHBG-bound and non-SHBG-bound steroid levels. There is, in my opinion, no need to further fractionate into albuminbound and free dialyzable steroids.

With regard to your question on sulfates and the enterohepatic circulation, I had the privilege to read Dr. Goldzieher's manuscript on this subject, and perhaps Dr. Goldzieher would comment on the sulfates of ethinylestradiol which he has studied extensively in the baboon.

DR. GOLDZIEHER: In a paper which should appear very shortly in the American Journal of Ob/Gyn, we synthesized the three possible sulfates of ethinylestradiol and studied them intravenously and orally in the baboon. To our great surprise, their half-life is much faster than we anticipated possibly because we thought the sulfates might be a reservoir from which free ethinylestradiol could be regenerated. That turns out not to be the case because the efficiency is very poor.

We have found, but not yet confirmed in the human, that the 17-sulfate is not deconjugated following intravenous administration in the baboon. If it is given orally, the gastrointestinal tract can cleave the sulfate in the 17 position. So, once the 17-sulfate is circulating, it is no longer of biological significance.

DR. DICZFALUSY: Actually, that is also true for phosphates of estradiol. The 17-phosphate ester cannot be cleaved in the circulation.

DR. EASTERLING: This raises questions about esterification in these various animal species and I would like Drs. Goebelsmann, Humpel, and Goldzieher to express their views on the implication of these added variables as we look at animal models.

DR. GOEBELSMANN: If we would draw a parallel to natural steroids, especially estradiol, estradiol glucuronides (the 3- and the 17-glucuronide) are rapidly excreted as we know from Hobkirk's study. Estradiol sulfate appears to have a long half-life, being bound to albumin. A portion of the estradiol sulfate is metabolized largely to estrone sulfate and from estrone sulfate we have conversion back to estrone and estradiol.

However, the return to estradiol proceeds at a very slow rate; the transfer constants are minute. I would not expect that too much ethinylestradiol glucuronide should be returned into biologically active ethinylestradiol which is consistent with what Dr. Goldzieher has already mentioned.

DR. KATZENELLENBOGEN: Some target tissues, such as mammary gland and endometrium, can convert some of the estrogen sulfate to active estrogen. I think that while the blood level may not be a very important proportion of total estrogen, perhaps it may be of greater significance at the target tissue level.

DR. GOEBELSMANN: Yes. That is absolutely correct. It has been shown by Dr. Gurpide, and more recently by others, that the endometrium, can take up estrone sulfate and can actually generate estradiol. Perhaps other target tissues may be able to do the same.

DR. HUMPEL: It is a simplification of the total problem to measure plasma levels, but insofar as it is impossible to routinely make measurements in humans, we have to be content with that.

I personally don't care very much about glucuronides and sulfates because when we measure the active ingredient levels in plasma we will also see the results of any conjugate hydrolysis.

DR. FOTHERBY: We have studied ethinylestradiol sulfates and there is no doubt that in the human the concentration of this metabolite in plasma is roughly ten times the concentration of unconjugated ethinylestradiol. Now, if you measure the various pharmacokinetic parameters for ethinylestradiol and for its sulfate, you will find that these are identical. The correspondence is really quite remarkable and I think one of the main conclusions is that the sulfate is serving as a reservoir for ethinylestradiol. This may be where there is some disagreement with Dr. Goldzieher. This would then mean that there was a large amount of circulating ethinylestradiol in the circulation that was potentially available for exerting biological activity.

The sulfates of the contraceptive steroids are quite important as Dr. Goebelsmann showed from Dr. Gerhardt's work on the levels of norethisterone in plasma as opposed to the levels of radioactivity after giving labeled norethisterone enanthate.

We've also shown that there are very large amounts of norethisterone sulfate and norgestrel sulfate in plasma. Although we don't know what the various pharmacokinetic parameters and transfer constants for the gestagens are, I would suggest they could be of biological importance.

DR. DICZFALUSY: Is this not following oral administration? Isn't it true that if you deliver, for instance, estradiol percutaneously, there is relatively little estrone sulfate circulating? Meanwhile, after oral administration, the bulk, more than 90 percent, is estrone sulfate?

DR. GOEBELSMANN: I think eventually we will find that the bulk of circulating estrogens is made up of estrone sulfate, irrespective of the route of administration. If we give estradiol orally, we have very rapid conversion on the first pass into estrone and estrone sulfate. If we give it percutaneously, we have a higher serum estradiol to estrone ratio than we would have with estradiol tablets. But as metabolism takes place, we will have a rapid conversion of circulating estradiol to estrone and to estrone sulfate and estrone sulfate in the circulation will be bound to albumin. This will actually represent the bulk of estrogen circulating as estrone sulfate.

DR. DICZFALUSY: Thank you, and the last question is, you indicated some very interesting dissociation times from SHBG for endogenous steroids. Have you seen those, for instance, for levonorgestrel?

DR. GOEBELSMANN: No. I think it would be most important to obtain these. These data were obtained in the rat and are not human data. It would be interesting to have human data and to include synthetic and particularly contraceptive steroids as well.

DR. DICZFALUSY: Then I would like to thank Professor Goebelsmann for covering such an extremely complex field in such a lucid way.

SPECIES DIFFERENCES IN METABOLISM OF CONTRACEPTIVE STEROIDS

Kenneth Fotherby

University of London
Royal Postgraduate Medical School
Hammersmith Hospital
London, England

It has been known for a long time that species differ in the way they metabolise various drugs. An example which has some reference to steroid metabolism is that of the synthesis of glucuronide conjugates, which is an important metabolic pathway in humans and many other species, whereas in the cat this pathway is of little importance due to a deficiency of glucuronyl transferase. Even when there are no enzyme deficiencies, there are marked variations between species in the rate at which they metabolise the same compound. This could have important effects since if a particular metabolic reaction is much slower in one species than in another either the drug will persist for a longer time and hence exert a more marked biological effect or alternatively the slow metabolism will provide an opportunity for other metabolic reactions to occur. The synthetic contraceptive steroids show many structural differences, often including the introduction of novel substituents, from the naturally occurring sex hormones and by analogy with the metabolism of other drugs, marked species differences in the metabolism of the contraceptive steroids might be expected. This review summarises information regarding the in vivo and in vitro metabolism of the contraceptive steroids in various species.

A summary of the in vivo metabolism of contraceptive steroids in various animal species is shown in Table 1. In most species, many of the steroids undergo an enterohepatic circulation and values given in Table 1 for the proportion of the dose appearing in bile relate to animals in which the bile duct has been cannulated. There are marked differences between the species in the excretion via urine or faeces. For the gestagens, rat and dog appear to excrete the dose predominantly in the faeces whereas for rabbit and baboon the predominant route is urine. Ethynyloestradiol appears to differ from the gestagens, particularly in the rabbit where it is excreted mainly in the faeces. For many of the steroids considerable metabolism occurs in the intestinal wall and liver (first-pass effect) and in most species, except possibly the baboon, the steroids undergo an enterohepatic circulation. Polar compounds, which have not been characterized, are produced in most species and since many of them appear not to be reabsorbed, they limit the extent of the enterohepatic circulation.

The main pathway of metabolism particularly for the 17α-ethynyl

Table 1. In vivo metabolism of contraceptive steroids.

Species	Steroid Administered	% Dose Recovered In			Remarks
		Urine	Faeces	Bile	
Rat	EE	2 mainly non-hydrolysable metabolites	60 polar metabolites, poorly absorbed	70 5% free, 50% glucuronides, some sulphates	
	NET	25 mainly non-hydrolysable metabolites	80	80 60% glucuronides mainly polar metabolites	Metabolised in intestinal wall and liver to 4-en-3ß-OH and 3α,5αTH-metabolites
	EDD	-	-	-	Hydrolysed at 3ß, then 17ß
	CMA	20 mainly free, polar metabolites	80	65 20% free, polar metabolites	
	MGA	10	50	-	
Guinea Pig	EE	40 mainly EE as glucuronide	60 unconjugated	-	
Rabbit	EE	20 mainly glucuronides	40	-	Evidence for EE, 2-methoxy EE D-homo E_1-17α D-homo E_2-17α (as N-acetyl glucosamine conjugates)
	NET	50 DH- and TH-NET, mainly glucuronides	5	80	Metabolised in intestinal wall and liver. Loss of ethynyl group

	NOG	55 DH- and TH-NOG, mainly glucuronides	5	-	
	LYN	35 DH- and TH-NET	-	-	
	CMA	-	-	-	DH-, 2-OH and 17,20,21-tri-OH metabolites, loss of 17-acetoxy and 6-chloro group
	MGA	30	8	-	Hydroxylation at C2 and C6 methyl
Baboon	EE	80 mainly glucuronides, some sulphates	-	-	Detected EE and at least 10 polar metabolites in urine
	EDD	40 glucuronides	-	40	Metabolised to NET No enterohepatic circulation
	MPA	30	-	30	Mainly glucuronide conjugates. No sulphates. Possibly loss of C-17-acetate.

EE = ethynyloestradiol, MEE = mestranol, NET = norethisterone, EDD = ethynodiol diacetate, LYN = lynestrenol, NOG = norgestrel, MPA = medroxyprogesterone acetate, MGA = megestrol acetate, CMA = chlormadinone acetate, DH- and TH- = dihydro- and tetrahydro-metabolites, E_1=estrone, E_2=estradiol

(continued)

Table 1 (Continued)

Species	Steroid Administered	% Dose Recovered In: Urine	Faeces	Bile	Remarks
Baboon (cont.)	MGA	40	3	-	
	CMA	16 glucuronides	16	-	Possibly loss of C-17-acetate. No enterohepatic circulation.
Dog	EE	21 unchanged EE present	-	-	Metabolised in intestinal wall, liver
	NET	-	-	-	Epoxide detected
	MPA	-	-	-	TH-metabolites in liver, bile and faeces
	MGA	10	80	-	Hydroxylation at C-6
	CMA	8	40	-	
Monkey Rhesus	EE	40 mainly glucuronides	9-17 50% not extractable with methanol	-	Evidence for EE, E_1 and E_2

Monkey Rhesus (cont.)	NOG	37 45-62% free, 13-27% glucuronides. No sulphates	-	-	Large number of metabolites in urine Major metabolite was D-homosteroid. Also identified 2α-OH, 16α-OH and 16β-OH-NOG, TH-NOG and 16β-TH NOG
	MCA	22	44	-	
	CMA	36	28	-	
Monkey African Green	NOG	37-51 48-62% free, 13-27% glucuronides. No sulphates	41-55	-	Large number of metabolites in urine Identified D-homosteroid 2α-OH, 16α-OH and 16β-OH NOG, TH-NOG and 16β-OH TH NOG. Large variation between animals in proportion metabolites.

EE = ethynyloestradiol, MEE = mestranol, NET = norethisterone, EDD = ethynodiol diacetate, LYN = lynestrenol, NOG = norgestrel, MPA = medroxyprogesterone acetate, MGA = megestrol acetate, CMA = chlormadinone acetate, DH- and TH- = dihydro- and tetrahydro-metabolites, E_1=estrone, E_2=estradiol steroids, is reduction of ring A producing dihydro- and tetrahydrometabolites although considerable hydroxylation of both types of gestagens occurs. There is very little information on the nature of metabolites of any contraceptive steroid in rat, guinea pig, dog and baboon and the only extensive studies reported are those of ethynyloestradiol[1] and chlormadinone acetate[2] in the rabbit and norgestrel in the monkey[3,4].

Norethisterone-4β,5β-epoxide was isolated from livers of dogs given norethisterone and was also produced by incubation of norethisterone with the supernatant fraction from liver of phenobarbital treated dogs[5]. The largest amount of the epoxide was found after only short incubation times since it appeared to be rapidly metabolised. A tight binding of norethisterone to rat liver microsomes which might be due to formation of the epoxide has been reported by Kappus and Remmer[6]. The role of epoxide has been studied in more detail by White[7] who showed that the epoxide was rapidly metabolised to the dihydrodiol by a rat liver microsomal fraction. In contrast with the other findings, when norethisterone was incubated with the microsomal fraction neither the epoxide nor the dihydrodiol was detected. Although it has been suggested that a similar epoxide is formed from norgestrel this appears to bind less tightly than norethisterone epoxide to proteins.

The binding of the epoxide appears to involve proteins containing sulphydryl groups and no binding occurs to DNA or RNA[8]. It also has been suggested[9] that the metabolism of ethynyloestradiol to hydroxylated metabolites such as 2-hydroxyethynyloestradiol also results in a tight binding of the metabolites to liver proteins. Another interesting characteristic of 4,5-epoxide is that it appears to be readily aromatised[10] and this would be one way by which norethisterone could be converted to ethynyloestradiol.

The 4β,5β-epoxide of norethisterone is reported to be toxic to Walker cells in tissue culture and, suprisingly in view of its rapid metabolism, to cause hepatic cell necrosis in rats[7]. In mice the epoxide has no gross toxicity, no effect on foetal development and no antifertility or uterotrophic action[5]. Much more work is necessary to determine the occurrence and importance of the epoxide in various species and in the human.

Other interesting transformations include formation of D-homosteroids from ethynyloestradiol in the rabbit and the human and similarly from norgestrel in monkeys and humans (the formation of D-homosteroids may account for the loss of the ethynyl grouping which has been reported to a variable extent in some species), loss of the chlorine atom from C6 chlormadinone acetate in the rabbit but not so far reported for other species, the hydrolysis of the acetate of the 17α-acetoxyprogesterone derivatives in rabbit, baboon and humans and further metabolism (hydroxylation) of the 17β-side chain, and hydroxylation at C2 of the progestogens.

Table 2 summarizes information regarding the in vitro metabolism of contraceptive steroids. Almost all the studies relate to rat and rabbit and there is obviously a need for more widespread studies as a complement to, and confirmation of, in vivo findings. The interesting findings of

Table 2. In vitro metabolism of contraceptive steroids.

Species	Steroid incubated	Tissue	Products and Remarks
Rat	MEE	Liver	Converted to EE, hydroxylated, binding to liver proteins
	NET	Liver and other tissues	DH-NET, TH-NET and polar metabolites, ? 4ß,5ß-epoxide
	EDD	Liver and intestine	NET
	MPA, MGA	Liver and instestine	Liver metabolism, progesterone>MPA>MGA. Intestinal contents, MGA MPA, DH and TH metabolites.
	CMA	Liver	3-OH and 2-OH metabolites
Guinea pig	EE	Liver	Little metabolism (but E_1 and E_2 formed are metabolised)
	NET	Liver	Reduction of ring A
Rabbit	NET	Liver and other tissues especially lung	TH-NET
	NOG	Liver and other tissues	TH-NOG. d-NOG > 1-NOG but 1-NOG not metabolised by tissues other than liver.
	LYN	Liver	NET, TH-NET
	EDD	Liver and kidney	NET
	MPA, MGA	Liver	Less readily metabolised than progesterone
	CMA	Liver	3-OH and 2-OH metabolites
Dog	NET	Liver	5α-3,i.e. 3,6 6-dione, polar metabolites, 4ß,5ß-epoxide ?
	MPA	Liver	DH and TH metabolites

C2 hydroxylation of 17α-acetoxyprogestogens in vivo by rat and rabbit is confirmed by in vitro studies.

Differences between species occur in the binding of the contraceptive steroids, particularly norgestrel and norethisterone[11]. In the baboon and rhesus monkey, as in humans, these two progestogens bind both to sex hormone binding globulin and to albumin although there are differences in the binding affinities in the three species. In the dog and rabbit more binding occurred to albumin and less to sex hormone binding globulin and the nature of this protein in these two species is known to differ from that in primates. In guinea pig and rat, binding occurred only to albumin. In six species studied, medroxyprogesterone acetate and ethynyloestradiol bound only to albumin[12] but variations were observed in the stability and apparent association constants for the steroid albumin complexes. These differences between the species in their binding of the contraceptive steroids are likely to imply differences in pharmacological activity.

It is obvious from the above summary that knowledge of the metabolism of most contraceptive steroids in most species is meagre. The available information however does show differences between the species in the pharmacokinetics, metabolism and protein binding of the steroids. No comparative investigation of different steroids in any species with the exception of two *in vitro* studies[13,14] and one *in vivo* study[15] has been performed and most investigations have utilized only a small number of animals so that a comparison between species and steroids is not possible. The metabolism of the contraceptive steroids in women is known to vary widely[16]; such wide variations probably also occur in animals and caution is needed in interpreting the results from small numbers of animals. No evidence is available regarding the changes in metabolism when animals are administered large doses over a prolonged period of time as occurs in many toxicological studies.

From the information summarised above, no species would appear to be suitable as a model for human studies and on this basis toxicological findings in animals must have dubious relevance to the use of the contraceptive steroids in humans.

REFERENCES

1. Abdel-Aziz, MT, Williams, KH: Metabolism of 17 -ethynylestradiol and its 3-methyl ether by the rabbit; an *in vivo* D-homoannulation. *Steroids*, 13:809, 1969.

2. Abe, T, Kambegawa, A: Urinary and biliary metabolites of 17 -acetoxy-6choloro-4,6,pregnadiene-3,20-dione in the rabbit. *Chem Pharm Bull*, 22: 2824, 1974.

3. Sisenwine, SF, Kimmel, HB, Liu, Al, Ruelius, HW: Stereoselective biotransformations of dl-norgestrel and its enantiomers in the African green monkey. *Drug Metab Disp*, 2:65, 1974.

4. Sisenwine, SF Kimmel, HB, Liu, AL, Ruelius, HW: The metabolic disposition of norgestrel in female rhesus monkeys. *Drug Metab Disp*, 7:1, 1979.

5. Cook, CE, Dickey, MC, Christensen, HD: Oxygenated norethindrone derivatives from incubation with beagle liver. Structure, synthesis and biological activity. *Drug Metab Disp*, 2:58, 1974.

6. Kappus, H, Remmer, H: Metabolic activation of norethisterone (norethindrone) to an irreversibly protein-bound derivative by rat liver microsomes. *Drug Metab Disp*, 3:338, 1975.

7. White, INH: Chemical reactivity and metabolism of norethindrone-4 ,5

-epoxide by rat liver microsomes in vitro. Chem-Biol Interactions, 29:103, 1980.

8. Bolt, HM: Structural modifications in contraceptive steroids altering their metabolism and toxicity. Arch Toxicol, 39:13, 1977.

9. Bolt, HM, Kappus, H, Kasbohrer, R: Metabolism of 17 -ethinylestradiol by human liver microsomes in vitro: aromatic hydroxylation and irreversible protein binding of metabolites. J Clin Endocr, 39:1072, 1974.

10. Morand, P, Lompa-Krzymien, L, Williamson, DG, Layne, DS, Labow, R, Salvador, J: The metabolism of the epoxide of testosterone by human placental microsomes. Steroids, 26:387, 1975.

11. Jenkins, N, Fotherby, K: Binding of the gestagens norethisterone and levonorgestrel in blood of various species. J. Steroid Biochem, 14:493, 1981.

12. Akpoviroro, JO, Mangalam, M, Jenkins, N, Fotherby, K: Binding of the contraceptive steroids medroxyprogesterone acetate, and ethynyloestradiol in blood of various species. J. Steroid Biochem, 14:493, 1981.

13. Cooke, BA, Vallance, DK: Metabolism of megestrol acetate and related progesterone analogues by liver preparations in vitro. Biochem J, 97:672 1966.

14. Khan, FS, Fotherby, K: In vitro metabolism of 17 -ethynylsteroids. J. Steroid Biochem, 10:437, 1979.

15. Ghatei, MA, Fotherby, K: Comparative study of ethynyloestradiol metabolism in the rabbit, guinea pig and rat. Hormone Res, 10:320, 1979.

16. Fotherby, K: Variability of pharmacokinetic parameters for contraceptive steroids. J Steroid Biochem, in press.

DISCUSSION

DR. DICZFALUSY: Thank you very much, Dr. Fotherby. May I invite questions, comments? Dr. Blye?

DR. BLYE: Dr. Fotherby, assuming there is a relationship between liver metabolism and hepatotoxicity, is there any way to quantify it for a given drug?

DR. FOTHERBY: Not that I know of.

DR. BLYE: Do you agree with the assumption that there is a relationship?

DR. FOTHERBY: I don't think I would agree with that. We don't have any current evidence that bears on that question. It has been raised in connection with the epoxide and the 2,3 catechols formed from ethinylestradiol. These might interact with liver proteins, bind very tightly to them and exert an undesirable effect, however evidence for this is almost nonexistent. It is entirely an assumption.

DR. HUMPEL: I don't think that knowledge of steroid metabolism in animal species is meagre. You are correct in terms of the number of metabolites finally identified, but we know how difficult it is to isolate and identify 0.1 percent of a given drug as a metabolite.

What I tried to point out in my conclusion is that while the principle routes of biotransformation are known, i.e., reduction, hydroxylation at different sites, and conjugation. They vary between species but do occur in all animals and in man.

DR. FOTHERBY: I would agree with that as a general statement but I still believe our knowledge is meagre in most species for most contraceptive steroids. While in most cases we are able to identify only a very small percentage of the dose, we can account for much of the dose in terms of radioactivity in urine and faeces, but we have no idea what that radioactivity is associated with.

DR. GOLDZIEHER: I would like to make two points. It is entirely possible that the nature of the metabolites may be more important than we realize, and I believe Dr. Clark will refer to some our the studies we have done on the potential importance of the epoxides and catechols. The baboon, for example, is excellent in forming C2-hydroxy compounds and is even more active in that regard than the human, and should the catechol compounds have biological importance, would be a useful model.

The other point I also wish to make is that we are not considering trivial metabolites when we study, for example, medroxyprogesterone acetate. I don't think 10 percent of the metabolites have been identified yet. The compound has been around for decades. This reflects, a serious deficiency in our knowledge of that substance.

DR. FOTHERBY: Is there any evidence that generally what happens with a particular steroid in animal species is remotely similar to what happens with that steroid in the human? I hope you agree from that what I have shown you that we don't really have enough data to make a firm conclusion. The existing data suggest that none of the species studied are really very suitable as animal models for the human. The most we can hope for is that in the test species the rate of metabolism of the steroid and its major metabolites are similar to the human, but we still require additional information before we can make such statements. When I emphasized the baboon, I did so because at the moment it is the only species which shows a correspondence in certain respects with the human. However, I suspect that with more data in the baboon, probably the differences rather than similarities will become apparent.

STEROIDS OF ONE CLASS CAN MIMIC, INHIBIT AND POTENTIATE THE BIOLOGICAL EFFECTS OF OTHER STEROID CLASSES WHEN ADMINISTERED AT HIGH DOSES

C. Wayne Bardin and Olli A. Janne

Center for Biomedical Research
The Population Council
New York, New York

INTRODUCTION

Over the past 20 years, it has been customary to use up to 50 times the human dose of progestins and estrogens in chronic toxicity studies of contraceptive steroid formulations. It was anticipated that large doses administered for relatively short periods might be predictive of toxicological effects produced by smaller doses administered over many years, analogous to the predictive value of the cumulative effect of small doses of ionizing radiation. When these guidelines were established, there was almost no understanding of the mechanism by which hormones exert their effects on responsive tissues. Subsequently, an enormous body of information has broadened our understanding of the mechanism by which steroid hormones stimulate tissue specific protein synthesis, cell division, hyperplasia and neoplasia. It is now clear that steroids are not genotoxic agents (direct carcinogens) as is ionizing radiation. Rather, they exert their effects on cells that contain effector molecules which recognize and bind the steroid molecules of a particular class when present at or above physiological concentrations in body fluids.

These effector molecules have been termed steroid receptors and there is a receptor for each class of steroid hormone. For example, there is a progestin receptor for progesterone, estrogen receptor for estradiol, androgen receptor for testosterone, etc. Once a steroid such as testosterone binds to the androgen receptor, the steroid receptor complex elicits a biological response attributed to that class of steroids. The response, therefore, of a given tissue to a specific steroid not only depends upon the presence of physiological concentrations of the steroid hormone in blood, but upon a receptor that is capable of binding the hormone and eliciting the subsequent tissue specific response. It was also appreciated that the effects of supraphysiological concentrations of naturally occurring steroid hormones were manifest by other than homologous receptors. For example, high doses of testosterone produced changes on the endometrium that mimicked progesterone and these effects were mediated via the progestin receptor. Such effects were not viewed as physiologically important since they were only observed *in vivo* in association with steroid hormone producing tumors.

A large body of evidence indicates that all of the potent naturally occurring steroids of each class have relatively short half-lives in blood, are not active orally, and are inactivated in the splanchnic circulation. To produce steroids which were orally active and which could be infrequently administered required extensive modification of naturally occurring steroid structures. While these changes retained the desired biological activity, they also retained, and in some cases enhanced the ability of some synthetic steroids to interact with multiple receptors and thus exert more than one biological activity, especially when administered at the high doses used in classical toxicology studies. This phenomenon is particularly well illustrated by the spectrum of biological actions exhibited by synthetic progestins and androgens. The present report will review evidence indicating that superphysiological doses of progestins or androgens can have a variety of effects which cannot be attributed alone to their action by way of the progestin and androgen receptors, respectively. We have in most part restricted this analysis to a detailed discussion of progestins that have effects via the androgen receptor and androgens that act via the progestin receptor. The principles illustrated, however, apply to the action of other steroids that have effects by the "wrong" receptor when administered at high doses.

PROGESTINS MIMIC, INHIBIT, AND POTENTIATE THE EFFECTS OF ANDROGENS

Synthetic progestins are defined according to their biological activities. Among the most important of these are effects on the endometrium which permit implantation and subsequent maintenance of pregnancy. In addition to their effects on the uterus, large doses of some progestational steroids are known to stimulate the growth of the male reproductive tract and to virilize the external genitalia of the female fetus[1]. In this respect, progestins that behave like androgens and compounds structurally related to 19-nortestosterone are, in general, more androgenic than those that are derivatives of progesterone. In addition to their inherent androgenic potential, progestins may also potentiate and inhibit the actions of testosterone[2,3,4]. These modifying effects of progestins have been termed their synandrogenic and antiandrogenic actions which, like the androgenic effects of this class of steroids, depend on dose, steroid structure, and the responsiveness of individual tissues. Present evidence suggests that progestins may require a functional androgen receptor to initiate their androgenic, synandrogenic, and antiandrogenic actions[4,5]. In the experiments that have defined how progestins mimic or modify androgen action through involvement of steroid metabolic and receptor mechanisms, the kidney, submaxillary gland, prostate and seminal vesicle have been used extensively. The mouse is of particular interest since there are a number of well-defined genetic mutants in this species in which the actions of androgens and progestins are modified.

<u>The Effect of Androgens and Progestins on Specific Kidney Proteins</u>

The androgen induced hypertrophy of the cells of Bowman's capsule and of the proximal convoluted tubule of the mouse is associated with an increase in many kidney constituents and has been summarized in recent reviews[6,7]. Of the androgen responsive renal proteins, β-glucuronidase and ornithine decarboxylase (ODC) are perhaps the best studied[6,8,9,10]. All androgens tested to date stimulate the activities

Table 1. The Relative Androgenic, Antiandrogenic and Synandrogenic Activities of Progestational and Nonprogestational Agents.

Steroid		Relative biological activities[1]			
uctural name	Trivial name	Progestational	Androgenic	Antiandrogenic	Synandrogenic
C–21 Steroids					
1. 17α-acetoxy-6-chloro-1,2α-methylene-4,6-pregnadiene-2,30-dione	Cyproterone acetate	very potent	0	+++	+++
2. 17α-hydroxy-6-chloro-1,2α-methylene-4,6-pregnadiene-3,20-dione	Cyproterone	0	0	++	0
3. 17α-acetoxy-6α-methyl-4-pregnene-3,20-dione	Medroxyprogesterone acetate (MPA)	2000	+++	0	++
4. 17α-hydroxy-6α-methyl-4-pregnene-3,20-dione	17α-hydroxy-6α-methylprogesterone	...	0	0	+
5. 6α-methyl-4-pregnene-3,20-dione	6α-methylprogesterone	150	++	+++	+++
6. 17α-acetoxy-4-pregnene-3,20-dione	17α-acetoxyprogesterone	2500	++	0	0
7. 17α-hydroxy-4-pregnene-3,20-dione	17α-hydroxyprogesterone	1	0	0	0
8. 17α-acetoxy-6α-methyl-6-dehydro-4-pregnene-3,20-dione	Megestrol acetate	2500	+	+	+
9. 17α-caproxy-4-pregnene-3,20-dione	Progesterone caproate	100	0	0	+
10. 11β,17α,21-trihydroxy-4-pregnene-3,20-dione	Hydrocortisone	0	0	0	0
C–18 Progestins					
1. d-13β-ethyl-17α-ethynyl, 17β-hydroxy-4-gonen-3-one	d-norgestrel	375	++	0	++
2. 17α-ethynyl-17β-hydroxy-4-estren-3-one	Lynestrenol	155	++	0	+
3. 17α-ethynyl-17β-hydroxy-5(10)-estren-3-one	Norethynodrel	75	+	0	+
Others					
1. 6α-bromo-17β-hydroxy-17α-methyl-4-oxo-5α-androstan-3-one	BOMT	0	0	++	0
2. 3-trifluoromethyl-4-nitro-isobutyranilide	Flutamide	0	0	+++	0

1 Relative progestational activities (48, 49, 50; progesterone = 100). The relative androgenic, antiandrogenic and synandrogenic activities (3,4).

A+++ response was the maximal seen for any progestin listed.

+ was a response that could just be distinguished from 0 usually with 1 dose of steroid.

0 indicates no response at the doses tested (6).

of these enzymes, and the androgen receptor is necessary for these effects[8,9]. These increases in enzyme activities are preceded by rises in mRNA and enzyme synthesis[11,12,13,14]. Although these enzymes comprise much less than one percent of total kidney protein when fully induced, they are useful for the study of hormone action inasmuch as androgens produce 20- to 600-fold increases in their specific activities. In addition, several genetic loci have been identified that modify the androgen induced response of β-glucuronidase and ODC genes[6,15,16]. Recent studies have indicated that ODC exhibits a rapid response to androgen treatment. For example, this enzyme increases rapidly within hours after testosterone administration whereas days are required for β-glucuronidase[9].

Experiments by several investigators[4,16,17] indicated that certain progestins such as medroxyprogesterone acetate (MPA) also stimulate β-glucuronidase, ODC, and other renal proteins. These observations prompted an examination of a series of steroids to determine the relationship between steroid structure and the ability to stimulate these proteins. The studies on β-glucuronidase (Table 1) may be summarized as follows: progesterone itself was inactive, but was agonistic (androgenic) following the addition of a 6α-methyl group. The activity of this latter steroid (6α-methylprogesterone) was further modified by the addition of functional groups at the 17α-position; a 17α-hydroxyl group inhibited whereas a 17α-acetoxy group increased the androgenic activity of the 6α-substituted progestin. The introduction of a

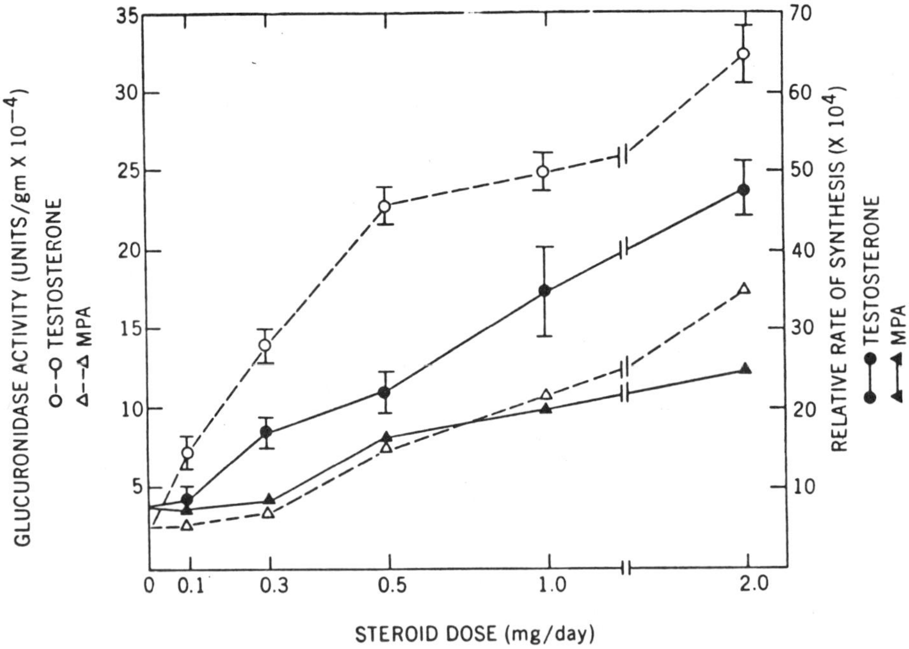

Figure 1. The effect of testosterone or medroxyprogesterone acetate (MPA) on β-glucuronidase activity per gram wet weight and on the relative rate of β-glucuronidase synthesis in mouse kidney. The five animals in each group were treated for six days. Mean ± SEM (from 19).

double bond at the C-6 position of MPA also reduced the androgenicity of this progestin. In addition to the C_{21} steroids, C_{18} progestins were also androgenic. Besides β-glucuronidase and ODC, the androgenic activities of progestins have been shown on other kidney proteins, including alcohol dehydrogenase, 3-keto reductase, and the T proteins found in kidney membrane fractions[3,6,17,18].

In order to investigate how progestins increase renal proteins, a procedure was used which measures the in vivo incorporation of ^{3}H-amino acid into immunoprecipitable β-glucuronidase[19]. This assay was then used to demonstrate that MPA increased β-glucuronidase activity by increasing the rate of synthesis of new enzyme molecules. The results

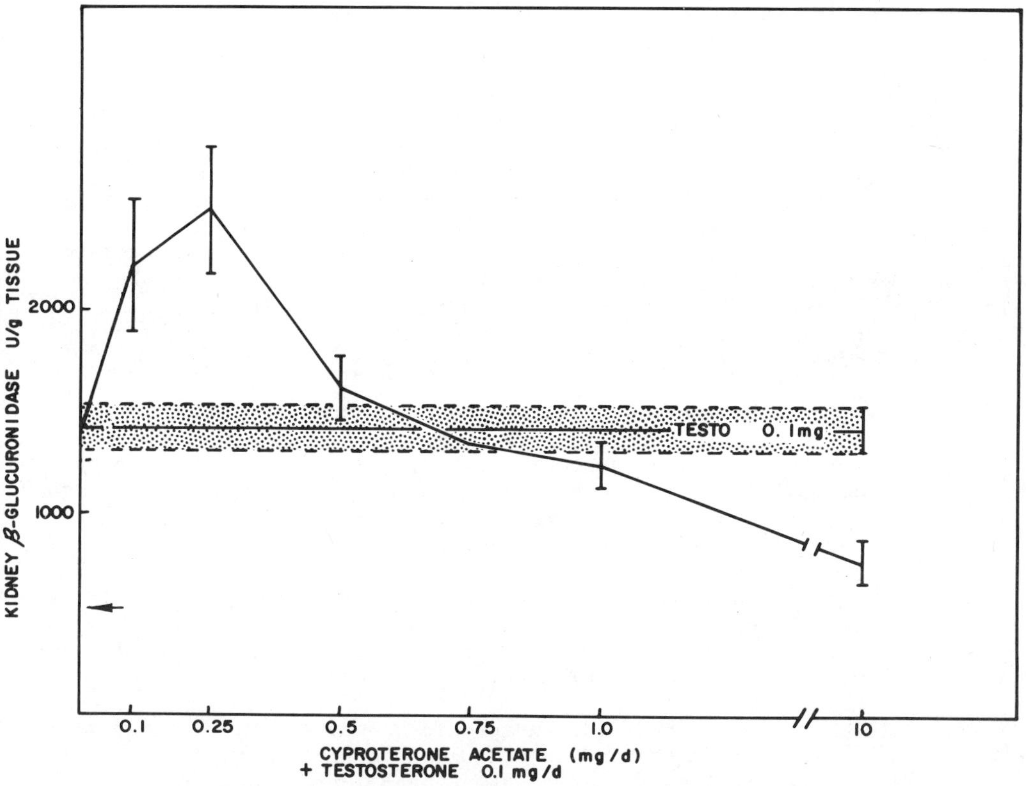

Figure 2. The syn- and antiandrogenic actions of cyproterone acetate on renal β-glucuronidase activity of female mice. Testosterone treatment (0.1 mg/day for 6 days) increased β-glucuronidase activity 2-fold in this study (horizontal shaded bar shows the mean ± SEM). When this treatment was combined with various doses of cyproterone acetate, the response was first potentiated and then inhibited (solid line). Cyproterone acetate alone produced no effect on β-glucuronidase activity. The arrow indicates the enzyme activity in untreated animals (from 4).

of these studies are summarized in Figure 1. These observations are consistent with the hypothesis that the androgenic action of progestins like that of testosterone requires gene activation and protein synthesis.

The Synandrogenic and Antiandrogenic Actions of Progestins on Mouse Kidney

Cyproterone acetate (CypAc) is known to be a potent progestin in the female reproductive tract and an effective antiandrogen in the male[20]. The effect of simultaneous administration of testosterone and CypAc on β-glucuronidase activity in kidney of female mice is shown in Figure 2. When the dose of CypAc was the same or up to 2-5 times higher than the dose of testosterone, androgen action was potentiated[4]. However, when increasing amounts of CypAc were given with a constant dose of testosterone, an antiandrogenic effect was observed (Figure 2). A similar pattern of response was observed when 5α-dihydrotestosterone was used instead of testosterone[3]. It is of note that CypAC alone had no androgenic activity on either the kidney or the other androgen responsive tissues of the mouse such as the submaxillary gland or male reproductive tract. In an experiment similar to that shown in Figure 2, MPA was given to female mice in place of CypAc. That is, a fixed dose of testosterone was administered alone and with various doses of MPA from 1 to 10 times that of the androgen; other groups of mice were treated with MPA alone. A low dose of MPA was inactive when administered alone but was synandrogenic when given with an equal mass of testosterone. Higher doses of this progestin mimicked testosterone when given alone (as noted above), and potentiated the androgen action when administered with testosterone. These observations indicated that both androgenic (MPA) and antiandrogenic (CypAc) progestins can potentiate the actions of testosterone on mouse kidney when the progestin:androgen ratio is appropriate[6].

A series of steroids was investigated to determine whether the synandrogenic property of progestins relates to steroid structure. Several different analogs of MPA were tested (Table 1). Many compounds with the 6α-methyl substitution showed synandrogenic activity. Although these observations suggested the importance of 6α-substitution, progesterone caproate and several other progestins without the 6α-methyl group were also synandrogenic. It may be significant, however, that the synandrogenic response of these latter steroids was produced only with very large doses. As a consequence, the mechanism by which they produce synergism may be different from those of the 6α-methyl series which synergise at lower progestin:androgen ratios[3,6].

In view of the fact that antiandrogenic progestational steroids such as CypAc were found to have synandrogenic activity, it was pertinent to investigate the actions of nonprogestational antiandrogens. Two steroidal (cyproterone and BOMT) and one nonsteroidal (flutamide) compounds were studied (Table 1). Flutamide and BOMT had no effect on kidney β-glucuronidase when administered alone, whereas cyproterone reduced the activity of this enzyme by 25 percent. None of these agents demonstrated synandrogenic activity when administered with testosterone, although all the compounds exhibited antiandrogenic activities on the male reproductive tract and the mouse kidney. This indicated that the synandrogenic and antiandrogenic activities are not strictly related. Although all but one of the androgenic progestins tested enhanced testosterone action to some extent, three synandrogens were not androgenic. Furthermore, all synandrogenic agents tested were potent progestins, but the reverse was not true. The results of the studies summarized in Table 1 indicate that the synandrogenic activity was best correlated with progestins which were substituted in the 6α-position[6]. The results of these and other studies suggest that the standard requirements for a synandrogen may be quite limited while those for an antiandrogen are quite diverse[21,22,23].

The potentiating effects of progestins like their agonistic actions were related to an increase in new enzyme molecules. Further studies did, in fact, indicate that MPA potentiated the action of testosterone at all doses tested when the rate of β-glucuronidase synthesis was used as an end point. Similarly, low doses of CypAc potentiated and high doses inhibited the testosterone stimulated rate of β-glucuronidase synthesis[19]. This later experiment confirmed the conclusions from the study shown in Figure 1 based upon the specific activity of the enzyme. When the synandrogenic effect of progestins was first reported, it was proposed that this activity might be exerted on several androgen responsive proteins in kidney. To date, however, the only ones which show this response are β-glucuronidase and 3-keto reductase. This is in marked contrast to the androgenic and antiandrogenic actions of progestins which are manifest on most androgen responsive proteins[6].

Interaction of Androgens and Progestins with the β-Glucuronidase Locus

As noted above, one of the best studied androgen-induced protein in the kidney is β-glucuronidase. A genetic analysis of β-glucuronidase activity in several strains of mice led to the identification of the complex locus, Gus. The structural gene, Gus-s, is the source of both the lysosomal and microsomal glucuronidases. The gene is located near the distal end of chromosome 5, and the mutations at this locus code for a thermolabile enzyme (Gus-s^h) and two electrophoretic variants of β-glucuronidase (Gus-s^a and Gus-s^b)[15].

Mouse strains generally fall into two groups according to their temporal and quantitative responses to androgens. In some β-glucuronidase activity increases rapidly to a high plateau, and in others the response is less rapid and of lesser magnitude. These different responses are defined by the regulatory locus, Gus-r, within the Gus complex. The A/J and the C57BL/6J mice are typical of high and low inducing strains, respectively[14]. Strain A/J is homozygous for the allele, Gus-r^a, and its glucuronidase can be induced to a level several times higher than in C57BL/6J, which is homozygous for the Gus-r^b allele as shown in Figure 3. The regulatory locus acts in a cis-manner on the structural gene[24] and, on the basis of breeding studies, is near or within the Gus-s structural gene[15].

Previous studies have shown that Gus-r determines the rate of enzyme synthesis from Gus-s during androgen treatment[15]. In view of the regulatory role of Gus-r on the androgen induction of β-glucuronidase, it was pertinent to determine if other classes of β-glucuronidase inducers would be recognized by the Gus-r^a and Gus-r^b alleles. Figure 3 shows the response of A/J and C57BL/6J mice treated for varying periods of time with MPA[6]. As was the case with testosterone, this progestin produced a greater stimulation of β-glucuronidase activity in animals carrying the Gus-r^a allele. It is significant, however, that MPA

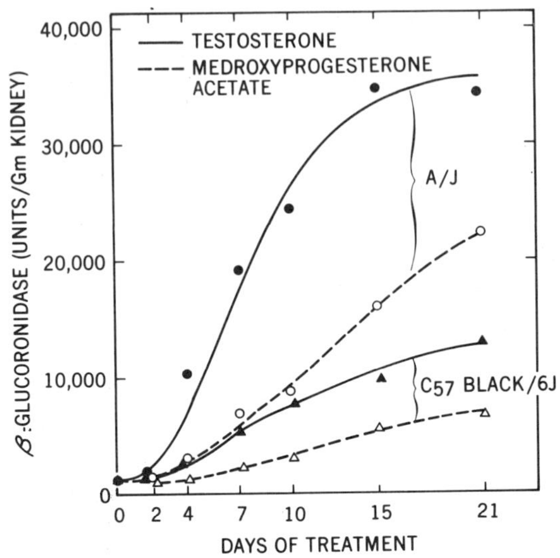

Figure 3. The effect of testosterone and medroxyprogesterone acetate on β-glucuronidase activity in the kidneys of female mice. A/J mice (○,●) are homozygous for the Gus-r^{a} allele and C57BL/6J animals (△ , ▲) are homozygous for the Gus-r^{b} allele (from 6).

was not as potent as testosterone in either of the strains (Figure 3). These studies demonstrate that both the steroid and the Gus-r locus determine the rate and magnitude of the steroid induced response from the β-glucuronidase gene. By analogy with other steroid responsive systems, it seems likely that Gus-r regulates glucuronidase synthesis in part by affecting the synthesis of its mRNA. Experiments using frog oocytes to measure mRNA activity or hybridization to complementary DNA to quantify mRNA sequences indicate that an increase in the rate of enzyme synthesis is preceded by an increase in β-glucuronidase mRNA activity[13,14]. However, the extent to which the appearance of new enzyme molecules in response to testosterone and progestin treatment reflects transcriptional, as opposed to posttranscriptional control remains to be established.

The influence of the Gus-r locus on the synandrogenic and antiandrogenic actions of progestins was also investigated. When administered with testosterone, low doses of CypAc produced a synandrogenic response in animals carrying the Gus-r^{a} allele. By contrast, little or no synandrogenic response was noted in animals carrying the Gus-r^{b} allele that were treated with a comparable dose. However, when testosterone and CypAc were administered in a 1:10 ratio, androgen action was inhibited in animals carrying both Gus-r alleles. It is of note that all the studies on the synandrogenic effects described above (Table 1) were performed in mice with the Gus-r^{a} allele. In summary, progestins may mimic or modify the action of androgens on the mouse kidney. The synandrogenic effects are most easily demonstrated using β-glucuronidase as an endpoint in animals with the Gus-r^{a}, but not the Gus-r^{b} allele; this effect is not readily observed on most other androgen responsive renal proteins. By contrast, the antiandrogenic and androgenic actions of progestins have been observed on almost all kidney proteins examined to date[7]. In view of this, we have reviewed how some of these varied effects of progestins are manifest in other tissues.

The Effects of Progestins on Other Androgen Responsive Organs

The mouse submaxillary glands, like the kidneys, are dimorphic structures in male and female animals. In females and castrated males, testosterone increases the activity of several enzymes, as well as the concentration of epidermal and nerve growth factors (EGF and NGF) in this organ[2]. Of the progestins studied, MPA caused the greatest androgenic response when given alone, with large doses producing a 40-fold increase in EGF concentration. Progesterone and megestrol acetate also had weak androgenic activities. CypAc had no activity when administered alone and acted as a potent antiandrogen when given with testosterone. The only synandrogenic response elicited was with a high dose of progesterone caproate. This is in striking contrast to the mouse kidney in which 100-fold lower doses of a variety of progestins, such as MPA, CypAc and megestrol acetate, were synergistic with testosterone[2].

In the rat, progesterone stimulates preputial gland growth by an androgen receptor dependent mechanism[8]. When the action of several progestins was tested using mouse preputial gland weight as the end point[4], the response was similar to that in the mouse submaxillary gland[2]. Of the progestational agents tested, only MPA had a significant effect on preputial gland weight in the absence of testosterone. When progestins were administered with testosterone, only high doses of progesterone caproate were synandrogenic. High doses of CypAc and megestrol acetate were antiandrogenic but the synandrogenic activity produced by low doses of these steroids on kidney was not observed in the preputial gland. Thus, the action of progestins on the preputial gland is strikingly different from that on the kidney[4,8].

Progestins are known to be potent inducers of hepatic microsomal enzymes. The effect of several of these steroids on mouse liver was studied to determine their inherent potency and ability to modify the biologic activity of testosterone. When increased hepatic ethylmorphine demethylase activity and cytochrome P-450 content were used as end points, the biological potencies of progestins *per se* on the liver were ranked as follows: CypAc $>$ progesterone $>$ MPA $>$ progesterone caproate $\cong$ controls[25]. The induced alterations of these parameters were, therefore, unrelated to the reported progestational or androgenic activities of these steroids on the uterus and male reproductive tract. A similar conclusion was reached when hepatic weight and microsomal protein contents were used as end points. When various doses of these progestins were administered with testosterone, the effects were additive. No synergistic or antagonistic actions of progestins were noted. This is in contrast to their actions on the kidney, submaxillary, and preputial glands[26]. It is of note that the nonprogestational antiandrogen, flutamide, was able to inhibit some of the actions of testosterone on the liver[27]. Since progestins alone are better inducers of hepatic proteins than testosterone, the ability to demonstrate their modifying effect on the action of androgens will be difficult[28].

The effects of progestins on the male reproductive tract have been studied by many investigators (for review see 1,6,7). As a consequence, the ability of these steroids to mimic the action of androgens is widely recognized. When progestins are assayed in the adult castrate rat, progesterone and its derivatives have only minimal androgenic effects, whereas compounds structurally related to 19-nortestosterone stimulate the male reproductive tract. By contrast, both progesterone and 19-nortestosterone derivatives masculinize the external genitalia of female fetuses. Some agents, such as MPA, are as potent as testosterone propionate on the fetus, whereas megestrol acetate, which is structurally related to MPA, has much less androgenic activity and then only on selected parts of the reproductive tract[29,30]. In addition to these structure-function differences, there are species dependent variations in responsiveness. This point is particularly well illustrated by studies indicating that CypAc virilizes the external genitalia of guinea pigs but not the rat. The antiandrogenic actions of progestins such as CypAc are evident to a variable extent on the reproductive tract in external genitalia of many species[20]. The synandrogenic action of this class of steroids is much more difficult to demonstrate, however. When an experiment similar to that shown in Figure 2 was performed in castrated male mice, an antiandrogenic without a synandrogenic effect was observed on the weight of prostate and seminal vesicles[4]. By contrast, Coffey and associates noted a marked increase in prostatic DNA synthesis over that expected for testosterone alone when CypAc was administered to rats several hours before testosterone; when CypAc was given simultaneously with testosterone it was inhibitory[31]. Similarly, CypAc also potentiated the androgen induced carnitine accumulation by epididymis[32]. In addition, low doses of megestrol acetate which have no effect on their own acted synergistically with estradiol in stimulating epithelial growth in the prostate[29]. In organ culture of rat prostate CypAc appeared to have a different effect: when used alone in low doses this steroid stimulated growth, whereas higher doses were inhibitory; when CypAc was administered with testosterone, marked hyperplasia occurred[33]. The reason for the discrepancy between the *in vivo* and *in vitro* results is not known. It is clear, however, that progestins can have similar effects on the male reproductive tract as on mouse kidney, depending on the conditions used.

EVIDENCE THAT THE ANDROGEN RECEPTOR IS INVOLVED IN THE ACTION OF PROGESTINS

The Action of Progestins in the Androgen-Insensitive Mouse (Tfm/Y): Tfm/Y mice have inherited end organ insensitivity to androgens. Several studies indicate that mice with this gene defect have defective androgen receptors[34,35]. As a consequence, testosterone does not stimulate androgen responsive tissues as it does in normal littermates. Since MPA and other androgenic progestins stimulate many of the same proteins as testosterone, it was pertinent to examine the effect of this class of steroids in Tfm/Y mice. Several experiments demonstrated that progestins do not increase renal or submaxillary gland proteins in the absence of a functional androgen receptor[2,4]. A similar conclusion was made from studies on androgen insensitive rats[8] and in humans with testicular feminization[36]. These observations suggested that some of the androgenic actions of progestins can be mediated by the androgen receptor.

As noted above, progestins are stimulators of many hepatic proteins and their potencies were not correlated with their androgenic or progestational activities. In Tfm/Y mice, the dose dependent increase in some proteins was not distinguishable from that of normal littermates with a full complement of androgen receptor[25,27]. These observations suggest that many progestin mediated effects on liver are not mediated via the androgen receptor as is the case in other organs.

In Vivo and In Vitro Binding of Progestins to Androgen Receptors: The inference that the androgen rather than the progesterone receptor mediates the responses of progestins on some androgen sensitive tissues was tested in a series of in vivo experiments in rats and mice. The specific nuclear uptake of [^{3}H]MPA or ^{3}H-androgens in prostate and seminal vesicle, kidney, and submaxillary glands was more readily blocked by the simultaneous administration of androgens than by MPA or other progestins[5,37]. In addition, there was no evidence of nuclear uptake of either [^{3}H]MPA or ^{3}H-androgens in Tfm/Y mice[5]. These observations imply that the androgen (rather than progestin) receptors are involved in the nuclear [^{3}H]MPA. The hypothesis that androgens and progestins may share the same receptor was also supported by ultra-centrifugal analysis of progestin and androgen binding to mouse kidney cytosol[5]. [^{3}H]MPA and [^{3}H]testosterone were both bound with high affinity to macromolecules with sedimentation coefficients of 8S. This binding was displaced by a nonradioactive MPA or T in a dose dependent fashion and by a 100-fold excess of other progestins and estradiol, but no dexamethasone. There was no detectable binding of [^{3}H]MPA or [^{3}H]testosterone to 8S components in kidney cytosol from Tfm/Y mice. These observations, along with the biological studies mentioned above, strongly support the conclusion that the androgenic, like the antiandrogenic, effects of progestins are mediated via the androgen receptor. The significance of these experiments was increased by the inability to demonstrate a binding protein in the mouse kidney with the same steroid specificity as the progesterone receptor from the uterus (unpublished, O. Janne).

The ability of progesterone, CypAc, and other progestins to bind to the androgen receptor has been demonstrated by many investigators. In fact, progestin binding is now accepted as one of the features that distinguishes androgen receptor from extracellular androgen binding proteins such as ABP and TeBG.

The relative binding affinities of various progestins for [^{3}H]testosterone binding sites on the androgen receptor in mouse kidney cytosol was studied using equilibrium binding analysis. The apparent affinities of several progestins for the androgen receptor were not directly correlated with the magnitude or direction (agonist or antagonist) of their effects on renal β-glucuronidase[5,37]. In addition, when kidney slices were incubated with [^{3}H]testosterone in the presence or absence of unlabeled progestins, the relative binding affinities to the nuclear androgen receptor differed from those obtained with the cytosol assay mentioned above[37]. The results from the in vitro nuclear uptake assay were similar to in vivo studies of the relative potency of progestins to inhibit nuclear testosterone uptake by mouse kidney. Results from these latter experiments suggest that the nuclear uptake of progestins relative to testosterone correlates with their androgenic but not their antiandrogenic and synandrogenic actions. Similar results were obtained in studies in which binding of various progestins to pyridoxal

5'-phosphate-extracted nuclear androgen receptors was examined _in vitro_[38]. From these considerations we conclude that the multiple actions of progestins in mouse kidney cannot be accurately predicted from a simple analysis of their affinities to androgen receptors. As a consequence, the binding curves were examined with a more complex model.

A Steric-Allosteric Model for Androgen-Progestin Interaction: Unlike the classic allosteric model for interaction between identical or dissimilar ligands, the steric-allosteric model includes the competitive binding of similar ligands to the same site, as well as their effects on the putative equilibrium between active and inactive states of the receptor[5]. The observation that the relative affinities for the receptor are unrelated to the direction of their physiological effects was compared with the predictions of the model for combined steric and allosteric interactions. According to this model, the response elicited by a mixture of steroids is determined by the combined effects of an equilibrium between an active and inactive state of the receptor. Each steroid influences this allosteric equilibrium according to the ratio of its dissociation constants for the two states. The observation that androgen binding to mouse kidney cytosol was similarly inhibited by progestins with disparate physiological effects (androgenic, antiandrogenic, and synandrogenic or undetectable) was consistent with the prediction of the steric-allosteric model.

It should be noted that the computations from the model were based on the assumption that steroid receptors have two binding sites. The steric-allosteric model predicted that a monomeric receptor could also mediate a range of responses produced by progestins. In contrast, a cooperative response to one steroid or a synergistic response to a mixture of steroids is consistent with the model only if two or more binding sites are involved in the allosteric transition. Thus, the synandrogenic action or certain progestins may involve either a coordinated transition between states of a steroid receptor with two or more subunits, or a cooperative interaction at a later stage of the hormone response such as a concerted effect of several steroid receptor complexes on the genome. Although the individual effect of progestins on androgen responsive tissue (androgenic, antiandrogenic, and synandrogenic activity) could be predicted for the steric-allosteric model, it was difficult for the model to predict how a synandrogenic effect could be produced by one dose of a given progestin, and an antiandrogenic effect by a higher dose. These considerations led to the conclusion that the interaction of the steroid receptor complex with the nucleus, as well as steroid binding to the receptor, must be important in determining the biological response observed[5].

Androgens Mimic the Actions of Progestins

Both natural and synthetic androgens can interact with three separate receptor systems in the uterine tissue including those from androgens[39], estrogens[40,41] and progestins[42,43]. In the latter two instances, superphysiological androgen concentrations were required for the interaction with these "wrong" receptors which led to expression of the biological action characteristic of the receptor rather than the androgen. In order to illustrate these observations, we have reviewed results on the interaction of androgens with the uterine progestin receptor.

Table 2. Relative binding affinity of physiological and synthetic androgens to the cytosol progestin receptors from human and rabbit uteri.

Compound	Relative binding affinity[a] Human receptor	Rabbit receptor
Progesterone	100.0	100.0
Testosterone	1.6	1.6
5α-Dihydrotestosterone	3.3	3.3
19-Nortestosterone	8.9	11.8
6α-Methyl-19-nortestosterone	15.5	19.6
17α-Methyltestosterone	4.6	3.4
17α-Ethyl-19-nortestosterone	130.0	70.1
7β,17α-Dimethyltestosterone	8.6	6.4
7α,17α-Dimethyl-19-nortestosterone	148.0	176.0

[a]The relative binding affinity was determined according to 48 with cytosol progestin receptor preparations partially purified by $(NH_4)_2SO_4$ precipitation. Adapted from 42.

Interaction of Androgens with the Progesterone Receptor

Table 2 summarizes the studies in which the relative binding affinities of androgens to human and rabbit progestin receptors were investigated[41]. All androgens tested, including testosterone and 5α-dihydrotestosterone, blocked the binding of progesterone to its receptor. In general, 19-nortestosterone derivatives seemed to bind to the progestin receptor better than derivatives of testosterone (Table 2). Two of the androgens, 17α-ethyl-19-nortestosterone and 7α, 17α-dimethyl-19-nortestosterone, bound to the progestin receptors to the same or greater extent than progesterone.

Progestational Actions of Androgens

To determine whether or not the interaction of the androgens with the cytoplasmic progestin receptor had biological consequences, the ability of these steroids to induce uteroglobin, a progesterone-regulated protein in rabbit uterus, was examined[42,44,45]. All the androgens induced uteroglobin secretion *in vivo* (Table 3) and in good agreement with their *in vitro* binding affinity for the rabbit or human progesterone receptors (cf. Tables 2 and 3). It is of note that physiological androgens such as testosterone and 5α-dihydrotestosterone, brought about a clear stimulation of uteroglobin synthesis which was 1-3 percent of that elicited by progesterone, when the response was calculated on the molar basis of the steroid administered. Additional

Table 3. Relative progestational activity of physiological and synthetic androgens as determined by their ability to induce uteroglobin synthesis in the rabbit uterus.[a]

Compound	Relative biological activity
Progesterone	100.0
Testosterone	0.9
5α-Dihydrotestosterone	1.9
19-Nortestosterone	5.2
6α-Methyl-19-nortestosterone	9.6
17α-Methyltestosterone	0.6
17α-Ethyl-19-nortestosterone	114.9
7β,17α-Dimethyltestosterone	5.3
7α,17α-Dimethyl-19-nortestosterone	215.6

[a]The animals were treated for 5 days with daily subcutaneous injections of 2 mg each steroid. Uteroglobin content in the uterine flushing was measured by radioimmunoassay. The values are relative to progesterone which was set at 100. Adapted from 14.

studies indicated that testosterone and progesterone had similar slopes in their dose dependent curves[42], suggesting a common mechanism of action.

Although all the previous data strongly suggested that androgen and estrogen receptors were not involved in the androgenic regulation of uteroglobin secretion, additional experiments were performed to substantiate this postulate. First, synthetic androgens such as 7α, 17α-dimethyl-19-nortestosterone were able to translocate uterine progesterone receptors to nuclei[42]; this effect was not inhibited by a concomitant administration of flutamide that prevents ligand binding to the androgen receptors[46]. Second, flutamide and another nonsteroidal antiandrogen, RU 23908[47], were not able to inhibit induction of uteroglobin synthesis[42,44] or accumulation of uteroglobin-mRNA[44,45] elicited by androgens in the rabbit uterus (Table 4). These results make it very unlikely that androgen receptors were involved, as the nonsteroidal antiandrogens specifically prevent androgen receptor mediated events[46,47]. Finally, administration of estradiol with androgens prevented androgen induced uteroglobin secretion and uteroglobin-mRNA accumulation[44,45] in a manner similar to the estrogen mediated inhibition of the action of progesterone on uteroglobin synthesis[45].

These data illustrate that androgens can modulate endometrial functions through interacting with the uterine progesterone receptor. Physiological androgens seemed to do it only when administered at pharmacological doses. By contrast, some synthetic androgens (e.g., 17α-ethyl-19-nortestosterone and 7α, 17α-dimethyl-19-nortestosterone)

Table 4. Influence of a non-steroidal antiandrogen on 5α-dihydrotestosterone elicited accumulation of uteroglobin and uteroglobin-mRNA activity in the rabbit uterus.

Treatment	Luminal fluid Uteroglobin (μg)	Uteroglobin-mRNA activity[a]
Vehicle	0.7 ± 0.2 (4)	4.1 ± 1.6 (4)
5α-Dihydrotestosterone (5mg)[b]	314.8 ± 127.5 (4)	56.7 ± 6.0 (4)
RU 23908 (25 mg)	1.0[c] (2)	1.1[c] (2)
5A-Dihydrotestosterone (5 mg) + RU 23908 (25 mg)	295 ± 151.7 (4)	80.3 ± 26.7 (4)

[a]Expressed as pmoles of L-[^{35}S]methionine incorporated to immunoprecipitable preuteroglobin during cell-free translation of total poly(A) -containing uterine RNA.

[b]Daily doses of the compounds administered for 5 days.

[c]Mean of two observations.

Adapted from 45.

were as potent as progesterone itself. This was not surprising in that many of the structural modifications in the androgens that render them biologically more active (addition of double bonds or hydrophobic substituents, removal of the 19-CH_3 group) are very similar to the modifications of the progesterone molecule required for its improved biological potency and receptor-binding affinity[48]. It is of particular note that the rabbit and human progesterone receptors have almost identical steroid binding specificities[43,48] and consequently, physiological and synthetic androgens are expected to interfere with the human endometrial functions in a manner similar to the rabbit.

SUMMARY AND CONCLUSIONS

Progestins can mimic, inhibit or potentiate the action of androgens. These responses have been termed the androgenic, antiandrogenic and synandrogenic action of progestins, respectively. The androgenic and antiandrogenic action of this class of steroids are manifest on many tissues and on many endpoints within a given organ. These effects are believed to involve an early step(s) of androgen action which is common to all sensitive tissues. Results to date suggests that this early step involved the androgen receptor. By contrast, the synandrogenic action of progestins is limited in that it is not observed on all tissues, and not even on all endpoints within a single organ. In the mouse kidney, the synandrogenic actions of progestins has been most extensively studied on β-glucuronidase. With this enzyme this unusual response to progestins can be demonstrated in only mice which carry the Gus-r^a allele. This observation suggests that the potentiating action of progestins on β-glucuronidase is manifest directly on the Gus gene complex. It is not certain at this time whether a similar mechanism is involved in the potentiation of androgen action on other organs such as the prostate. The androgenic action of progestins is believed to be similar to that of other androgens. Androgenic progestins such as MPA bind to the androgen receptors and translocate them to nuclei. This is followed by a dose dependent increase of proteins similar to what is observed after testosterone administration. In addition, the regulatory genes which modulate androgen action have the same effect on the androgenic effect of progestins. The fact that the potency of progestins such as MPA is less than that of testosterone is believed to relate in part to their lower affinity for the androgen receptors.

To date, the mechanism of action of antiandrogens is less certain. These compounds bind androgen receptor with lesser affinity than testosterone, and in competitive binding assays cannot be distinguished from androgenic progestins. It is assumed therefore, that they bind to the androgen receptor and hold it in a state whose conformation is different from that of the testosterone receptor complex. The main reason for this assumption is that antiandrogens usually have little if any androgenic activity in relation to the amount of receptor that they bind and transfer to the nucleus. Preliminary data suggest that the antiandrogen receptor complex can be retained in the nucleus but never to the level attained by the androgen receptor complex.

At present it is not possible to postulate a single mechanism that will explain the synergistic action of progestins on all tissues. This is, in part, due to the fact that this action is limited to a few end-points. Another reason is because the synergistic action of progestins is highly dose and time dependent. In addition, the progestins which produce this effect may also be androgenic, antiandrogenic, or both.

The progestational action of androgens is believed to be similar to that of other progestins. Progestational androgens bind to the progestin receptor and facilitate binding of the steroid receptor complex to nuclei. This is followed by an increase in mRNA synthesis which, in turn, directs specific protein synthesis. The potency of a given androgen for inducing progestational effects on the uterus is believed to be related to its affinity to the progestin receptor.

The examples presented in this review, progestin action via the androgen receptors and androgen action via the progestin receptors, are but two of the phenomena of hormone action via the "wrong" receptor. These effects are observed with large doses of hormone and are not observed when the amount of the progestin or androgen administered is just sufficient to stimulate the uterus or the male reproductive tract, respectively. As a consequence, toxicology studies which employ large doses up to 50 times that to be used in humans will certainly observe biological effects which will not be observed with the physiological dose.

ACKNOWLEDGEMENTS

This work was supported in part by NIH Grants HD-13541 and HD-16105.

REFERENCES

1. Bullock, LP, Bardin, CW: Androgenic, synandrogenic, and antiandrogenic actions of progestins. Ann NY Acad Sci, 286:321, 1977.

2. Bullock, LP, Barthe, PL, Mowszowicz, I, Orth, DN, Bardin, CW: The effect of progestins on submaxillary gland epidermal growth factor: Demonstration of androgenic, synandrogenic and antiandrogenic actions. Endocrinology, 97:189, 1975.

3. Gupta, C, Bullock, LP, Bardin, CW: Further studies on the androgenic, antiandrogenic, and synandrogenic actions of progestins. Endocrinology, 102:736, 1978.

4. Mowszowicz, I, Bieber, DE, Chung, KW, Bullock, LP, Bardin, CW: Synandrogenic and antiandrogenic effect of progestins: comparison with nonprogestational antiandrogens. Endocrinology, 95:1589, 1974.

5. Bullock, LP, Bardin, CW, Sherman, MR: Androgenic, antiandrogenic, synandrogenic actions of progestins: Role of steric and allosteric interactions with androgen receptors. Endocrinology, 103:1768, 1978.

6. Bardin, CW, Brown, TR, Mills, NC, Gupta, C, Bullock, LP: The regulation of the β-glucuronidase gene by androgens and progestins. Biol Reprod, 18:74, 1978.

7. Bardin, CW, Catterall, JF: Testosterone: a major determinant of extragenital sexual dimorphism. Science, 211:1285, 1981.

8. Bardin, CW, Bullock, LP, Sherin, RJ, Mowszowicz, I, Blackburn, WR: Part II: Androgen metabolism and mechanism of action in male pseudohermaphroditism: A study of testicular feminization. Recent Prog Horm Res, 29:65, 1973.

9. Pajunen, AEI, Isomaa, VV, Janne, OA, Bardin, CW: Androgenic regulation of ornithine decarboxylase activity in mouse kidney and its relationship to changes in cytosol and nuclear androgen receptor concentrations. J Biol Chem, 257:8190, 1982.

10. Isomaa, VV, Pajunen, AEI, Bardin, CW, Janne, OA: Ornithine decarboxylase in mouse kidney: purification, characterization, and radioimmunological determination of the enzyme protein. J Biol Chem, 258:6735, 1983.

11. Kontula, KK, Torkkeli, TK, Bardin, CW, Janne, OA: Androgen induction of ornithine decarboxylase mRNA as studied by complimentary DNA. Proc Natl Acad Sci USA, 81:731, 1984.

12. Janne, OA, Kontula, KK, Isomaa, VV, Torkkeli, TK, Bardin, CW: Androgen receptor-dependent regulation of ornithine decarboxylase gene expression in mouse kidney. In: Gustafsson, J-A, Erikson, H (eds): Steroid Hormone Receptors: Structure and Function, Amsterdam, Elsevier/North Holland Biomedical Press, 1983.

13. Catterall, JF, Leary, SL: Detection of early changes in androgen-induced mouse renal β-glucuronidase messenger ribonucleic acid using

cloned complimentary deoxyribonucleic acid. Biochemistry, 22:6049, 1983.

14. Paigen, K, Labarca, C, Watson, G: A regulatory locus for mouse β-glucuronidase induction, Gus, controls messenger RNA activity. Science, 203:554, 1979.

15. Swank, RT, Paigen, K, Davey, R, Chapman, V, Labarca, C, Watson, G, Ganshow, R, Brandt, EJ, Novak, E: Genetic regulation of mammalian glucuronidase. Recent Prog Horm Res, 34:401, 1978.

16. Bullock, LP: Androgen and progestin stimulation of ornithine decarboxylase activity in the mouse kidney. Endocrinology, 112:1903, 1983.

17. Mowszowicz, I, Bardin, CW: In vitro androgen metabolism in mouse kidney: High 3-keto-reductase (3β-hydroxysteroid dehydrogenase) activity relative to 5α-reductase. Steroids, 23:793, 1974.

18. Lin, YC, Bullock, LP, Bardin, CW, Jacob, ST: Effect of medroxyprogesterone acetate and testosterone on solubilized RNA polymerases and chromatin template activity in kidney from normal and androgen-insensitive (Tfm/Y) mice. Biochemistry, 17:4833, 1978.

19. Gupta, C, Mills, NC, Bullock, LP, Bardin, CW: The effects of testosterone and progestins on the rate of β-glucuronidase synthesis in mouse kidney as studied with an immunoprecipitation assay. Int J Androl, 4:342, 1981.

20. Neumann, F, Berswordt-Wallrabe, R, Elger, W, Steinbeck, H, Hahn, JD, Kramer, M: Aspects of androgen-dependent events as studied by antiandrogens. Recent Prog Horm Res, 26:337, 1970.

21. Starka, L, Hampl, R, Kasal, A, Kohout, L: Androgen receptor binding and antiandrogenic activity of some 4,5-secoandrostanes and ring B cyclopropano-androstanes. J Steroid Biochem, 17:331,1982.

22. Yates, J, King, RJB: Antiandrogen effects on androgen-responsive mammary tumour cells in culture. J Steroid Biochem, 14:819, 1981.

23. Brown, TR, Rothwell, SW, Sultan, C, Migeon, CJ: Inhibition of androgen binding in human foreskin fibroblasts by antiandrogens. Steroids, 37:635, 1981.

24. Lusis, AJ, Chapman, VM, Herbstman, C, Paigen, K: Quantitation of cis versus trans regulation of mouse β-glucuronidase. J Biol Chem, 255:8959, 1980.

25. Brown, TR, Greene, FE, Bardin, CW: The additive effects of progestins on testosterone-stimulated hepatic ethylmorphine metabolism and cytochrome P-450 content. Steroids, 30:805, 1977.

26. Brown, TR, Bardin, CW, Greene, FE: Hormonal control of cytochrome P-450-dependent ethylmorphine N-demethylase activity of the mouse: In: Garattini, S, Berendes, HW (eds): Pharmacology of Steroid Contraceptive Drugs, New York, Raven Press, p 237, 1977.

27. Brown, TR, Greene, FE, Bardin, CW: Androgen receptor dependent and independent activities of testosterone on hepatic microsomal drug metabolism. Endocrinology, 99:1353, 1976.

28. Brown, TR, Greene, FE, Bullock, LP, Bardin, CW: Effect of the Tfm locus on the hepatic ethylmorphine N-demethylase system in mice. Endocrinology, 103:1374, 1978.

29. Salander, H, Tisell, L-E: Effects of megestrol on oestradiol induced growth of the prostatic lobes and the seminal vesicles in castrated rats. Acta Endocrinol, 82:213, 1976.

30. Tisell, L-E, Salander, H: Androgenic properties and adrenal depressant activity of megestrol acetate observed in castrated male rats. Acta Endocrinol, 78:316, 1975.

31. Coffey, DS: The effects of androgens on DNA and RNA synthesis in sex accessory tissue. In: Brandes, D (ed): Male Accessory Sex Organs. Structure and Function in Mammals, New York, Academic Press, p 307, 1974.

32. Bohmer, T, Hansson, V: Androgen-dependent accumulation of carnitine by rat epididymis after injection of [^{3}H]butyrobetaine in vivo. Mol Cell Endocrinol, 3:103, 1975.

33. Lasnitzki, I, Robel, R: Effects of cyproterone on the rat prostate gland grown in organ culture. Adv Biosci, 3:175, 1969.

34. Bullock, LP, Bardin, CW: Androgen receptors in testicular feminization. J Clin Endocrinol Metab, 35:935, 1972.

35. Bullock, LP, Bardin, CW: Androgen receptors in mouse kidney: A study of male, female and androgen-insensitive (tfm/Y) mice. Endocrinology, 94:746, 1974.

36. Perez-Palacios, G, Chavez, B, Escobar, N, Vilchis, F, Larrea, F, Lince, M, Perez, AE: Mechanism of action of contraceptive synthetic progestins. J Steroid Biochem, 15:125, 1981.

37. Brown, TR, Bullock, L, Bardin, CW: In vitro and in vivo binding of progestins to the androgen receptor of mouse kidney. Correlation with biological activities. Endocrinology, 105:1281, 1979.

38. Isomaa, V, Pajunen, AEI, Bardin, CW, Janne, OA: Nuclear androgen receptors in the mouse kidney: validation of a new assay. Endocrinology, 111:833, 1982.

39. Giannopoulos, G: Binding of testosterone to cytoplasmic components of the immature rat uterus. Biochem Biophys Res Commun, 44:943, 1971.

40. Ruh, TS, Wassilak, SG, Ruh, MF: Androgen-induced nuclear accumulation of the estrogen receptor. Steroids, 25:257, 1975.

41. Garcia, M, Rochefort, H: Androgens on the estrogen receptor. II. Correlation between nuclear translocation and uterine protein synthesis. Steroids, 29:111, 1977.

42. Janne, O, Hemminki, S, Isomaa, V, Kokko, E, Torkkeli, H, Torkkeli, T, Vierikko, P: Progestational activity of natural and synthetic androgens. Intl J Androl Suppl, 2:162, 1978.

43. Janne, O, Kontula, K, Vihko, R, Feil, PD, Bardin, CW: Progesterone receptor and regulation of progestin action in mammalian tissues. Med Biol, 56:225, 1978.

44. Kopu, H: 5α-Dihydrotestosterone-induced uteroglobin synthesis in rabbit uterus is not inhibited by antiandrogen administration but is prevented by estradiol. Biochem Biophys Acta, 654:293, 1981.

45. Janne, OA, Isomaa, VV, Torkkeli, TK, Isotalo, HE, Kopu, HT. Hormonal regulation of uteroglobin synthesis in the rabbit uterus. In: Bardin, CW, Milgrom, E, Mauvais-Jarvis, P (eds): Progesterone and Progestins, New York, Raven Press, p 33, 1983.

46. Liao, S, Howell, DK, Chang, TM: Action of a non-steroidal antiandrogen, flutamide, on the receptor binding and nuclear retention of 5α-dihydrotestosterone in rat ventral prostate. Endocrinology, 94:532, 1974.

47. Raynaud, J-P, Bonne, C, Bouton, M-M, Lagace, L, Labrie, F: Action of a non-steroidal antiandrogen, RU 23908, in peripheral and central tissues. J Steroid Biochem, 11:93, 1979.

48. Kontula, K, Janne, O, Vihko, R, deJager, E, deVisser, J, Zeelen, F: Progesterone-binding proteins: in vitro binding and biological activity of different steroidal ligands. Acta Endocrinol, 78:574, 1975.

49. Boris, A, DeMartino, L: The utilization of uterine weight as an adjunct to histology in the evaluation of progestational steroids. Steroidologica, 2:57, 1971.

50. Smith, HE, Smith, RG, Toft, DO, Neergaard, JR, Burrows, EP, O'Malley, BW: Binding of steroids to progesterone receptor proteins in chick oviduct and human uterus. J Biol Chem, 249:5924, 1974.

DISCUSSION

DR. DICZFALUSY: Thank you very much indeed. May I invite questions or comments on Dr. Bardin's presentation?

DR. ZBINDEN: A lot was said about protein binding of steroids and that only the free steroids are active. What about protein binding in the plasma or in tissue as compared to the binding affinity of receptors?

DR. BARDIN: I don't agree with the assumption that only the free steroid in serum is biologically active. I think there is an enormous amount of data suggesting it is the free plus albumin-bound steroid that can enter cells. In addition, there is the long held assumption that serum binding proteins, like TeGB and CBG, do not enter cells. The evidence is now overwhelming that these binding proteins which were thought of as solely extracellular, can enter cells, particularly in tissues that respond to steroids.

In view of these findings, I think we are only now beginning to face the very interesting role of binding proteins in the modulation of hormone action.

DR. CLARK: It is true that these proteins enter cells, but they have never been shown to function in that intracellular location. In fact, all the data are against this possibility in that the free level, is in some way equated to the biological activity. All the old cell studies done with CBG and free corticoids indicated that this was true.

DR. BARDIN: I don't really agree. I think even if you don't like the idea about the intracellular activity of the protein, you must at least still recognize that it could influence steroid availability in the cell.

DR. CLARK: Well, that may be. But the localization of CBG, or whatever, within the cell has not been demonstrated to be associated with biological activity of the steroid.

DR. BARDIN: Well, this protein certainly does not function as a receptor, but I think it can certainly partition steroids between enzymes. There are data that show this.

DR. CLARK: Well, yes, that's possible.

DR. GOEBELSMANN: With regard to the problem of androgen excess in hirsutism, a lot of this work is very pertinent. When you look at the hirsute female, Free testosterone, or non-SHBG bound, in hirsute females, is only elevated in a certain percentage (60-70 percent) depending on the particular study. However, the metabolite which is uniformly elevated in hirsute women, irrespective of ovulatory status, is 5-alpha-dihydroxyandrostane glucuronide.

So it may be that the pathway by which the androgen is metabolized within the cell may be determined to some extent by the intracellular binding proteins such as TeBG. There are published data on this topic.

MECHANISM OF ACTION OF ESTROGEN AND ITS RELATIONSHIP TO TOXICOLOGICAL ASSESSMENT

James H. Clark

Department of Cell Biology

Baylor College of Medicine

Houston, Texas

INTRODUCTION

Estrogens are steroid hormones, produced primarily by the ovary, which are necessary for normal reproductive function in the female of the species. Yet, estrogens may also be toxic substances under certain circumstances. The fine line between normal physiological function and toxicological outcome has made testing of such compounds a difficult task. The purpose of this paper is to relate the normal physiological actions of estrogens to their toxicological assessment.

Steroid Hormone Action and Model Studies

Steroid hormones, such as estradiol and progesterone, are thought to act at the cellular level by binding to macromolecules called receptors (Figure 1)[1]. This binding interaction results in an accumulation of receptor steroid complexes in the nucleus where the complexes bind tightly to nuclear constituents. Nuclear binding appears to stimulate transcriptional events which result in increased levels of various classes of RNA. Elevated levels of RNA result in increased protein synthesis which alters cellular functions and may cause cellular hypertrophy. Eventually these multiple cellular events lead to cellular proliferation.

Although there are many details of the above interactions that are not fully understood most investigators would agree on this general scheme. Therefore, if this is the way steroid hormones work, can this information be used in the design of more meaningful animal studies? The answer is yes, if it can be shown that a given response pattern is associated with reproductive dysfunction or abnormalities. For example, if a drug binds to the estrogen receptor, causes it to accumulate in the nucleus of target cells, and stimulates mRNA patterns which differ from those stimulated by a physiological hormone; and if these anomalous patterns can be correlated with reproductive dysfunction, then the supposition can be made that the drug may be a hazardous substance.

If such were the case, drugs could readily be screened, probably with cell culture techniques, for patterns of synthetic activity which differed from the normal. Such experiments could be done with human cells in culture or in the immunodeficient nude rodent model.

The difficulty with this scheme is being able to show that a particular response pattern is associated with reproductive dysfunction. This, of course, requires that model systems be established to examine such relationships. Once anomalous patterns of drug stimulated events are described and shown to correlate with the development of dysfunction or abnormalities, screening systems which do not involve long term studies could be established.

At the present time studies similar to these have not yielded many differences. For instance, estrogenic toxins, such as DES, kepone, and o,p'DDT, have been shown to bind to estrogen receptors, and to stimulate many of the same biosynthetic events and growth responses as physiological estrogens[2,3,4,5]. Even androgenic steroids will act as estrogens if they are given in amounts sufficient to cause estrogen receptor binding[6]. An exception to this general scheme may be the action of triphenylethylene antiestrogens such as clomiphene which will be discussed later. Thus, the question arises: Is the reproductive toxicity of an agent simply a function of its estrogenicity? The answer to this question is still forthcoming; however, it is clear that all estrogenic agents, whether physiological or non-physiological, act as reproductive toxins if administered at critical periods of development in a continuous fashion in the adult. Therefore, it is likely that estrogenicity and toxicity are closely related. Indeed, estradiol (one of the physiologically occurring estrogens) will cause mammary cancer in rats if administered by pellet implant over several months[7] (Clark and Markaverich, unpublished observation). Such data would surely have been used by the FDA to suggest that the ovary is a hazardous organ and should be banned, if it were not for its obvious importance to normal reproductive function.

Such results and concepts lead to the conclusion that you can't tell one estrogen from another, and thus, the development of screening tests for anomalous hormone induced synthetic patterns would be futile. Perhaps so, at least with our current level of technological application. What is needed, if this avenue is pursued, is to put the recent advances in biochemistry and molecular biology to work. That is, the differences induced by deleterious substances may be small and difficult to detect; however, with modern methods for identification of such differences, it may be possible to devise such a screen.

Even if it were shown that all estrogens are alike, this knowledge is valuable because short term toxicological tests are already in use which detect estrogenic toxins very readily. Such procedures can signal the potential estrogenic hazards of drugs and can be used to greatly reduce the need for long term animal studies.

Steroid Hormone Interactions

The concepts discussed above relate to the actions of a single hormone; however, it is well known that hormones interact and such interactions should be considered in any drug testing scheme. The continuous occupancy of estrogen receptors by estrogen will cause reproductive dysfunction and abnormalities in various species including humans. However under normal physiological conditions, continuous occupancy of estrogen receptors does not occur. Instead, the actions of estrogens are usually modified and decreased by the presence of progesterone. Progesterone decreases estrogen receptors in the cytoplasm of target cells and elevates the activity of enzymes which convert active estrogens to less active metabolites[9,10]. Both of these actions decrease the ability of estrogen to stimulate cell growth. Progesterone is present during the second half of the menstrual cycle in the human, and transforms an estrogenized uterus into a secretory one which is capable of supporting pregnancy if conception occurs. This monthly exposure to progesterone may be a very important modular of estrogen action and may act to protect against continuous exposure to estrogen. This protective effect of progesterone can be visualized as a monthly fluctuation in the effectiveness of estrogen which results in normal female function. Without this protective effect of progesterone, estrogen is free to act in an unopposed way which could lead to abnormal development and neoplasia of estrogen sensitive tissues.

These considerations lead to the conclusion that drug testing should include protocols which utilize combinations of test substances as they will be used in the human.

Developmental and Pharmacokinetic Differences Between Species

The general scheme for steroid hormone action which is shown in Figure 1 is probably applicable to all species. However, developmental and pharmacokinetic properties may differ greatly between species, and alter the interpretation of this scheme with respect to extrapolations from rodent to human. A good example of this problem is the induction of reproductive tract abnormalities in young women whose mothers were treated with DES during pregnancy[11,12]. Since high levels of physiological estrogens are present during pregnancy, why don't they cause adverse effects? Is there something special about DES? Are estrogens different in their action after all?

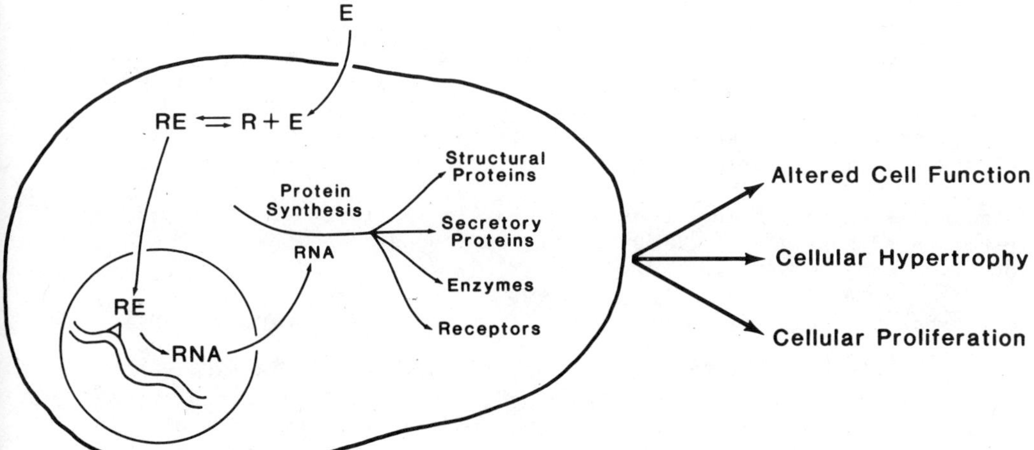

Figure 1: Generalized scheme of the mechanism of action and effects of estrogen on a target cell. Abbreviations: E, estrogen; R, receptor.

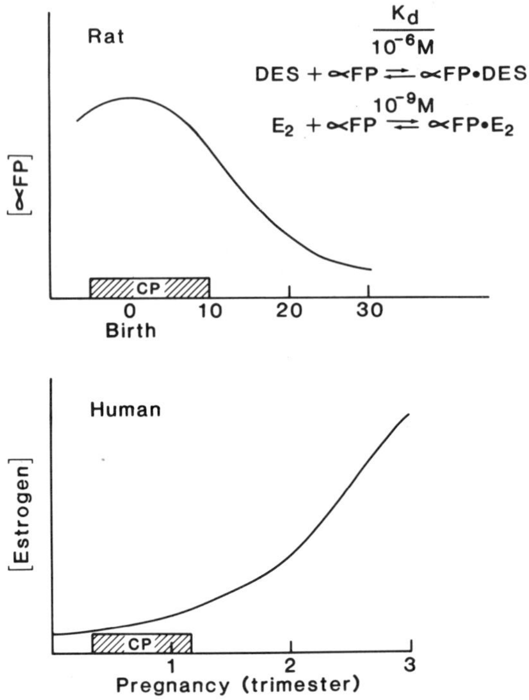

Figure 2. Relationship of the critical period (CP) for urogenital tract development and estrogen exposure. Abbreviations: α FP, alpha-fetoprotein; DES, diethylstilbestrol; k_d, dissociation constant, E_2, estradiol.

The answer to these questions probably involves several developmental and physiological considerations. The critical period for the development of vaginal adenosis is during the early months of pregnancy, a period during which the urogenital tract is differentiating, and is characterized by relatively low levels of physiological estrogens (Figure 2). DES exposure during these early months increases the estrogenic load of the mother and fetus and causes an inappropriate stimulation of the developing urogenital tract, which predisposes the fetus to subsequent development of vaginal abnormalities. If physiological estrogens were administered (instead of DES) during these early months of pregnancy similar adverse effects might have been observed. Thus, it is likely that critical period exposure to high levels of estrogenic compounds is the cause of the observed adverse effects.

Rodent models have been used to examine estrogen exposure during the critical period, and such studies are good examples of the difficulties which can be encountered with interspecies variation. In rats the critical period is between 14 days of pregnancy through 8-10 days after birth (Figure 2). DES is more potent than estradiol in causing reproductive tract abnormalities when the hormones are administered during this critical period[13]. This effect is not due to differences in the inherent estrogenicity of these two compounds but rather to the presence of alpha-fetoprotein (AFP) which binds estradiol with high affinity but does not bind DES very effectively. Therefore, the amount of free DES is much greater than estradiol following an injection, and since the level of free hormone determines the amount of hormone available for receptor binding, the response is greater with DES than with estradiol. Although these concepts seem to be valid for rodent models, they may not be directly applicable to the human. In the human, AFP does not bind physiological estrogens very tightly and cannot be readily called a protective protein[14]. In addition, as mentioned above, it may not be necessary to involve an AFP to protect the human fetus because, during the critical period in the human, physiological estrogens are relatively low.

These differences between the rodent and human exemplify the need for a more complete understanding of the pharmacokinetics and developmental functions in these species. More meaningful animal studies can be designed only when a more complete understanding of these basic species differences is at hand.

Metabolism

A principal contribution to the pharmacokinetic properties of any drug or hormone is made by the metabolic alterations which it may undergo. It is well known that many substances are not toxic unless they are metabolized to active metabolites. This concept has led some investigators to suggest that estrogens act as toxins by such activation mechanisms. It has been proposed that the carcinogenic potential of DES results from its metabolic conversion to active intermediates such as E-DES-3,4-oxide[15]. This compound is very active in the sister chromatid exchange assay and is estrogenic. Since E-DES-3,4-oxide also binds to the estrogen receptor, it has been proposed that the receptor transports E-DES-3,4-oxide to the nucleus where it may become covalently bound to DNA. The presumed covalent interaction would lead to altered genomic function and the development of abnormal cell growth.

Although these suggestions concerning E-DES-3,4-oxide are important, it must be shown that the formation of active DES metabolites occurs under conditions which are similar to those that result in abnormal development. The doses of [^{14}C]-DES which have been administered range from 50 μg i.p. (neonatal mice) to 500 μg i.p. (adult mice). These doses are well above those which will cause reproductive tract abnormalities, and therefore, it becomes important to demonstrate that lower doses also result in the formation of such metabolites. It will also be necessary to show that other estrogens also form active intermediates, since it is well known that other estrogens, such as estradiol, estrone and estriol, will also cause reproductive tract abnormalities.

Along these lines of reasoning, it has been suggested that estrogens, such as estradiol-17β, manifest their deleterious effects because they are metabolized to epoxide or quinone intermediates[16]. These authors have measured the ability of various steroids to cause the transformation of Balb/c 3T3 cells in culture. They concluded that DES, estrone, ethynyl estradiol and estradiol will cause transformation while moxestrol and estriol will not. Since the first four compounds are good substrates for catechol estrogen formation and the latter two are not, these authors conclude that transformation is linked to the formation of active intermediates and not to the estrogenicity of these hormones. As in the case of DES metabolism discussed in the previous paragraph, this is an interesting and potentially important concept; however, it will be necessary to show that transformation and metabolism occurs at concentrations of hormone which are expected under *in vivo* exposure conditions. The observed cell transformations were seen only when the concentration of estrogen was in the μM range and no effects were seen below this level of exposure. Such high concentrations are 100-1000 times those which would be expected for hormone exposure *in vivo*. In addition, it has been demonstrated that estriol will cause adverse effects on reproduction, including mammary cancer, and yet estriol is a poor substrate for conversion to catechol estrogens[7]. Such observations will require further examination before the metabolic conversion concept can be accepted as valid.

Structure-Function Relationships

At the present time the relationships between structure and function are not completely understood. For example, no one would have predicted from the structure of kepone that it would bind to the estrogen receptors and stimulate estrogenic responses. Obviously, there is much to be learned about what constitutes an estrogenic molecule. However, kepone would have been detected as an estrogen by a screening test for estrogenic substances, and indeed, if we had known more about structure-function relationships its estrogenicity might have been suspected before any tests were performed.

It may be possible to establish an estrogenic toxicity profile, similar to those discussed earlier, that will enable predictions to be made from the chemical structure of a molecule. For example, standard estrogens, such as DES or estradiol, stimulate vaginal opening in neonatal rats, uterine growth and estrogen receptor binding. These actions are typical responses induced by estrogenic substances. Clomiphene, a triphenylethylene drug which is used to induce ovulation in anovulatory women, is also active in these tests, but with important differences[8]. The affinity of the estrogen receptor for clomiphene is much below that of estradiol, yet it manifests long-term nuclear binding[1]. Long term nuclear retention is also observed with estradiol and DES; however, it is reduced when compared to clomiphene. All three compounds stimulate epithelial cell hypertrophy; however, only estradiol and DES stimulate extensive hyperplasia. These differences may relate to a difference in nuclear processing of the compounds or to metabolic clearance rates. Regardless of the reason, all triphenylethylenes have similar properties and their function can be predicted from their structure.

The establishment of reproductive toxicological profiles and structure function prediction models has only just begun[17]. Much basic information is required before such a system could be realized. Therefore, support for basic research in reproductive toxicity with a major emphasis on establishing such models is needed. Such model systems which use acute *in vivo* or *in vitro* tests can go a long way in reducing the need for long term animal tests.

Pharmacology and Species Differences

The extrapolation of data obtained in animals to the human has been mentioned earlier and we need to know more about the basic pharmacology and physiology of animals and humans. In addition, we need to examine the differences that are already known, in light of their relevance to toxicology. For example, exposure of female rats to androgens or estrogens during fetal or neonatal life results in the disruption of the mechanisms that control cyclic secretion of the various hormones. This leads to the development of the persistent estrous syndrome, which is characterized by a lack of reproductive cyclicity and infertility. Such animals may display masculine behavior and masculinized external genitalia.

This effect of estrogen or androgen takes place only if the animal is exposed during the critical period of development that extends from day 18 of pregnancy to days 8-10 of life in the rat. During this period, the hypothalamic structures believed to be involved in control of normal cyclic hormone secretion are undergoing neuronal maturation. Disruption or modification of hypothalamic maturation has a permanent effect that results in a male like or acyclic pattern of hormone release and infertility[18,19]. It should be noted that species vary greatly in their susceptibility to hormonal insult during development, and that extrapolation of data in the rodent to other species must be done with caution. This point will be discussed further below.

In the rat and other rodent species, the persistent estrous syndrome appears to result from the action of estrogens on hypothalamic development. Even the effects of androgens are thought to occur by their metabolic conversion to estrogens[18]. Physiological estrogens, such as estradiol, estriol, and estrone, and nonphysiological estrogens such as diethylstilbestrol (DES), kepone, o,p'-DDT, and clomiphene are known to cause this acyclic syndrome in the rat[3,20,21]. Thus, it appears that the estrogenicity of an agent is correlated with the toxic effect.

In contrast, these hormonal interactions which control gonadotropin secretion do not occur in humans and other primates. Testosterone administered to pregnant monkeys beginning during the early periods of gestation does not alter the ability of the hypothalamus to release gonadotropins in a cyclic fashion[22]. Yet, the external genitalia and sexual behavior are masculine like. In human females with congenital virilizing adrenal hyperplasia, or in females exposed to androgens _in utero_, administration of gonadotropin releasing hormone causes a female type gonadotropin release[23]. Furthermore, in castrate men and male monkeys, an ovulatory like surge of LH can be observed following administration of estradiol, which is similar to that seen in women[24,25]. These findings suggest that in primates the potential for cyclic gonadotropin secretion is intact and that androgen induced differentiation of the mechanism which controls gonadotropin secretion in the primate is different from that of the rodents.

These differences between species make it impossible to extrapolate findings in the rodent directly to the human when one is concerned with drug effects on the hypothalamic control of gonadotropin secretion. However, it is clear that perinatal exposure of rodents or humans to androgens will cause masculinization of other structures (external genitalia and secondary sex characteristics) and these effects appear to be quite comparable[22,26,27]. Therefore, it is easy to detect potentially hazardous substances which will masculinize females by perinatal screening tests. Such tests are acute and require relatively short time periods. The current long term studies which detect differences in behavior and fertility could be replaced with procedures which involve administration of the test substance during the perinatal period. Animals can then be examined for the masculinizing effects of such exposure within the first few days of life.

Initiation and Promotion Effects of Estrogens

In addition to the effects on the reproductive cycle discussed above, exposure of rats and other rodents to sex steroids during neonatal life also causes development of various abnormalities in the reproductive system. Neonatal or chronic exposure of mice, rats, and hamsters to estrogens of various types results in preneoplastic and neoplastic changes in the vagina, uterus, pituitary, and mammary gland[28-36]. Neonatal androgen treatment causes squamous metaplasia and reorientation of stromal collagen in rat uteri[37] and persistent vaginal estrus in mice[38]. These effects of androgen may either result from the conversion of androgens to estrogens during the neonatal period or from the continuous exposure to ovarian estrogens during adult life (Figure 3).

Nonphysiological estrogens, such as DES and clomiphene, will also cause the development of reproductive tract abnormalities in rodents[21,31,36,39]. Other estrogenic agents, such as kepone and o,p'-DDT, are known to have adverse effects on reproductive function[3,20], however, little is known about the teratogenic effect of these agents.

Thus, in the rodent, neonatal exposure to estrogens appears to predispose the animal to the development of abnormalities. Although this probably is true, it should be noted that the development of such abnormalities depends on the presence of abnormal ovarian function. That is, the ovary of the animal in persistent estrus is producing a continuous level of estrogen which is unopposed by progesterone (Figure 3). Similar adverse effects can be observed in the neonatally exposed animal which has been ovariectomized and treated with estrogen[36]. If estrogen is not given to the animal after ovariectomy no adverse effects develop. Therefore, it can be concluded that the situation is somewhat similar to the classical initiation-promotion concept of carcinogenesis. That is, the neonatal or critical period exposure to estrogen acts as an initiator

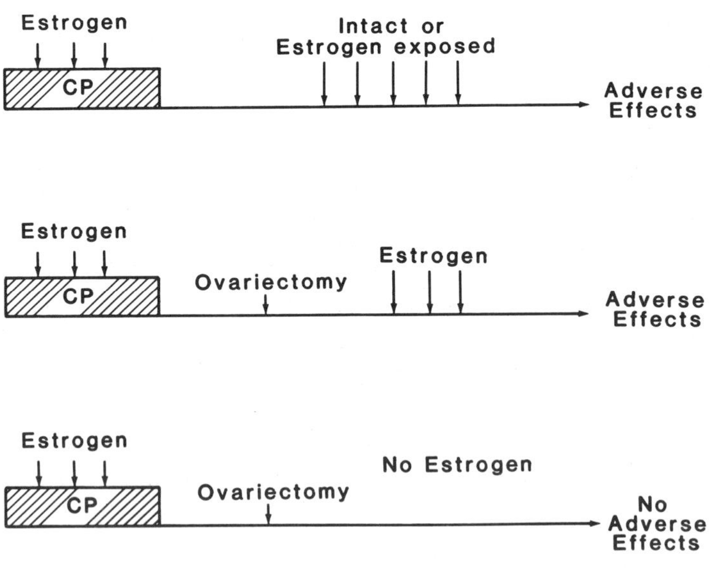

Figure 3. Initiation and promotion concept as it relates to estrogen induction of adverse reproductive effects.

of events which predispose the tissue to the promotional effects of subsequent estrogen exposure in adult life.

Whether this will be the case in DES exposed humans is not yet known. Menstrual irregularity and possible subfertility have been noted by some investigators[40,41,42], but not by others[43]. Since the hypothalamic centers which control cyclic secretion of gonadotropins in humans are not affected to any great extent by inappropriate estrogen exposure, as previously pointed out, it seems likely that women will not suffer from the persistent estrus ovary and will not develop abnormalities and neoplasia to the extent that rodents do. The vaginal abnormalities which have been observed in DES exposed individuals probably result from the disruption of normal Mullerian duct development.

Mode of Administration

The method of administration can obviously influence the action of drugs and hormones. There are many examples of such effects and only one will be presented here. Some estrogens, such as estriol, dimethystilbestrol, and estradiol-16α, have been classified as short-acting estrogens because they are rapidly cleared from the body and from estrogen receptor sites following a single injection[1,41]. Consequently, these hormones fail to elicit full estrogenic responses in organs such as the uterus. However, if such hormones are supplied to receptor sites in a continuous fashion, either by a series of injections or implants, they stimulate full estrogenic responses. Hence, these short-acting estrogens, previously called weak or impeded estrogens, are fully competent to elicit estrogenic responses. This concept is important because some investigators consider estriol to have protective effects against the adverse effects of estradiol[45,46,47]. This proposal is based on the concept that estriol is a weak or impeded estrogen that is in turn based on the evidence derived from experiments that employ a single injection of hormone. However, since estriol is continuously present during either the luteal phase of the cycle or during pregnancy, it is unlikely that this hormone has any power to reduce the effectiveness of other estrogens, and, in fact, only adds its additional estrogenicity to the system. In addition it is known that estriol exposure during the neonatal period causes reproductive dysfunction and is equal to estradiol in its ability to facilitate the onset of mammary cancer in mice[48,49]. Likewise, both estradiol and estriol implants in adult rats will cause multiple abnormalities of the reproductive tract and other related systems[7].

Therefore, the ability of estriol to express its toxicity is related to the way in which it is administered and simply reflects the pharmacokinetic and receptor dynamics of this compound. These properties should obviously be considered in the evaluation of the reproductive toxicological potential of any compound.

Target Organs

Drug safety studies should consider the responsiveness of the end organ (target organ) in question. This statement is based on the assumption that target organ stimulation results in the eventual development of an adverse effect. This point has been discussed earlier. It is possible that an adverse effect may be indirect and not associated with direct stimulation of the target organ. Such indirect effects would only occur at very high doses and not be relevant to testing under conditions which mimic drug use.

Hormones and drugs bind receptors and produce their effects at concentrations which can be predicted from the dissociation constant (K_d) of the receptor hormone interaction. Deviations from this rule will occur due to metabolism of the injected hormone, pharmacokinetic differences and blood binding proteins.

The extrapolation of animal studies for the prediction of hazards to humans is the most difficult question of all. As pointed out earlier in this paper, species differences in pharmacokinetic and metabolic functions hamper such extrapolations. Thus, it appears that valid prediction of human hazard from animal studies will only occur when sufficient information is available concerning species differences to make such extrapolations. We simply do not know enough at the present time to make accurate predictions. More research is needed to establish model systems which can be used.

Relationship of Response Profiles to Abnormal Function

Hormone or drug stimulation of target organs results in a response profile which is characterized by the elevation of various cellular constituents or functions (Figure 1). If such response profiles can be related to abnormal functions then the ultimate predictor will be at hand. As discussed earlier, there are many difficulties involved in such analyses; however, it is conceivable that distinctive patterns could be ascertained. Therefore it is recommended that research be begun which would test this concept.

In conjunction with this proposal the relationships shown in Figure 4 should be examined. The dose-reponse curve given in this figure is typical of many obtained with hormones and represents the stimulation of

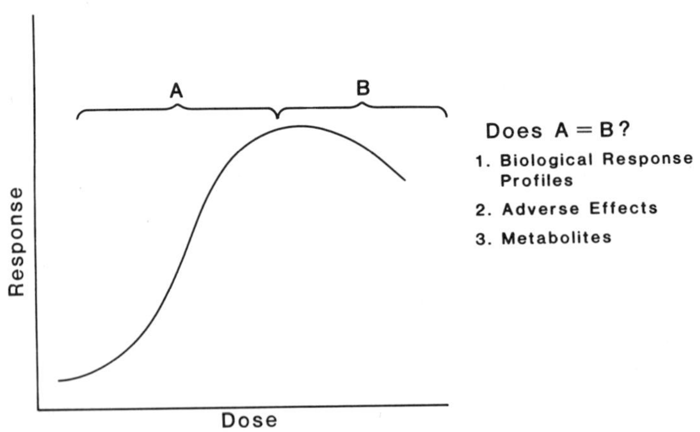

Figure 4. Relationship between physiological or therapeutic (A) and pharmacologic (B) dose of hormone and biological response.

a response by low to relatively high doses of the hormone (A-range) and the inhibition of the response by high to very high doses (B-range). Does the response profile observed with hormone doses in the A-range of the dose-response curve equal that seen with doses in the B-range? This is an important question because drugs would ordinarily be administered in the A-dose range. Therefore, deviations noted in the B-range may not be relevant to the prediction of hazard.

Differences in adverse effects could also exist between dose ranges A and B. It is conceivable that no adverse effects might be observed with drugs tested in the A-range while B-range testing would result in abnormalities. Such results could relate to indirect effects of very high doses of drug which would be unrelated to doses used in the therapeutic range (A-range).

Likewise, the relationship between the production of deleterious intermediates via drug metabolism should be shown to be equal in dose ranges A and B. As previously pointed out, thus far only high doses or high concentrations of estrogens have been shown to form active intermediates and it needs to be demonstrated that this occurs at lower therapeutic doses (A-range).

The similarities or differences with respect to the above considerations in dose ranges A and B need to be resolved. Therefore, it is recommended that such research be established.

Hormone and Drug Interactions

It is well known that estrogen and progesterone interact to bring about their effects. Understanding such interactions is important to our basic knowledge concerning toxicological assessment of contraceptive drugs. These interactions involve analyses of steroid receptors (both qualitative and quantitative measurements), nuclear binding and processing of steroid receptors, response profile analysis as influenced by both hormone types and the biochemistry and molecular biology of these interactions. The understanding of the basic cellular mechanisms could provide very important insight into toxicological assessment.

Structure Function Relationships and Prediction

The ideal toxicological test would be one that could predict potential hazards by the examination of the structure of the molecule in question. This is otherwise known as the toxicologist's dream. Such a dream can come true only if we know considerably more than we do now about structure function relationships. The results of the research proposed in the previous section will go a long way in reaching this goal. That is, it may become apparent after the analysis of many drug and hormone structures, that certain specific response profiles are associated with specific chemical structures. Such information could be used in conjunction with data on pharmacokinetic and metabolic interactions to form a structure-function data bank which would be of great importance. The integration and establishment of such a data bank will require a great deal of research and effort, however, it seems well worth the expenditure.

Basic Biology of Animals Used in Prediction Model Systems

The differences in the biological functions between animals used in model test systems and humans constitutes one of the most important factors in extrapolation of these model systems to human hazard. Some of these differences have been discussed in previous sections of this paper and many more exist, both known and unknown. Continued research in these areas is needed to establish adequate prediction models.

REFERENCES

1. Clark, JH, Peck, EJ, Jr.: Female Sex Steroids: Receptors and Function. Berlin, Heidelberg, New York, Springer-Verlag, 1979.

2. Clark, JR, McCormack, SA, Kling, R, Hodges, D, Hardin, JW: Effect of clomiphene and other triphenylethylene derivatives on the reproductive tract in the rat and baboon. In: Iacobelli, S. et al (Eds.): Hormones and Cancer, New York, Raven Press, 1980, p 295.

3. Eroschenko, VF, Palmiter, RD: Estrogenicity of kepone in birds and mammals. In: McLachlan, J (Ed): Estrogens in the Environment, New York, Elsevier/North Holland, 1980, p 305.

4. Kupfer, D, Bulger, WH: Estrogenic properties of DDT and its analogs. In: McLachlan, J (Ed): Estrogens in the Environment, New York, Elsevier/North Holland, 1980, p 239.

5. Sheehan, DM, Branham, D, Medlock, K, Olson, M, Zehr, D: Uterine response to estradiol in the neonatal rat. Endocrinology, 109:76, 1981.

6. Rochefort, H, Garcia, M: The estrogenic and antiestrogenic activities of androgens in female target tissues. Pharmac Ther, 23:193, 1983.

7. Noble, RL, Hochachka, BC, King, D: Spontaneous and estrogen-produced tumors in Nb rats and their behavior after transplantation. Cancer Res, 35:766, 1975.

8. Clark, JH, Markaverich, BM: The agonistic-antagonistic properties of clomiphene: a review. Pharma Ther, 15:467, 1982.

9. Hsuch, AJW, Peck, EJ, Jr, Clark, JH: Control of uterine estrogen receptor levels by progesterone. Endocrinology, 98:438, 1976.

10. Tseng, L, Gurpide, E: Estradiol and 20 alpha-dihydroprogesterone dehydrogenase activities in human endometrium during the menstrual cycle. Endocrinology, 94:419, 1974.

11. Herbst, AL, Ulfelder, H, Poskanzer, DC: Adenocarcinoma of the vagina. Association of maternal stilbestrol therapy with tumor appearance in young women. N Engl J Med, 284:878, 1971.

12. Herbst, AL, Poskanzer, DC, Robboy, SJ, Friedlander, L, Scully, RE: Prenatal exposure to stilbestrol. A prospective comparison of exposed female offspring with unexposed controls. N Eng J Med, 292:334, 1975.

13. Sheehan, DM, Branham, WS, Medlock, KL, Olson, ME, Zehr, D: Estrogen

plasma binding and regulation of development in the neonatal rat. Teratology, 21:68A, 1980.

14. Nunez, EA, Benassayag, C, Savu, L, Vallette, G, Jayle, MF: Purification and comparative estrogen binding properties of different forms of rat, mouse, and human alpha fetoproteins. In: Fishman, WH, Sell, S (Eds): Onco-Developmental Gene Expression, New York, Academic Press, 1976, p 365.

15. Metzler, M, Gottschlich, R, McLachlan, JA: Oxidative metabolism of stilbene estrogens. In: McLachlan, J (Ed): Estrogens in the Environment, New York, Elsevier/North Holland, 1980, p 283.

16. Purdy, RH, Goldzieher, JW, LeQuesne, PW, Abdel-Baky, S, Durocher, CK, Moore, PH, Jr, Rhim, JS: Active intermediates and carcinogenesis. In: Lipsett, M, Merriam, GR (Eds): International Workshop on Catechol Estrogens, New York, Raven Press, 1982, p 123.

17. Clark, JR, Guthrie, SC: The estrogenic effects of clomiphene during the neonatal period in the rat. J Steroid Biochem, 18:513, 1983.

18. MacLusky, NJ, Naftolin, F: Sexual differentiation of the central nervous system. Science, 211:1294, 1981.

19. McEwen, BS: Neural gonadal steroid action. Science, 211:1303, 1981.

20. Gellert, RJ, Heinrichs, WL, Swerdloff, R: Effects of neonatally administered DDT homologs on reproductive function in male and female rats. Neuroendocrinology, 16:84, 1974.

21. Clark, JH, McCormack, S: Clomid or Nafoxidine administered to neonatal rats causes reproductive tract abnormalities. Science, 197:164, 1977.

22. Goy, RW, Resko, JA: Gonadal hormones and behavior of normal and pseudohermaphroditic nonhuman female primates. Rec Prog Horm Res, 28:707, 1972.

23. Reiter, EO, Grumbach, MM, Kaplan, SL, Conte, FA: The response of pituitary gonadotropes to synthetic LRF in children with glucocorticoid-treated congenital adrenal hyperplasia; lack of effect of intrauterine and neonatal androgen excess. J Clin Endocrinol Metab, 40:318, 1975.

24. Karsch, FJ, Dierschke, DJ, Knobil, E: Sexual differentiation of pituitary function: apparent difference between primates and rodents. Science, 179:484, 1973.

25. Barbarino, A, DeMarinis, L, Lafuenti, G, Muscatello, P, Matteucci, BR: Presence of positive feedback between oestrogen and LH in patients with Klinefelter's syndrome and Sertoli-cell-only syndrome. Clin Endocrinol, 10:235, 1979.

26. Grumbach, MM, Ducharme, JR, Moloshok, RE: On fetal masculinizing action of certain oral progestins. J Clin Endocrinol Metab, 19:1369, 1959.

27. Grumbach, MM, Ducharme, JR: The effects of androgens on fetal sexual development: androgen-induced female pseudohermaphrodism, Fertil Steril, 11:157, 1960.

28. Cramer, W, Hornig, ES: Experimental production by oestrin of pituitary tumours with hypopituitarism and of mammary cancer. Lancet, 1:247, 1936.

29. Allen, E, Gardner, WU: Cancer of the cervix and of the uterus in hybrid mice following long-continued administration of estrogen. Cancer Res, 1:359, 1941.

30. Gardner, WU, Pfeiffer, CA, Trentin, JJ: Hormonal factors in experimental carcinogenesis. In: Homburger, F (Ed.): The Physiopathology of Cancer, New York, Harper & Row, 1959, p 1529.

31. Dunn, TB, Green, AW: Cysts of the epididymis, cancer of the cervix, granular cell myoblastoma and other lesions after estrogen injection in newborn mice. J Natl Cancer Inst, 31:425, 1963.

32. Takasugi, N, Bern, HA: Tissue changes in mice with persistent vaginal cornification induced by early postnatal treatment with estrogen. J Natl Cancer Inst, 33:855, 1964.

33. Forsberg, J-G: Estrogen, vaginal cancer and vaginal development. Am J Obstet Gynecol, 113:83, 1972.

34. Forsberg, J-G: Late effects in the vaginal and cervical epithelium after injections of diethylstilbestrol in neonatal mice. Am J Ob Gyn, 121:101, 1975.

35. Furth, J, Ueda, G, Clifton, KH: Pathophysiology of pituitaries and their tumors; methodological advances. In: Busch, H (Ed.): Methods in Cancer Research, New York, Academic Press, 1973, Vol. 10, p 201.

36. Leavitt, WW, Evans, RW, Hendry, WJ III: Etiology of DES-induced uterine tumors in the syrian hamster. In: Leavitt, WW (Ed.): Hormones and Cancer, New York, Plenum Publishing Co., 1981, p 63.

37. Lobl, RT, Maenza, RM: Androgenization: alterations in uterine growth and morphology. Biol Repro, 13:255, 1975.

38. Takasugi, N: Cytological basis for permanent vaginal changes in mice treated neonatally with steroid hormones. Int Rev Cytol, 44:193, 1976.

39. Forsberg, J-G: Cervicovaginal epithelium: its origin and development. Am J Ob Gyn, 115:1025, 1973.

40. Pomerance, W: Post-stilbestrol secondary syndrome. Obstet Gynecol, 49:1, 1977.

41. Bibbo, M, Gill, WB, Azizi, F, Blough, R, Fang, VA, Rosenfield, RL, Schumacher, GF, Sleeper, K, Sonek, MG, Wied, GL: Follow-up study of male and female offspring of DES-exposed mothers. Obstet Gynecol, 49:1, 1977.

42. Haney, AF, Hammond, CB, Soules, MR, Creasman, WT: Diethylstilbestrol induced upper genital tract abnormalities. Fertil Steril, 31:142, 1979.

43. Barnes, AB: Menstrual history of young women exposed in utero to diethylstilbestrol. Fertil Steril, 32:148, 1979.

44. Clark, JH, Paszko, A, Peck, EJ, Jr: Nuclear binding and retention of the receptor estrogen complex: relation to the agonistic and antagonistic properties of estriol. Endocrinology, 100:91, 1977.

45. Wotiz, HH, Shane, JA, Vigersky, R, Brecher, PI: The regulatory role of oestriol in the proliferative action of estradiol. In: Forrest, APM, Kunkler, PB (Eds): Prognostic Factors in Breast Cancer, Edinburgh, Livingston Press, 1968, p 368.

46. Cole, P, MacMahon, B: Oestrogen fractions during early reproductive life in the aetiology of breast cancer. Lancet, 1:604, 1969.

47. Lemon, HM, Miller, DM, Foley, JF: Competition between steroids for hormonal receptor. Natl Cancer Inst Monogr, 34:77, 1971.

48. Kincl, FA, Folch, PI, Maqueo, M, Lasso, LH, Oriol, A, Dorfman, RI: Inhibition of sexual development in male and female rats treated with various steroids at the age of five days. Acta Endocrinol, 49:193, 1965.

49. Rudali, G, Apiou, F, Muel, B: Mammary cancer produced in mice with estriol. Eur J Cancer, 11:39, 1975.

DISCUSSION

DR. DICZFALUSY: Thank you very much, Dr. Clark. Are there questions and comments.

DR. SCHUPPLER: You mentioned information on the epoxides. Have you any evidence that suggests that the epoxides actually do anything? Have you any practical examples of a correlation between epoxide formation and, say, protein binding and a specific effect of the protein binding?

DR. CLARK: The work on epoxides is not mine. It has been reported that epoxides bind to various cellular constituents, however, this was done *in vitro* under conditions which are far from physiological.

DR. SCHUPPLER: As far as I am aware, one of the points that would be necessary would be that there be covalent binding of the epoxide to DNA.

DR. CLARK: Yes, that has not been shown *in vivo* under appropriate pharmacological or physiological conditions.

DR. SCHUPPLER: That has not been shown either *in vitro* or *in vivo* for any species?

DR. CLARK: Not that I know of. It has been demonstrated under nonphysiological circumstances with millimolar concentrations of estrogens.

DR. SCHUPPLER: There were, at the time most of those papers were written, a lot of technical difficulties including procedures for purification.

DR. VON EICKSTEDT: May I just comment on Dr. Schuppler's question. Bremer and Bolt published papers concerning the nuclear binding of epoxides. The nonphysiologic model used demonstrated that these doses were not relevant to any clinical use of steroids, such as estrogens.

You showed the dose-dependent activities of the estrogens, the more estrogen you give in many models, the more estrogenic activity observed. But with other steroids, like medroxyprogesterone acetate, higher doses result in different effects not observed at lower doses, i.e., MPA's corticoid-like activity and NET enanthate's estrogenic activity. I think we should take into account these differences between sex steroids that can not be determined and tested in the same manner.

DR. CLARK: I think that is relevant to Dr. Bardin's discussion. At those high doses you produce effects that have nothing to do with either the physiologic or therapeutic action of these drugs and are

therefore irrelevant, because the human will never be exposed to it.

DR. GOLDZIEHER: Jim and I have discussed this many times, certainly agree that the concentrations used for in vitro studies are nowhere near the physiological range. On the other hand, what is used in vitro is simply a model, that is all it is intended to be. What the in vitro studies show is that an epoxide is ten times as potent in producing malignant transformation of a cell line, as a catechol, or as estradiol. A catechol is five times as potent as the free compound.

You see a sequence of events at very high concentrations. I don't consider this irrelevant to human physiology, because you do not know what the concentration is at the active sites or within a cell. Until we know that, I don't think discussing about gross concentrations in solvents, mixtures, or intestines is all that important.

I am not saying that this experiment is relevant to human physiology but I think it is a model which may point the direction in which further investigations can go which elucidate mechanisms.

DR. CLARK: I agree, because one can always argue that especially in the liver, even small quantities of an undetectable epoxide could be very important. However, it must be shown empirically before any conclusions can be drawn.

The one point I didn't make but which is discussed in the paper that you provided on this compound, is that estriol is not a good catechol former and does not form epoxides readily. But estriol is a carcinogen, it will cause mammary cancers, as well as other types of neoplasia as Nobel showed several years ago.

DR. DICZFALUSY: We have time for three questions and two answers.

DR. KATZENELLENBOGEN: I wanted to comment on dose response relationships. In looking at the maintenance of tumors that may be hormone-dependent for their growth, a physiological concentration of estrogen seems optimal. If one actually increases the hormone levels obtained following physiological estrogen doses, then one might consider estrogen as an anticancer agent, because pharmacologic doses will extinguish certain hormone-dependent tumors and are used in high dose estrogen treatment of breast cancer.

So certainly the dose response relationships are very important and must be considered.

DR. BARDIN: I think with regard to epoxides, it is worthwhile pointing out that the body makes them all the time from everything. It is the normal way that the body detoxifies everything, and there are mechanisms to handle epoxides and only when there is a genetic abnormality of one of these detoxifying mechanisms do we really see an effect. It is a normal pathway of metabolism of hepatic microsomes. This is not unique to steroids, it is a normal intermediate of hydroxylation. I think it is worthwhile to remind ourselves of this.

DR. LIPSETT: Jim, I liked your sermon, I guess for a couple of reasons including that it agrees with my own prejudice.

DR. CLARK: I knew it did.

DR. LIPSETT: About 15 years ago we wrote a paper in which we said an estrogen is an estrogen is an estrogen. One of the arguments, though, about epoxides that no one has mentioned is that they are considered to be direct carcinogens, and you would expect to see the dose response curves observed with radiation, viruses and so forth. However, hormones, including estrogens, apparently don't have this effect, because we have no evidence for it. It would be very hard to invoke the epoxide argument for the DNA adduct.

DR. CLARK: Yes, I agree.

ENDOCRINE EFFECTS OF SYSTEMIC, STEROIDAL CONTRACEPTIVES

Richard A. Edgren

Director of Scientific Affairs
Syntex Laboratories, Inc.
Palo Alto, California

INTRODUCTION

Contraceptives are mechanical devices, locally acting chemicals or systemic drugs, usually steroids, that may be employed for long periods by otherwise healthy people. As such they must, in addition to assured efficacy rates, have high levels of safety. In recent years, particular attention has been devoted to the systemic drugs and some thirty years of accumulated experience is now available on the steroidal contraceptives used by women.

Currently, systemic steroidal contraceptives are of three types: the oral combination products containing progestational and estrogenic components, the so-called minipills containing only a progestational agent, and the long-acting injectable progestagens. Since their introduction over two decades ago, their use has been surrounded by a bedlam of controversy concerning safety; fortunately, efficacy has never been seriously questioned.

Since the marketing of OCs they have been subjected to a surveillance unprecedented in medical history. As a result, it is now possible to view these agents from the perspective of extensive experience and to examine our early concerns dispassionately to determine how they fared in the light of new knowledge and whether preclinical pharmacological and toxicological studies based on these concerns were justified.

I propose to examine these agents from the frame of reference of an endocrine pharmacologist, while others at this workshop will consider different aspects of the problem. It should be emphasized that the mass of safety data on steroidal contraceptives deals with combination products, each containing an estrogen and a progestagen. These, therefore, are complex drugs with biological effects resulting from independent actions of each component and from their synergistic interactions. I shall initially focus on the independent actions of the separate components, with specific reference to the predictive value of animal endocrine pharmacology to clinical effects, follow with some consideration of interactions, and finally discuss some specific safety issues and recommendations. With respect to the pharmacological studies, the data presented were generated in my own laboratories or in those with which I have been closely associated.

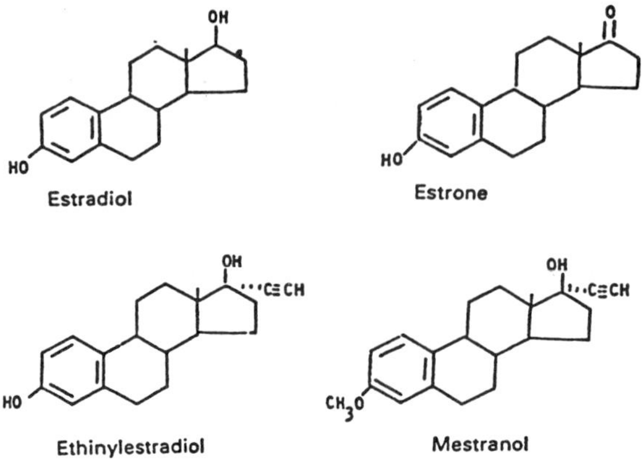

Figure 1. Structural formulae of representative estrogens. Only ethinyl estradiol and mestranol are used in oral contraceptives.

ENDOCRINE PHARMACOLOGY OF ESTROGENS

Only two estrogens, ethinyl estradiol (EE) and mestranol (ethinyl estradiol-3-methyl ether) are employed as components of the oral contraceptives (Figure 1). These agents are 17α-ethinyl derivatives of the natural human estrogen, estradiol; the substitution contributes to oral efficacy, presumably by retarding hepatic inactivation of the material.

In mammals, estrogens are the predominant substances that control the attainment of female sexual maturity and that dominate the follicular phase of estrous and menstrual cycles. In the human female, they terminate growth of the uterus, particularly of the preovulatory endometrium, and control cyclic changes in the vagina; through effects on the hypothalamus and pituitary they regulate the sexual cycle. Their absence, as in natural or surgical menopause, leads to vasomotor instability, bony degeneration and, perhaps, to an increased risk of cardiovascular problems.

These wide-ranging effects are easily predicted from a few simple laboratory assay procedures. Allen and Doisy employed spayed female rats in the original extraction and identification of estrone (Figure 1). Removal of the ovaries from laboratory rodents abolishes the cyclic changes in the vaginal epithelium. These can be mimicked by administration of estrogen. In ovariectomized or immature rats and mice, estrogens cause growth of the uterus, and these systems have been adapted to simplified assay techniques. The uterine growth assays are not specific for estrogens in that androgens and progestagens also cause growth of this organ, particularly in rats.

I have personally employed both tests for evaluation of estrogencity. Vaginal smear tests have been the more specific while the uterine growth tests are the more quantitative.

Both effects are mediated through cytoplasmic receptors as are many effects in humans. Specific high affinity estrogen receptors have been demonstrated in the uterus, vagina, breast and hypothalamus of a range of animal species. To the best of my knowledge, receptors have not been identified in bone or vascular tissues.

Table 1. Potency comparisons in various tests for estradiol-17β and 18-homoestradiol. From Edgren, Jones, and Peterson[1].

Compound	Vaginal smears Rat 1 day	2 day	Mouse	Uterine growth Rat 3 day	7 day	Mouse	Vaginal opening	Oviduct growth
Estradiol-17β	100%	100%	100%	100%	100%	100%	100%	100%
18-Homoestradiol	30	1	1.25	?	67	< 0.1	10	< 100

* From Edgren, Jones, and Peterson (1).

Projection of estrogenic effects from animal assay systems to the clinic has been quite successful. If a material were shown to have estrogenic effects in the pharmacology laboratory, estrogenic activity has consistently been demonstrated clinically, and this extends to nonsteroidal estrogens as well. Quantitative projection, however, has been a more serious problem. Slight variations in assay protocol may lead to major differences in potency estimates (Table 1); note the wide variation in relative potencies cited for 18-homoestradiol. Also, since slopes of dose-response curves differ, potency estimates may be technically impossible. Furthermore, the end point to be evaluated clinically can rarely be defined. Ethinyl estradiol is normally employed at a dose of 30-50 μg daily in oral contraceptive formulations, while doses in the range of 20-50 μg are recommended for menopausal control. In the latter use, however, individualization of dose is normal and may vary widely from patient to patient. In neither case are exact end points isolated for comparison.

It seems quite clear that, although animal assay techniques may be employed to evaluate relative potency with great precision, clinical potency may not be assessed as critically. This leaves one in doubt of the utility of such highly precise evaluations.

One final point on the estrogens. I know of no qualitative difference between oral and parenteral administration. Although oral potency is consistently lower than parenteral where a material is examined by both routes, the spectrum of effects is similar.

ENDOCRINE PHARMACOLOGY OF PROGESTAGENS

The progestational agents employed in oral contraceptives are more diversified than the estrogens although most are related to 19-nortestosterone (Figure 2). The acetoxyprogesterone derivatives are no longer employed as components of combination products in the U.S.; more recently they have been used mainly as minipills (chlormadinone acetate) and long-acting injectables (medroxyprogesterone acetate). However, the IPPF Directory of Contraceptives (1981 edition) lists only combination and sequential products containing chlormadinone acetate, while Depo-Provera (MPA) appears only to be used as an injectable[2]. Quingestanol acetate, desogestrel and norgestrienone are employed in certain products outside of the U.S. as are norethindrone enanthate (as an injectable) and combination products containing dihydroxyprogesterone acetophenide and estradiol enanthate.

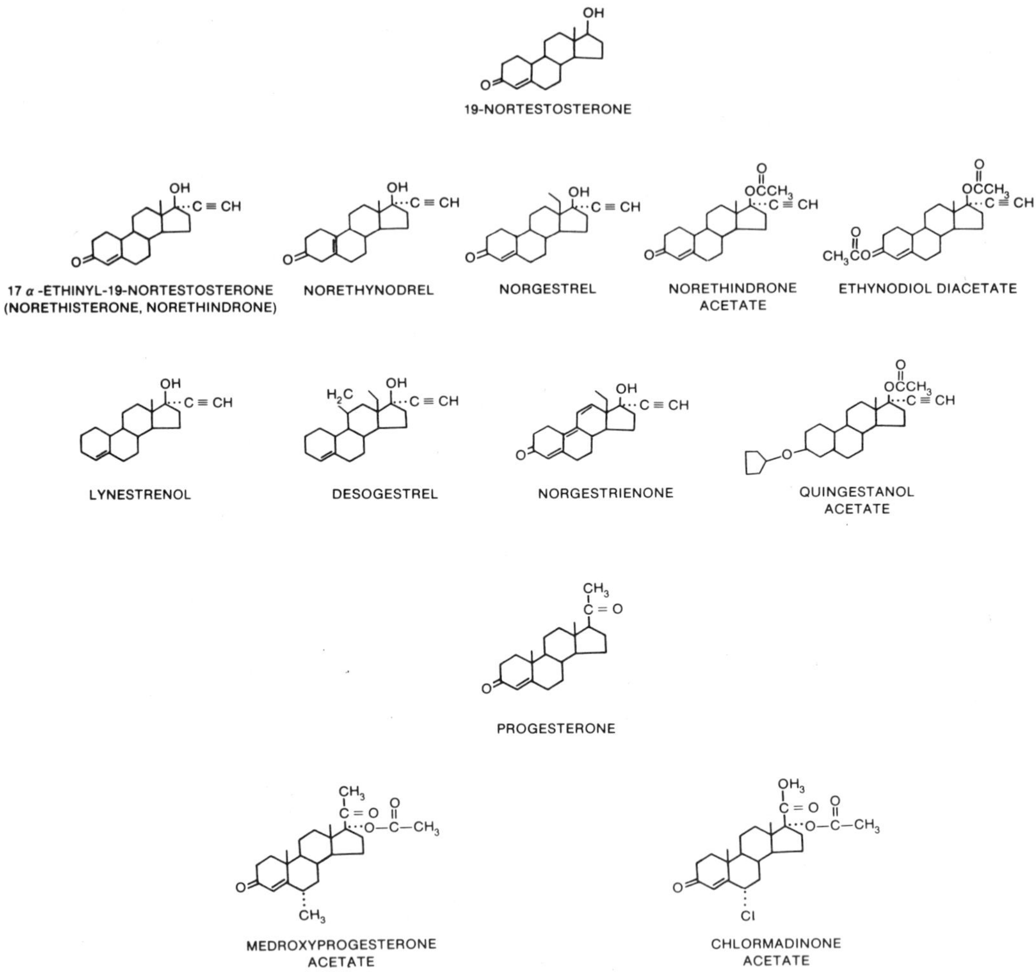

Figure 2. Structural Formulae of selected progestagens used as contraceptives or as components of contraceptives.

PROGESTATIONAL EFFECTS

The biological properties of these drugs are also heterogenous, although I do not have satisfactory comparative data on a number of the agents. Binding to the endometrial progesterone receptor is demonstrable with most of the products (Table 2). However, certain active progestagens of the 19-nortestosterone series fail to bind to the receptor leading one to believe that they exert their actions after metabolic conversion to norethindrone.

The most commonly employed measure of progestational activity in the laboratory is the Clauberg or the McPhail test (Table 3) in which estrogen-primed rabbits receive the progestagen. The drug effect is measured by histological evaluation of arborization of uterine glands. With certain

Table 2. Steroid binding to human uterine progesterone receptors.*

COMPOUND	RELATIVE AFFINITY (% + SE) ENDOMETRIUM	MYOMETRIUM
Progesterone	100 + 2	100 + 2
Levonorgestrel (d-norgestrel)	95 + 2	96 + 3
Norethindrone	85 + 5	87 + 4
Medroxyprogesterone acetate	78 + 7	79 + 9
dl-Norgestrel	49 + 3	48 + 4
Chlormadinone acetate	28 + 6	31 + 5
Norethindrone acetate	6 + 5	6 + 4
Norethynodrel	5 + 4	3 + 2
Ethynodiol diacetate	5 + 3	4 + 3
Lynestrenol	4 + 3	3 + 2
l-Norgestrel (dextrorotatory)	2 + 1	1 + 1
Mestranol	2 + 1	2 + 1
Ethinyl estradiol	2 + 1	2 + 1

*Data of Briggs (3).

exceptions, this measure correlates with such other measures of progestational activity as observed in as the McGinty test, where the progestagen is administered directly into the lumen of the uterus of estrogen-primed rabbits, the maintenance of pregnancy in female rats spayed after implantation, and the delay of parturition in pregnant rats. Human effects, such as secretory transformation of the uterus, delay of menses and efficacy as an oral contraceptive when admixed with estrogen, have been employed for comparative purposes.

Inspection of the data in Table 3 indicate that there is no simple, direct, quantitative correspondence between the animal studies and the human. Qualitatively, predictability is good, but precise quantitative correspondence are lacking.

ESTROGENIC EFFECT

Since uterine growth assays are not specific for estrogens, I shall restrict my comments to vaginal smears and receptor binding assays (Table 4). Of the progestagens that have been studied using reasonably comparable techniques, norethindrone, norethynodrel, and ethynodiol diacetate bind to estrogen receptors and have some measurable estrogenic effect on the

Table 3. Comparative activities of various progestagens in a series of assay procedures.

		ASSAY							
		LABORATORY ANIMAL				HUMAN			
COMPOUND	BINDING (%)*	CLAUBERG**	MCGINTY**	PREGNANCY MAINTENANCE**	DELAY OF PARTURITION‖	DELAY OF MENSES a	DELAY OF MENSES b	MINIMUM BLEEDING DOSE***
Progesterone	100	100	A	A	100	-	-	-
Levonorgestrel	95	1,800	-	A	-	-	-	
Norethindrone	85	8	I	I	100	4(?)	0.9	2
Medroxyprogesterone acetate	78	3,500	A	A	300	22.5	-	-
dl-Norgestrel	49	900	A	A	1,000	0.125	0.35	0.5
Norethynodrel	5	?	I	I	A	5.3	-	5
Ethynodiol diacetate	5	240	-	-	-	1.5	2+	1

* Data of Briggs (3).

+a With 100μg mestranol; figures are ED_{50} values in milligrams. Data of Swyer and Little (4) -- or b with 50μg of EE. Data of Swyer (5).

*** With 50μg of ethinyl estradiol or 100μg of mestranol; oral contraceptive values are given in milligrams Data of Edgren (6).

** Data of Edgren (7).

‖ Data of Edgren and Peterson (8).

A = active; I = inactive.

vaginal epithelium. In man, only norethynodrel and ethynodiol diacetate appear to have potent estrogenic activity as judged by effects on vaginal epithelium or cervical mucus.

Again there would appear to be good qualitative correlation between animal and human effects, but no quantification seems possible with available data.

ANDROGENIC EFFECTS

Like testosterone, a number of the progestagens bind to the testosterone receptor (Table 5), and exhibit androgenic effects in laboratory animals and man. The acetoxyprogesterone derivatives, medroxyprogesterone acetate (MPA) and chlormadinone acetate appear to be exceptions; they bind to the receptor, but lack marked androgenic activity in castrated male rats (Hershberger test). I have never seen convincing published evidence of clinical androgencity. The masculinization of female rat fetuses by MPA may reflect this activity but this is not seen clinically.

ANTI-ESTROGENIC ACTIVITIES

Most of the progestagens will alter the effects of estrogens on the uterus or vagina when administered simultaneously. Various assay procedures have been employed and close correspondence between mouse uterine

Table 4. Estrogenic effects of progestagens.

	BINDING CONSTANT FOR ESTROGEN* RECEPTOR	ALLEN-DOISY VAGINAL SMEAR (RAT)**	LONG-TERM VAGINAL CHANGES (RAT)***	HUMAN EFFECTS
Progesterone	I	I	I	I
Medroxyprogesterone acetate	I	I	I	
Levonorgestrel	I	I	I	I
Norethindrone	6×10^{-7}	I	0.3%	I
Norethynodrel	2.8×10^{-8}	7%	2.1%	A
Ethynodiol diacetate	9.9×10^{-8}	4%	0.4%	A

* Data of Terenius (9).

** Data of Edgren (unpublished) and Elton, and Nutting (10). Figures express potency relative to estrone.

*** Data of Jones and Edgren (11), and Edgren (unpublished). Figures represent potency relative to ethinyl estradiol, 100%; all by oral route.

A = active; I = inactive.

weight and vaginal smear assays have been defined. How this anti-estrogenic action is manifested clinically is not well defined. The mid-cycle liquifaction of human cervical mucus appears to be an estrogen-controlled response that is reversed by progestagens, and may be the basis of the minipill prevention of sperm migration. At any rate, there is a qualitative relationship between these measures, and a suggestion of a quantitative correlation between antiestrogenic potency as measured by the mouse vaginal smear assay and that observed with use of the minipill (Table 6).

GLUCOCORTICOID EFFECTS

Some years ago the routine toxicological evaluation of medroxyprogesterone acetate showed that two week treatment with the drug produced atrophy of the adrenal gland. These observations were then extended to a number of measures of corticoid activity. More recently, these materials have been shown to bind to the glucocorticoid receptor and considerable evidence indicates clinical corticoid action[14]. These effects do not appear to extend to the use of Depo Provera as a contraceptive.

Table 5. Receptor binding and prostatic growth effects of various progestagens.

COMPOUND	DISPLACING POTENCY (%)*	PROSTATIC GROWTH, RELATIVE POTENCY**	CLINICAL ANDROGENICITY
Testosterone	100	100	A
Levonorgestrel	42	15.0	A
dl-Norgestrel		7.5	A
Norethindrone	23	1.6	A
Ethynodiol diacetate	< 1	1.0	I
Norethynodrel	< 1	I	I
Medroxyprogesterone acetate	23	I	I
Chlormadinone acetate	7	I	I
Progesterone	< 1	I	I

* Data of Labrie (12).

** Data of Edgren (7).

A = active; I = inactive.

COMMENTS

It should be apparent from the foregoing, summarized in Table 7, that I believe we did a good job in predicting clinical activities from animal models when classical definitions of progestational, estrogenic and anti-estrogenic effects are employed. I do not believe that these techniques projected more than extremely crude quantitative estimates. It is my opinion that quantification can only be satisfactory when carried out in the species for which the drug is intended and on the end-point for therapeutic use. Even comparative pharmacology can only provide estimates as to whether initial doses should be small or large and rough indications of what small and large may mean. In the final analysis, the identification of the optimum dose must be based on human data.

SOME REMARKS ON INTERACTIONS

When one specifically examines the complex oral contraceptive drug combinations, the problem of steroid interactions becomes critical, and unfortunately, the results are largely unpredictable from the properties of either component. It has been known for decades that progestagens act poorly on the uteri of mammals unless primed with estrogen. We know that generation of the progesterone receptor is estrogen-controlled, explaining the priming phenomenon. We also have evidence that progestagens reverse

Table 6. Antiestrogenic and minipill contraceptive dose for various progestagens.

COMPOUND	ANTIESTROGENIC POTENCY*	MINIPILL DOSE**
Progesterone	100%	
Chlormadinone acetate	130	500µg
Norethindrone	700	350
Norgestrel (racemic)	7,400	75
Medroxyprogesterone acetate	A	
Ethinodiol diacetate	A	500µg
Norethynodrel	I	

* Potencies based on ED_{50} levels in mouse vaginal smear antiestrone assay.

** Dose for Pearl index of 2-3 in large-scale studies.

A = active; I = inactive.

Based on data from Edgren (13).

the effects of estrogens on certain targets. Further, large doses of estrogen will inhibit the effects of progesterone on the proliferation of uterine glands.

We certainly lack adequate data to predict the composite effect of interactions for any combination of estrogen and progestagen or how the estrogenic, progestational, anti-estrogenic and anti-progestational effects activity and synergistic interactions will be expressed is unpredictable. Clinically, Swyer and Little have shown that in the Swyer-Greenblatt delay-of menses test, the simultaneous employment of norethynodrel and 0.1 mg. of mestranol, increases the potency of the progestagen about four-fold, while the potency of norgestrel is increased about 30 times. More recently Swyer has published data suggesting a ten-fold increase in potency of norgestrel when EE is employed as the estrogen at 0.05 mg.

It is unlikely that any measure of interaction in animal systems will project directly to human effects of contraceptive steroids. This conjecture is most critical in assessing activities of combination preparations, but is similarly important in evaluating effects of drugs which fail to shut down the ovary completely.

ROUTE OF ADMINISTRATION

The mass of clinical safety experience with steroidal systemic contraceptives is based on orally administered combination preparations, raising questions concerning the applicability of these data to injectable materials. Natural steroids, such as estradiol-17β, testosterone and

Table 7. Comparative biological effects of progestational agents in laboratory animals and humans.

COMPOUND	EFFECT									
	Progestational		Estrogenic		Androgenic		Anti-Estrogenic		Glucocorticoid	
	Lab Animal	Human	Lab Animal	Human	Lab Animal	Human	Lab Animal	Human	Lab Animal	Human
Progesterone	+	+	-	-	-	-	+	+	?	?
Norethindrone	+	+	+*	-	+	+	+	+	-	-
Norethindrone acetate	+	+			+	+				
Ethynodiol diacetate	+	+	+	+	+	+	+	+		
Norgestrel	+	+	-	-	+	+	+	+	-	-
Norethynodrel	+	+	+	+	-	-	-	-	-	-
Medroxyprogesterone acetate	+	+	-	-	+**	-	+		+	+
Chlormadinone acetate	+	+	-	-	-	-	+	+		

* Long-term studies only

** Fetal masculinization only

progesterone are poorly active by the oral route, presumably due to hepatic degradation. Similarly, semisynthetic estrogens and progestagens tend to be less effective orally than parenterally. This generalization would suggest that orally administered materials are more rapidly converted into less effective metabolites than when given parenterally. This concept is supported by quantitative studies performed with known or presumed metabolites of the 19-norsteroidal progestagens and the ethinyl estrogens, all of which are of low potency.

Such logic suggests that oral studies actually reflect the effects of a broader range of materials, parent and metabolites, than parenteral routes. One would surmise that a dangerously toxic metabolite of a steroid, if such exists, would be more likely to be observed in oral toxicity studies than with parenteral administration. In my opinion, on the basis of probable metabolites, the oral toxicity studies that have supported the individual components of oral contraceptives are largely adequate to support injectable materials.

I know of only one qualitative change among the groups of steroids under consideration. I have never seen a clear estrogenic effect of parenteral norethindrone. When given orally for several days, however, characteristic vaginal keratinization is seen in spayed female rats[11]. I know of no evidence for this phenomenon in humans.

SOME HISTORICAL CONSIDERATIONS

When oral contraceptives were first studied and marketed, concern was expressed by many physicians and scientists about potential dangers.

Predominant among these was the fear of possible steroid induced cancer. Studies carried out shortly after steroid hormones were isolated suggested the possibility that estrogens, in particular, were carcinogenic in target tissues. These studies, many in highly sensitive strains of mice and often with massive doses of hormone (frequently diethylstilbestrol rather than steroidal estrogens), should be reevaluated using modern standards. They should also be interpreted with caution, particularly since the carcinogenesis studies for OC's and their components required in Great Britain did not suggest any significant danger[15].

Concern was revived during the middle to late 1960's when first MK-665 and later acetoxyprogesterone derivatives were associated with increased incidences of mammary nodules in beagle bitches. These findings led to the requirements for long-term dog and monkey studies which have done so much to dampen industrial interest in new steroids in general and systemic contraception in particular. The initial observations in the dogs have been repeatedly confirmed, at great expense in time and money. The monkey studies appear to have failed to provide evidence of mammary tumor induction, and human data again and again indicate that the response seen in the dog lacks a human counterpart. The 10-year monkey studies were also designed in the heat of recrimination following the disclosure of the dog nodules. They have also failed to predict deleterious human effects.

Long term OC use would also, it was feared, result in permanent sterility. Although current data suggest some delay in return of fertility in OC users, a recovery of full reproductive potential after one to two years after termination of use, leaves those fears unfounded[16].

Closely linked with fertility was the possibility that OC use would affect the conceptus as measured by increased prevalence of congential malformations. As I interpret the mass of literature that has accumulated on this question, there is no acceptable evidence that OC's used as OC's and terminated prior to impregnation lead to abnormalities. When employed inadvertently during early pregnancy or when used as a pregnancy test, there is only minimal evidence to suggest an increase in abnormalities. Most publications show no increase. The data implicating the progestational compounds as teratogens when they are used in compromised pregnancies is also weak. The endocrine effect, masculinization of the female fetus with androgenic progestagens, is clearly restricted to exposure during pregnancy[17]. Again the OC's appear to be vindicated and early fears have not been substantiated.

Finally, OC's have been associated clinically with abnormal blood clotting and thrombotic episodes. Whether the risks are real or reflect artifacts of the epidemiological techniques employed for their evaluation remains to be demonstrated. However, it is clear that these problems were not predicted from animals studies, and to the best of my knowledge there is no acceptable model, animal or human.

In addition to the long-term dog and monkey studies, an extended range of toxicology for OC's is required that grossly exceeds those for other types of drugs. Time does not permit an exhaustive analysis of these requirements, but one must question their value in the face of the overall relative safety of OC's and failure to predict the putative vascular effects. Treatment of steroidal contraceptives as a special group of drugs seems unwarranted.

RECOMMENDATIONS FOR PRECLINICAL REQUIREMENTS

On the basis of these considerations I recommend that FDA:

1. Continue to require enough endocrine study to fully characterize any new steroid; to include, where appropriate:
   a. Progestational effects - receptor binding, Clauberg and pregnancy maintenance assays.
   b. Estrogenic effects - receptor binding, vaginal smear and uterine growth assays.
   c. Androgenic effects - receptor binding, prostatic growth assays.
   d. Antiestrogenic effects - vaginal smear or uterine growth assays.
   e. Corticoid effects - receptor binding, glucocorticoid and mineral-ocorticoid assays.
   f. Pituitary blocking effects.

2. Continue to require a range of standard pharmacological testing to fully characterize the drug before clinical use.
   To include:
   a. Cardiovascular/hypertensive assays
   b. Renal effects
   c. CNS/Behavior

3. Permit initiation of field trials with new steroids after six months of toxicity studies in two species.

4. Limit NDA toxicity requirements to those established for other classes of drugs.

5. Abandon 7-year dog and 10-year monkey studies as irrelevant to tumor development in humans.

REFERENCES

1. Edgren, RA, Jones, RC, Peterson, DL: The estrogenic effects of a series of 13-substituted compounds related to estradiol-17β. Eur. J. Steroids 2:19, 1967.

2. International Planned Parenthood Federation. Directory of Contraceptives. IPPF International Office, London, 1981.

3. Briggs, MH: Contraceptive steroid binding to the human uterine progesterone receptor. Curr. Med. Res. Opin. 3:95, 1975.

4. Swyer, GIM, Little, V: Clinical assessment of relative potency of progestagens. J. Reprod. Fertil., (suppl.) 5:63, 1968.

5. Swyer, GIM: Potency of progestagens in oral contraceptives--further delay of menses data. Contraception 26:23, 1982.

6. Edgren, RA: The biology of steroidal contraceptives, in Lednicer, D (Ed): Contraception: The chemical control of fertility. New York, Marcel Dekker, Inc., 1969.

7. Edgren, RA, Jones, RC, Peterson, DL: A biological classification of progestational agents. Fertil. Steril. 18:238, 1967.

8. Edgren, RA, Peterson, DL: Delay of parturition by various progestational steroids. Proc. Soc. Exp. Biol. & Med. 123:867, 1966.

9. Terenius, L: Affinities of progestogen and estrogen receptors in rabbit uterus for synthetic progestogens. Steroids 23:909, 1974.

10. Elton, RL, Nutting, EF: 17-ethynyl-4-estrene-3, 17-diol diacetate: a unique steroidal "progestin." Proc. Soc Exp. Biol. & Med. 107:991, 1961.

11. Jones, RC, Edgren, RA: The effects of various steroids on the vaginal histology in the rat. Fertil. Steril. 24:284, 1973.

12. Labrie, F, Ferland, L, Lagace, L, Drouin, J, Asselin, J, Azadian-Boulanger, G, Raynaud, J-P: High inhibitory activity of R5020, a pure progestin, at the hypothalamic-adenohypophyseal level on gonadotropin secretion. Fertil. Steril. 28:1104, 1977.

13. Edgren, RA: Progestogens as contraceptives. J. Reprod. Med. 13:79, 1974.

14. Sadeghi-Nejad, A, Kaplan, SL, Grumbach, MM: The effect of medroxyprogesterone acetate on adrenocortical function in children with precocious puberty. J. Pediatrics 78:616, 1971.

15. Carcinogencity tests of oral contraceptives. A report by the Committee on Safety of Medicines. Her Majesty's Stationary Office, London, 1972.

16. Vessey, MR, Doll, R, Peto, B, Johnson, B, Wiggins, P: A long term follow-up study of women using different methods of contraception--An interim report. J. Biosoc. Sci., 8:373, 1976.

17. The effect of female sex hormones on fetal development and infant health. Report of a WHO Scientific Group, Tech. Rep. Ser. 657, 1981.

The reader is referred to the following publications for additional information on assay systems.

Emmens, CW: Hormone Assay. New York, Academic Press, 1950.

Dorfman, RI (Ed): Methods in Hormone Research [Vol. II]. New York, Academic Press, 1962.

DISCUSSION

DR. DICZFALUSY: Thank you very much, Dr. Edgren. May I invite questions, comments?

DR. VON EICKSTEDT: I would like to add a fourth point to your last slide, that is inclusion of metabolic studies, including liver changes prediabetes and obese problems. Which species would you recommend for the six month studies?

DR. EDGREN: I am tempted to say I would leave that to the toxicologists, but I would certainly include rats because we know much more about what happens when we inject these materials into rats than any other animal. If any untoward effects occurs there is a fair likelihood of identifying it first in rats. Dogs or monkeys would be possibilities for the second species.

DR. VON EICKSTEDT: Mice?

DR. EDGREN: I would hesitate to use mice because they are another rodent. I would probably use the rat or another rodent and a nonrodent species. The dog or monkey would seem logical. The toxicologists would be better qualified to answer that.

DR. CLARKSON: Several things about your presentation were troublesome. I would like to comment on those. In terms of the ten-year monkey studies predicting the possibility of clinical problems associated with oral contraceptive use, I think a major mistake was to feed those monkeys monkey chow; monkey chow is unlike any diet in the world. There is no population of people that eat anything that is in any way like monkey chow. Monkey chow is very high in fiber and carbohydrates with miniscule amounts of fat, principally vegetable oil. Given that nutritional setting, it would be unlikely to see the kinds of complications that one might see in humans that would resemble thrombotic phenomena or cardiovascular diesase.

Another concern is use of the "monkeys" or even the term "baboons" as though they are not monkeys. There are very major differences among monkeys, and one must be more specific in making recommendations. There are over 100 species and over 15 species that are commonly used in laboratory investigations.

The question of diet will certainly have to be considered, as the subject of this conference goes on and cardiovascular and hemostasis questions become more important.

Now, the six-month testing period also concerns me. You mentioned cardiovascular assay. If you are talking about any diseases of the blood vessels, those are chronically developing problems, and one would not identify any significant advancements in arterial lesions, even with a very high risk situation during a six month period. It is upsetting to an atherosclerosis researcher to hear periods like six months.

DR. EDGREN: Thank you for pointing the "monkey" problem out. I meant Rhesus monkeys because I think it is the only primate in which we have the kind of background information and experience that would really be meaningful in this type of study. My apologies to Joe Goldzieher and his baboons, but I don't think we know quite as much about the baboon as we know about Rhesus monkeys.

Secondly, with regard to nutrition, I am not quite sure, what one would do here. The problem is that neither Rhesus monkeys nor, to the best of my knowledge, any other infrahuman primate has a diet comparable to the human diet.

Thirdly, with regard to the atherosclerosis, I agree with you. What I had in mind were acute pharmacological studies of cardiovascular effects to make sure that somebody's heart does not stop beating while using a steroidal contraceptive.

On the other hand, none of the completed long-term dog or monkey studies has been suggestive of atherogenesis. In addition, as one evaluates human studies, how good is the evidence for any type of real atherosclerotic heart disease developing in high incidence in women taking oral contraceptives? I don't know of any, but I am certainly concerned about the atherogenic potential of any of these substances.

DR. STADEL: You mentioned the difficulties in trying to make any sort of sensible classification of combined progestogen-estrogen oral contraceptives. One way of classification is in terms of their effects on lipoprotein patterns and perhaps antithrombin activity.

I share your reservations about these very long-term animal tests. Certainly the large epidemiological studies with oral contraceptives and cancer don't support any real problem. In fact, they show beneficial effects for several forms of cancer.

DR. SCHAFFENBERG: I would like to comment on Dr. Edgren's statement about the use of two species. As a former pupil of Hans Selye, I recall that he built a phenomenal structure based upon the disease of adaptation. Studies of the alarm reaction led to many discoveries applicable to man. However, when he began to build a total edifice with work in rats as a foundation, I told him that I was not aware that the arthritis he produced in rats with DOCA resembled human rheumatoid arthritis, or that nodule-like lesions in the rat hearts produced by the same procedure resembled known human disease, nor indeed, any other disease of adaptation be induced in rats resembled the human counterpart in any way.

While I am not a toxicologist, I participated in the development of many drugs and, after studying the acute toxicology in animals, literally chewed my fingernails during early clinical use. When nothing happened clinically you felt that you should go back and find a more appropriate animal model. The widespread use of the rat in drug safety studies is merely one of convenience, it is easily housed and reproduces quickly. But I believe it is the poorest selection for studies of the reproductive effects of drugs in the human. I wish we could choose another species but I don't know which one. Menstruating primates, while more expensive, do behave sexually more like humans.

Although I am with the FDA, I believe we should pull away from long-term animal studies, the results of which frequently completely misguide us. I am unaware of a single rat which developed stroke, deep vein thrombosis or heart attack following oral contraceptive treatment. What we must do is an acute experiment followed by cautious waiting for clinical adverse effects and then try to explain them with additional animal studies.

DR. EDGREN: Yes. I think I said very much the same thing. You eventually have to obtain full information in humans. The animal work is, at best, qualitative and certainly not quantitative.

DR. CLARK: I would like to defend the rat, although I agree to a large extent with the previous gentleman. For instance, the monkey is not susceptible to estrogen-induced uterine cancer, women apparently are. Rats, at least rodents and certainly mice, are a better model for that than are the primates themselves. So there is an exception to every rule, especially with respect to the reproductive tract.

Rats may not be good predictors for cardiovascular adverse effects, but they are pretty good predictors for reproductive phenomena.

DR. EDGREN: I might also point out that Rhesus monkeys are the last species you would ever inject with LHRH if you wanted a good pituitary response. The toxicology on native LHRH or Schally decapeptide was undertaken in Rhesus monkeys. I am fairly convinced it doesn't mean anything.

DR. BALAZS: I think the cardiovascular effect of oral contraceptives is beginning to be recognized, and perhaps these thromboembolic diseases are associated with long-term use. The manufacturer has an obligation to investigate and not dismiss the potential and significance of animal experiments. This is to discover and confirm adverse effects. One is continously moving back and forth between the clinic and the laboratory.

DR. EDGREN: In a forthcoming issue of International Journal of Fertility there is a paper by Reel amd Edgren describing a model for thrombotic problems associated with oral contraceptives. The model fell apart in the process of the study.

HEPATOTOXICITY OF ORAL CONTRACEPTIVES*

Kamal Ishak

Hepatic Pathology Department

Armed Forces Institute of Pathology

Washington, District of Columbia

INTRODUCTION

Hepatic effects of oral contraceptives (OCs) range from multiple biochemical changes[1,2] to structural alterations. The latter can be subcellular or may lead to a variety of diseases that mimic those related to diverse etiologies[3,4]. The adverse effects of OCs are most conveniently classified into those affecting the bile excretory system, vessels of the liver or hepatocytes; the latter are mainly hyperplastic and neoplastic processes. Miscellaneous effects of OCs on pre-existing liver disease, as well as the association of these agents with gallstones and pancreatitis, will also be discussed briefly.

INTRAHEPATIC CHOLESTASIS

The syndrome, which develops during the first or second cycle, is ushered in by pruritus, sometimes associated with malaise, anorexia and nausea[5-7]. Jaundice follows in one to two weeks. Total serum bilirubin levels are generally below 10 mg/dl. Alkaline phosphatase activity is only slightly or moderately increased and aminotransferase values are generally below 100 IU. Clinical recovery is usually prompt, but several weeks may elapse before all biochemical parameters return to normal. Chronic cholestasis, resembling that occasionally reported with the androgenic anabolic/steroids, does not occur.

Hepatic biopsy specimens obtained during the cholestatic phase reveal cytoplasmic and canalicular cholestasis that predominantly affects acinar zones 3 (Figure 1). There may be evidence of unicellular hepatocytic injury (acidophilic bodies, focal necrosis) and slight hypertrophy of Kupffer cells; portal inflammation is generally absent or very mild. The ultrastructural changes are not helpful in differential diagnosis since they resemble those of cholestasis of other etiologies[8,9].

---

* The opinions and assertions contained herein are the expressed views of the author and are not to be construed as official or as reflecting the views of the Department of the Army or the Department of Defense.

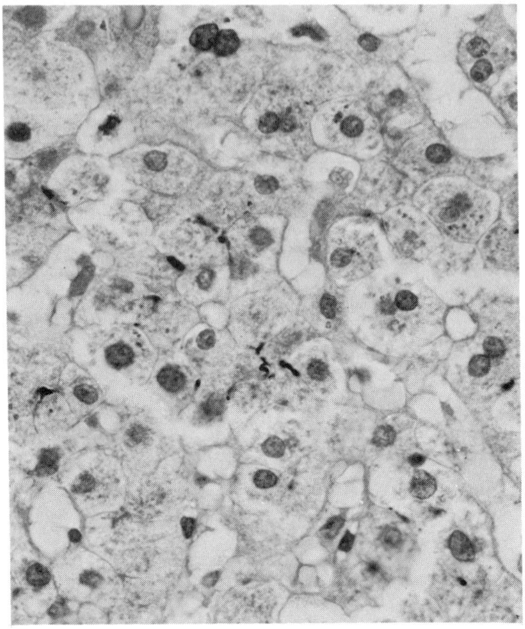

Figure 1. Intrahepatic cholestasis in 21 year old women who had used an oral contraceptive preparation containing norethindrone and mestranol for two weeks. The patient had developed jaundice during the last trimester of a past pregnancy (HE X630).

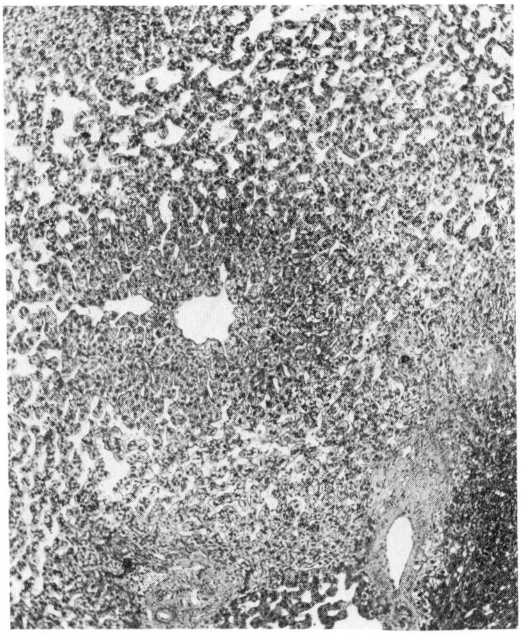

Figure 2. Sinusoidal dilatation with atrophy of liver cell plates involving acinar zones 1 and 2 (Masson X55).

The incidence of jaundice related to OCs is estimated to range from one in 4,000 to one in 10,000 users[5,6]. The frequency of the complication appears to be decreasing with decreasing potency of estrogens used in oral contraceptive preparations[10]. Its incidence is higher in Chile and Scandinavian countries. Affected patients give a history of pruritus or jaundice of pregnancy more often than controls, as do their mothers and sisters[11]. There is also a relationship between familial benign recurrent cholestasis, intrahepatic cholestasis of pregnancy and intrahepatic cholestasis associated with OCs[12]. With reference to intrahepatic cholestasis of pregnancy, the inheritance mode was found to be Mendelian dominant in type in a recent study[12]. No relationship between leukocyte histocompatibility antigens and intrahepatic cholestasis of pregnancy has been uncovered to date[13,14].

The cholestatic effects of the contraceptive steroids depend on C-17 alkylation and ring A unsaturation[15]. Extensive research has been performed with the synthetic estrogen ethinyl estradiol in an attempt to elucidate the mechanism of estrogen related cholestasis[2,16,17]. This compound depresses bile salt independent bile flow as well as the secretion of sulfobromophthalein and bile salts. The hypothesis that increased permeability of the biliary tract (with enhanced diffusion of water and bile constituents from bile to plasma) is involved in the pathogenesis of ethinyl estradiol induced cholestasis[18] is not supported by the results of recent research[17]. Current evidence supports the concept that changes in the lipid composition of liver cell membranes are responsible for estrogen induced cholestasis. Altered membrane fluidity resulting from an increase in the cholesterol ester content of liver plasma membranes has been demonstrated by several groups of investigators[19-21]. The effect of this membrane change would be decreased Na^+, K^+, adenosine triphosphatase activity, with diminution of bile salt independent bile flow and bile salt secretion rate.

VASCULAR COMPLICATIONS

Sinusoidal Dilatation. The majority of patients with this rarely reported complication are asymptomatic and come to medical attention because of hepatomegaly or mild biochemical abnormalities[22,23]. The duration of OC use prior to diagnosis ranges from one to several years. Angiographic studies in one case revealed multiple small accumulations of contrast material in the arterial phase that became more prominent in the parenchymatous and venous phases[24].

Microscopically, biopsies from patients with this disorder reveal moderate to marked dilatation of sinusoids with atrophy of liver cell plates. The change is more prominent in acinar zones 1 (periportal zones) (Figure 2).

No sequelae have been recognized and this change is not a precursor of peliosis hepatis. Improvement of biochemical abnormalities and return of liver size to normal have been reported[22].

Peliosis Hepatis. This lesion is a well documented complication of androgenic/anabolic steroid therapy. In the author's opinion, no acceptable cases related to OC use have been reported or are on file at this Institute.

Budd-Chiari Syndrome. An etiologic relationship between this entity and OC use is suggested by the preponderance of females over males in cases reported since 1969[25]. In a recent survey from France[26] the risk of the Budd-Chiari syndrome was found to be fourfold higher among OC users than among nonusers. The duration of oral contraception prior to development of the syndrome is variable, with a mean interval of 29.6 months[27]. The onset is usually insidious, with a prodromal phase lasting from a few weeks to several months[25,28]. Patients present with nausea, vomiting, abdominal pain, hepatomegaly, splenomegaly and ascites. An acute onset with a fulminant course associated with hepatic failure and death may ensue, or affected patients may recover only to subsequently develop portal hypertension[25,28]. Diagnosis is established by liver biopsy and hepatic venography; with the latter technique there is a characteristic "beaking" at the orifices of the hepatic veins, and the vena cava is often narrowed by the swollen or regenerated caudate lobe[25].

Twice as many patients with the Budd-Chiari syndrome related to OC use die as survive[28]; survival as long as five years has been reported[29]. In the review of Lewis et al[27], the mean survival for patients with the syndrome was found to be less than two years and fewer than 25 percent of patients survived beyond three years. A satisfactory response may accompany either medical or surgical management; however, patients with severe occlusive disease may benefit more from surgical decompression of the hepatic veins[27].

The liver grossly presents the "nutmeg" pattern characteristic of venous congestion. Thrombi may be identified grossly in the hepatic veins at their junction with the inferior vena cava (Figure 3), or in the large veins in the liver substance. Microscopically, rapidly fatal cases reveal recent thrombi. Veno-occlusive lesions have been rarely reported[30,31]. Accompanying the thrombosis is severe sinusoidal dilatation and congestion, as well as varying degrees of coagulative (ischemic) necrosis (Figure 4). Fibrosis, with central to central linkage, may be present in subacute and chronic cases.

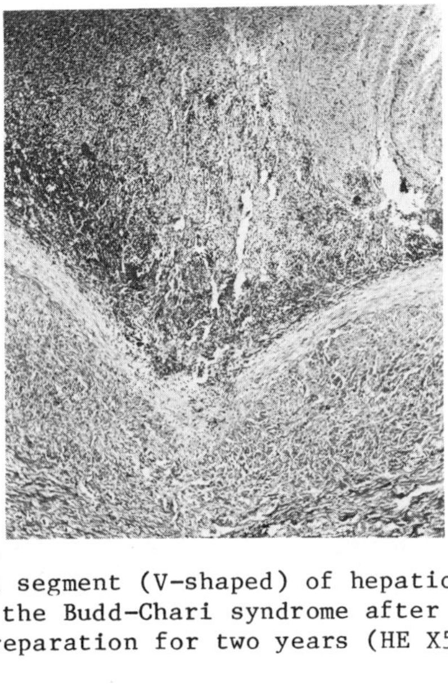

Figure 3. Thrombosed segment (V-shaped) of hepatic vein in patient who developed the Budd-Chari syndrome after using an oral contraceptive preparation for two years (HE X50).

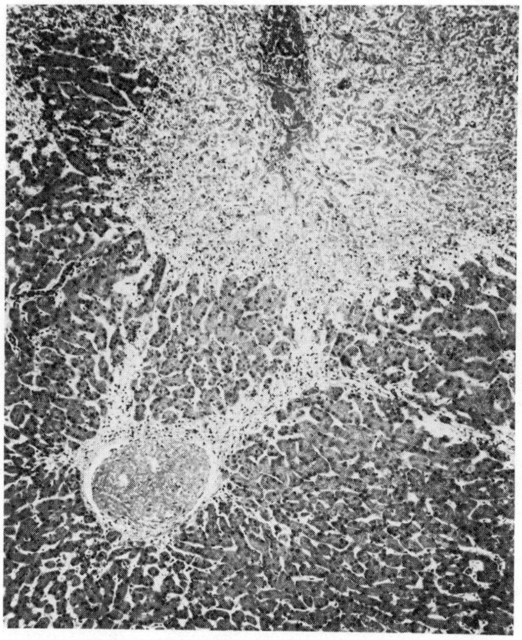

Figure 4. Recent thrombosis of efferent veins (arrows) in Budd-Chiari syndrome. There is necrosis of acinar zone 3 around one vessel (top) (HE X60).

The pathogenesis of the Budd-Chiari syndrome associated with OC use remains undetermined. Possible contributory factors include the hypercoagulable state and vascular intimal lesions[32] associated with the use of these agents.

BENIGN TUMORS

Hepatocellular Adenoma (HCA) The annual incidence of this tumor for long-term users of low potency OCs is estimated to be three to four per 100,000 in the United States[33]. About 320 cases are diagnosed per year[33]. Two case control studies have firmly established an association betwen HCA and long-term use of OCs[33,34]. There is an increased risk of development of HCA with increasing use of OCs. Rooks et al[33] found that the risk ratio increased steadily with increasing OC use for 85 or more months. Use of OCs with high hormonal potency and age over 30 years may further increase a woman's risk of developing HCA[33]. Besides use of OCs, the only variable found significantly more frequently in patients with HCA is a history of liver tumors in a close family member such as a sibling, parent or grandparent[33].

Experimental studies attempting to produce preneoplastic and neoplastic lesions in various animal species by synthetic steroid sex hormones will not be reviewed. Suffice it to say that there is overwhelming evidence supporting the concept that these agents act as tumor promoters and not as initiators[35-41].

The clinical aspects of HCA have been detailed in studies of several large series[42-44] and reviews[45,46]. The majority of patients come to medical attention in the childbearing period of life. The mean age at diagnosis in personally studied cases was 30.4 years[33]. A third to one-half of the patients present with an acute abdomen due either to rupture of the tumor with hemoperitoneum, or to hemorrhage or infarction within the tumor[31,33]. These complications may be associated with leukocytosis or mild to moderate increases in serum aminotransferase or alkaline phosphatase activities[31,44]. Pregnancy poses an increased hazard of rupture; consequently, it has been recommended that women with unresected tumors should avoid becoming pregnant[33,42]. Two thirds of women with HCA have an upper abdominal mass with or without associated gastrointestinal symptoms[46]. Serum alpha-fetoprotein values are within normal limits.

The radiographic aspects of HCA, including the differential diagnosis from focal nodular hyperplasia, are discussed in several reports[47-49]. Briefly, they include the finding of a defect by radioisotope scanning or computed tomography, and hypervascularity with areas of hypovascularity in angiographic studies.

Regression of HCA has been observed after discontinuation of oral contraceptive use[31,50,51]. The development of hepatocellular carcinoma in HCA has been documented in a few cases[31,52,53].

Hepatocellular adenoma should be resected because of the danger of rupture and the possibility, however small, of malignant transformation[54-56]. In the case of ruptured adenomas, the surgeon's efforts should be aimed primarily at controlling the bleeding; a sufficient amount of tumor should be resected to assure adequate hemostatic control[56].

The majority of hepatocellular adenomas (71 percent) are single and are most frequently (67 percent) located in the right lobe[46]. About half

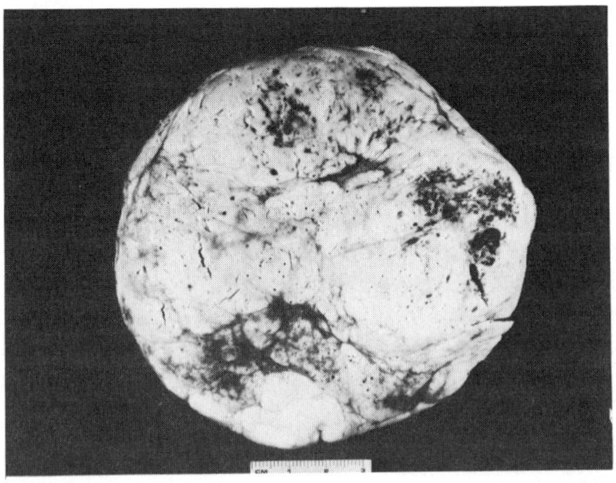

Figure 5. Cut surface of hepatocellular adenoma reveals a variegated pattern of light colored parenchyma alternating with dark hemorrhagic foci.

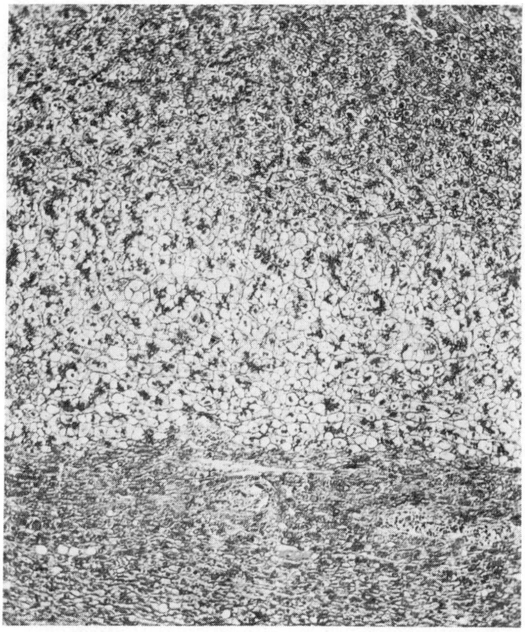

Figure 6. Sheet-like pattern of growth of hepatocellular adenoma. Tumor cells (upper two thirds of photograph) are large and more lightly stained than normal compressed liver cells below (HE X75).

are more than 10 cm in diameter[31]. They are more often soft than firm or hard. Cut sections usually present a variegated appearance areas of tan to light brown tumor parenchyma alternate with red-brown hemorrhages and grey-white areas of infarction (Figure 5). Large subcapsular hematomas or areas of rupture may be seen.

Histopathologically, HCA is composed of narrow trabeculae with inconspicuous sinusoidal spaces resulting in a "sheet-like" pattern of growth (Figure 6). Canaliculi may be identified between tumor cells. There is no fibrous stroma and reticulin fibers are absent. The largest feeding veins and arteries are observed at the periphery of the tumor (Figure 7). Cells of HCA are larger and paler than normal hepatocytes and have an increased content of glycogen and/or fat (Figure 6). Most cells contain one small nucleus with an inconspicuous nucleolus. Nuclear atypia, hyperchromasia and mitotic figures are not seen (Figure 8). The tumor cells can synthesize bile, which may be detected in the cytoplasm, or within dilated canaliculi surrounded by a ring of tumor cells (Figure 8). Uncommonly encountered features include hematopoietic activity in tumor sinusoids or the presence of noncaseating granulomas[46]. Vascular intimal lesions, similar to those described in women on OCs[32], may be seen in arteries in portal areas near the periphery of HCA[46]. The non-neoplastic hepatic parenchyma reveals no evidence of chronic liver disease or cirrhosis.

Focal Nodular Hyperplasia (FNH). No case-control studies of the relationship of this tumor to long term use of OCs has been conducted. It does occur with greater frequency in women, many of whom had taken

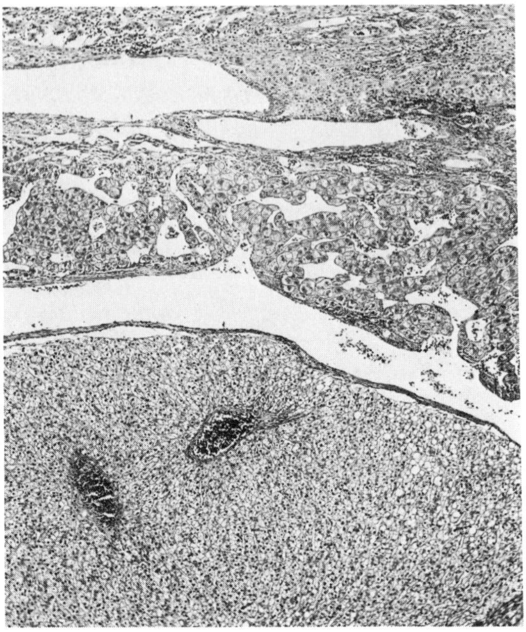

Figure 7. Large vessels (upper half of photograph) at surface of hepatocellular adenoma (HD X50).

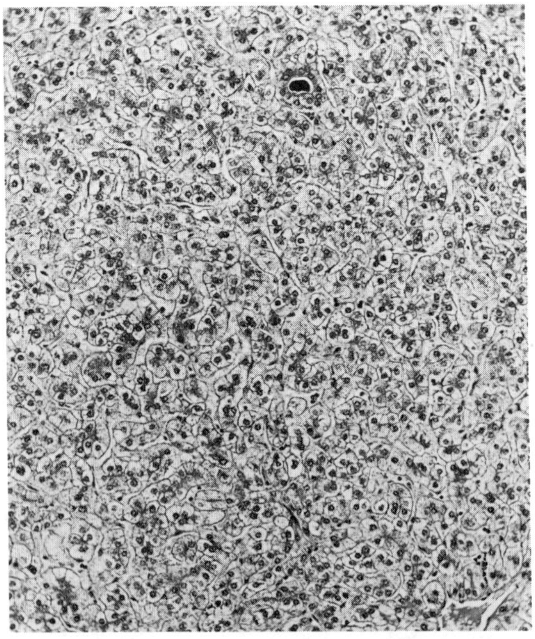

Figure 8. Cells of hepatocellular adenoma are uniform in size and shape and reveal no nuclear pleomorphism or mitoses. Note bile plug in dilated canaliculus (top) (HE X130).

OCs. In one recently reported series from the Mayo Clinic, 88 percent of the patients with FNH were female and 58 percent had used contraceptive steroids[31]. Despite these observations, however, an etiologic role for OCs in the induction of FNH is very unlikely[4,46,57]. Many cases of FNH were reported before the introduction of OCs in 1960, unlike HCA which was an exceptionally rare tumor prior to 1960. Focal nodular hyperplasia occurs in children of both sexes[58], in adult males and in females not using OCs. Rupture, a frequent complication of HCA, is an exceptionally rare event in FNH. Although initiation by OCs is unlikely, it has been suggested that these compounds may exert a "trophic" effect on a preexisting FNH[46]. This could explain the "regression" of some cases of FNH after discontinuation of oral contraception[59,60]. A brief discussion of FNH is considered relevant since it has often been confused with HCA.

Most cases of FNH are discovered incidentally at laparotomy or autopsy. About a fifth of the patients may have symptoms related to pressure on adjacent viscera and organs[44,46]. The majority of patients (83 percent) in one series had no physical signs[31]. Biochemical abnormalities attributable to the tumor are generally lacking.

Radionuclide imaging of FNH may show a focal defect but some tumors may have normal uptake of labeled colloid due to the presence of Kupffer cells[48]. Angiography reveals a hypervascular pattern with a dense capillary flush, visible septation during the capillary phase and marked arterial tortuosity[48,49]. There are no hypovascular areas comparable to those observed in HCA[31].

The treatment of choice for FNH is simple excision. Periodic follow-up by radiographic imaging techniques is advisable for patients whose tumors are unresectable. Long term follow-up of patients whose tumors were biopsied but not resected has revealed no change in the size or number of tumors, or any evidence of malignant transformation in cases reexamined histologically[31,44].

The majority of patients (78 percent) with FNH have a single tumor mass that most frequently measures less than 5 cm in diameter[46]. More

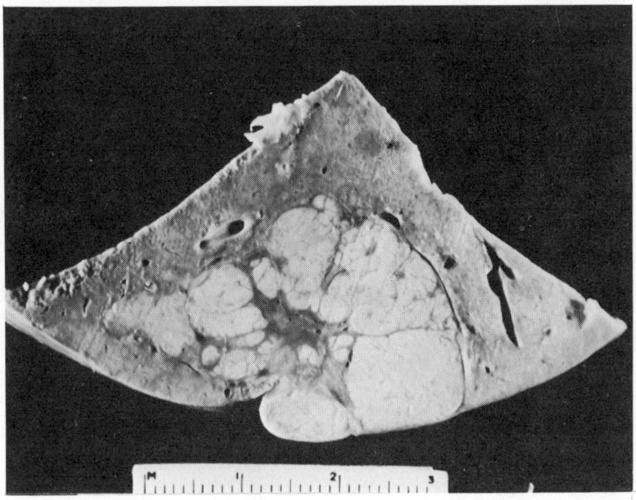

Figure 9. Cut surface of focal nodular hyperplasia. Note light color, central scar and septation.

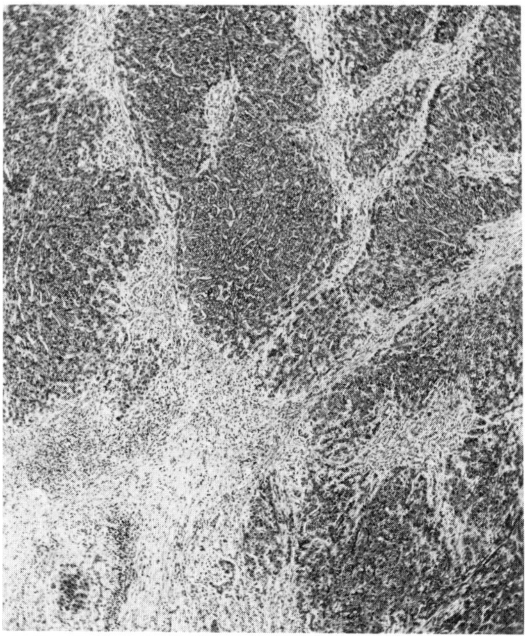

Figure 10. Thin septa are seen to converge on part of central scar in lower left hand corner of field (HE X50).

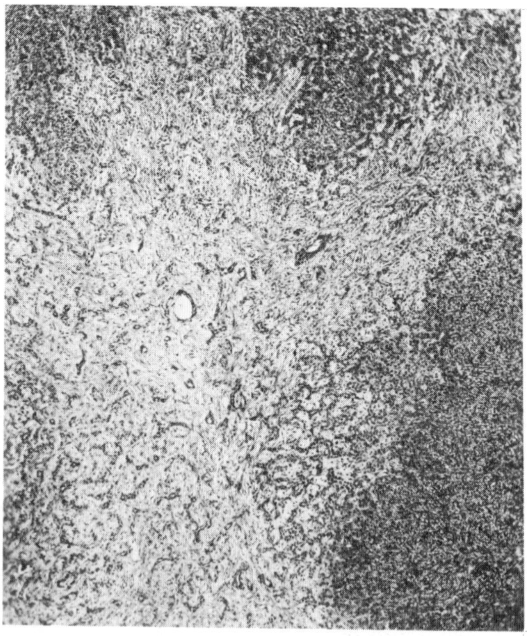

Figure 11. Fibrous tissue of focal nodular hyperplasia contains numerous small bile ducts (HE X50).

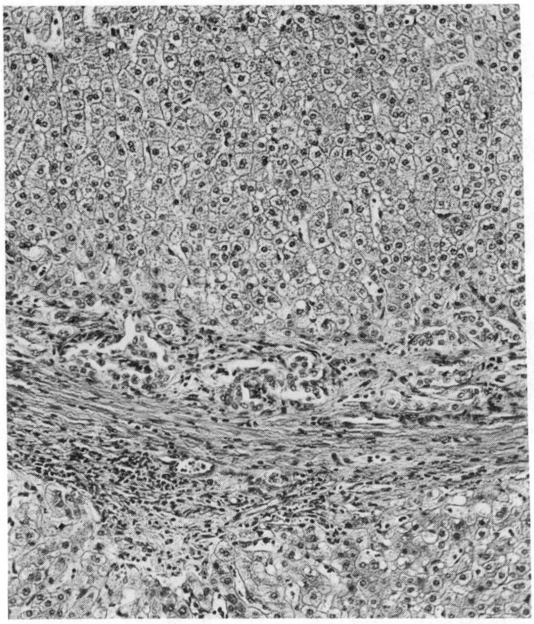

Figure 12. Cells of focal nodular hyperplasia resemble normal hepatocytes. Transverse septum (bottom) reveals bile ducts and is infiltrated by inflammatory cells (HE X115).

are located in the right than in the left or other lobes. Grossly, FNH is well demarcated, firm to rubbery in consistency and paler (tan to yellow) than the adjacent hepatic parenchyma (Figure 9). It is clearly subdivided into smaller lobules by fibrous septa which converge on a central depressed scar (Figure 9).

Microscopically, FNH differs from HCA in having a "substructure." The septa that subdivide the tumor are collagenous, carry a varying number of small bile ducts and are usually infiltrated by inflammatory cells (Figures 10 and 11). The largest vessels, often showing fibromuscular hyperplasia, are located in the central fibrous scar. The hepatocellular component of the tumor resembles normal hepatic parenchyma but lacks an acinar (lobular) architecture (Figure 12). It consists mainly of plates of hepatocytes that are two cells thick, with sinusoidal spaces in between and a well-formed reticulum framework. Bile production or areas of old hemorrhage or infarction, so typical of HCA, are not observed in FNH.

Nodular Transformation (NT). This condition, also known as nodular regenerative hyperplasia, has rarely been reported in women on OCs. In a series of 30 cases studied by the author, two patients had used OCs for three to several years prior to diagnosis[61]. It must be emphasized that the majority of cases of NT are idiopathic or associated with a variety of disease such as rheumatoid arthritis, Felty's syndrome, the CRST syndrome and myeloproliferative or lymphoproliferative disorders[61,62]. Symptoms and signs, when present, are related to portal hypertension. Proposed pathogenetic factors have included a proliferative reaction to long term use of a variety of drugs[61], or a response to an obliterative portal venopathy[62].

MALIGNANT TUMORS

Hepatocellular Carcinoma (HCC). In a survey of the literature up to 1982, Goodman and Ishak[63] found 98 cases of HCC associated with the use of OCs. Eleven other cases were on file at this Institute[63]. Since then, 11 other cases have been reported[31,64-69] bringing the total number to 120. Four of the reported cases of HCC had arisen in HCA[31,52-53].

Case-control studies to establish a relationship between HCC and OCs have not thus far been undertaken. The American College of Surgeons Survey of Liver Tumors[70] revealed that 31 percent of women with HCC between the age of 15 and 45 had used OCs. In a study from this Institute of 128 cases of HCC in women, 32 percent of patients in the same age group had used OCs. It is not at all clear that this represents an increased incidence of HCC since it is estimated that as many as 15 to 37 percent of women in the reproductive age group were using OCs in the 1970s[71-74]. As noted earlier, the widespread use of OCs since 1970 resulted in a marked increased in the number of hepatocellular adenomas in the United States; no such increase in the number of HCC has occurred. In fact, the incidence of primary liver cancer in the United States and Denmark has remained essentially constant from the 1950s to the 1970s[75].

In the personally studied series of 128 cases of HCC in women, 48 patients were under 40 years of age and 13 (27 percent) of them had used OCs[63]. An almost equal percentage of women with HCC under 40 years of age, who had or had not used OCs, had a recently recognized histologic variant of HCC known as fibrolamellar carcinoma[63]. This type of HCC occurs predominantly in young persons of both sexes. The conclusion was reached that the apparent increase in HCC in young women can be explained by the presence of cases of fibrolamellar HCC in this age group[63]. As noted earlier (see section of HCA), the weight of experimental evidence favors a promotional and not an initiating role for the induction of liver tumors by the synthetic sex steroids. One divergent view, proposing an initiating role for ethinyl estradiol and norethindrone in hepatocarcinogenesis in rats, has recently been published[76]. Clearly, additional epidemiologic and experimental studies are needed to shed light on the relationship between HCC and OCs.

Other Malignant Tumors. Several cholangiocarcinomas[77-79] and combined hepatocellular and cholangiocellular carcinomas[70,80] have been reported in users of OCs. There are also two tumors with malignant epithelial and sarcomatous elements[81,82] and two angiosarcomas of the liver[83,84] in women who had used contraceptive steroids.

MISCELLANEOUS EFFECTS

Effect of OCs on Pre-existing Liver Diseases. A well recognized effect of OCs is the unmasking of the Dubin-Johnson syndrome[85,86]. Pruritus and/or jaundice due to primary biliary cirrhosis may be manifested or aggravated by the use of OCs[87]. No detrimental effects of OCs have been observed in patients with acute viral hepatitis[88] or chronic active hepatitis[89]. On the other hand, hyperbilirubinemia and increased serum alkaline phosphatase activity have been recorded within three weeks of the administration of OCs to patients with postnecrotic cirrhosis[85].

Cholelithiasis and OCs. Pregnancy and use of OCs have been considered to be major risk factors for cholelithiasis[90-94]. Factors contributing to this are thought to be the hepatic secretion of lithogenic bile[92,93] and retention of bile in the gallbladder[95]. A recent study of the Royal College of General Practitioners[96] has concluded that the use of OCs is not associated with an overall increased risk in the long term. The previously demonstrated short term increase in risk is due to an acceleration of gallbladder disease only in women susceptible to it[96].

Pancreatitis and OC. This complication is only mentioned since it may secondarily affect the liver. It generally develops within three months of OC use[97]. The interested reader is referred to the reviews of Davidoff et al[98] and Mallory and Kern[97] for further information.

REFERENCES

1. Song, CS, Rifkind, AB, Gillette, PN, Kappas, A: Hormones and the liver: the effect of estrogens, progestins, and pregnancy on hepatic function. Am J Obst Gynecol, 105:813, 1969.

2. Anderson, KE, Kappas, A: Hormones and liver function. In: Schiff, L, Schiff, E (Eds): Diseases of the Liver, Philadelphia, Lippincott, 1982, p 167.

3. Ishak, KG: Morphological lesions associated with oral contraceptives (O.C.) and anabolic steroids (A.S.). Adv Pharmacol Therap, 8:185, 1978.

4. Ishak, KG: Hepatic lesions caused by anabolic and contraceptive steroids. Sem Liver Dis, 1:116, 1981.

5. Schaffner, F: The effect of oral contraceptives on the liver. JAMA, 198:1019, 1966.

6. Metreau, JM, Dhumeaux, D, Berthelot, P: Oral contraceptives and the liver. Digestion, 7:318, 1972.

7. de Pagter, AGF, van Berge-Henegouwen, GB, Brandt, KH, Bronkhorst, FB: Oral contraceptives and the liver. In: Davidson, CS (Ed): Problems in Liver Diseases, New York, Stratton International, 1979, p 121.

8. Larsson-Cohn, U, Stenram, U: Liver ultrastructure and function in icteric and non-icteric women using oral contraceptive agents. Acta Med Scand, 181:257, 1967.

9. Orlandi, F, Jezequel, A, Melliti, A: The action of some anabolic steroids on the structure and the function of human liver cells. Tidscher Gastroenterol, 7:109, 1964.

10. Sherlock, S: Hepatic effects of steroid sex hormones. In: Farber, E, Fisher, MM (Eds): Toxic Injury of the Liver, Part B. New York, Marcel Dekker, 1980, p 597.

11. Dalen, E, Westerholm, B: Occurrence of hepatic impairment in women jaundiced by oral contraceptives and in their mothers and sisters. Acta Med Scand, 195:459, 1974.

12. de Pagter, AGF, van Berge Henegouwen, GP, Huinink, JAT, Brandt, KH: Familial benign recurrent intrahepatic cholestasis: interrelation with intrahepatic cholestasis of pregnancy and from oral contraceptives. Gastroenterology, 71:202, 1976.

13. Holzbach, RT, Sivak, DA, Braun, WE: Familial recurrent intrahepatic cholestasis of pregnancy: a genetic study providing evidence for transmission of a sex-linked, dominant trait. Gastroenterology, 85:175, 1983.

14. Reyes, H, Wegmann, ME, Segovia, N, Cuchacovich, M, Jadresic, E, Contador, M, Fueutes, C, Melendez, M: HLA in Chileans with intrahepatic cholestasis of pregnancy. Hepatology, 2:463, 1982.

15. Zimmerman, HJ: Hepatotoxicity. New York, Appleton-Century-Crofts, 1978.

16. Schreiber, AJ, Simon, FR: Estrogen-induced cholestasis: clues to pathogenesis and treatment. Hepatology, 3:607, 1983.

17. Jaeschke, H, Krell, H, Pfaff, E: No increase in biliary permeability in ethinylestradiol-treated rats. Gastroenterology, 85:808, 1983.

18. Forker, EL: The effect of estrogen on bile formation in the rat. J Clin Invest, 48:654, 1969.

19. Davis, RA, Kern, F, Showalter, R, Sutherland, E, Sinensky, M, Simon, FR: Alterations of heptic Na^{+},K^{+}-ATPase and bile flow by estrogen: effects on liver surface membrane lipid structure and function. Proc Natl Acad Sci USA, 75:4130, 1978.

20. Keeffe, EB, Scharschmidt, BF, Blankenship, NM, Ockner, RK: Studies of relationships among bile flow, liver plasma membrane NaK-ATPase, and membrane microviscosity in the rat. J Clin Invest, 64:1590, 1979.

21. Simon, FR, Gonzalez, M, Sutherland, E, Accatino, L: Reversal of ethinyl estradiol-induced bile secretory failure with Triton WR-1339. J Clin Invest, 65:851, 1980.

22. Winkler, K, Poulsen, H: Liver disease with periportal sinusoidal dilatation: a possible complication to contraceptive steroids. Scand J Gastroenterol, 10:699, 1975.

23. Spellberg, MA, Mirro, J, Chowdhury, L: Hepatic sinusoidal dilatation related to oral contraceptives: a study of two patients showing ultrastructural changes. Am J Gastroenterol, 72:248, 1979.

24. Pliskin, M: Peliosis hepatis. Radiology, 114:29, 1975.

25. Langer, B, Stone, RM, Colapinto, RF, Meindok, H, Phillips, MJ, Fisher, MM: Clinical spectrum of the Budd-Chiari syndrome and its surgical management. Am J Surg, 129:137, 1975.

26. Valla, D, Poynard, T, Zucman, N, et al: Oral contraceptives and the Budd-Chiari syndrome. 18th Meeting of European Association for the Study of the Liver, Southampton, England, September 1983 (Abs).

27. Lewis, JH, Tice, HL, Zimmerman, HJ: Budd-Chiari syndrome associated with oral contraceptive steroids: review of treatment of 47 cases. Dig Dis Sci, 28:673, 1983.

28. Wu, S, Spurny, OM, Klotz, AP: Budd Chiari syndrome after taking oral contraceptives. A case report and review of 14 reported cases. Am J Dig Dis, 22:623, 1977.

29. Schramek, A, Better, OS, Brook, JC, et al: New observations on the clinical spectrum of the Budd-Chiari syndrome. Am Surg, 100:368, 1974.

30. Alpert, LI: Veno-occlusive disease of the liver associated with oral contraceptives. Case report and review of literature. Hum Pathol, 7:709, 1976.

31. Kerlin, P, Davis, GL, McGill, DB, Weiland, LH, Adson, MA, Sheddy, PF: Hepatic adenoma and focal nodular hyperplasia: clinical, pathologic and radiologic features. Gastroenterology, 84:994, 1983.

32. Irey, NS, Manion, WC, Taylor, HB: Vascular lesions in women taking oral contraceptives. Arch Pathol, 89:1, 1970.

33. Rooks, JB, Ory, H, Ishak, KG, Strauss, LT, Greenspan, JR, Paganini-Hill, A, Tyler, CW: Epidemiology of hepatocellular adenoma: the role of oral contraceptive use. JAMA, 242:644, 1979.

34. Edmondson, HA, Henderson, B, Benton, B: Liver-cell adenomas associated with use of oral contraceptives. N Engl J Med, 294:470, 1976.

35. Taper, HS: The effect of estradiol 17-phenylproprionate and estradiol benzoate on N-nitrosomorpholine-induced carcinogenesis in ovariectomized female rats. Cancer, 42:462, 1978.

36. Desser-Wiest, L: Promotion of liver tumors by steroid hormones. J Toxicol Environ Hlth, 5:203, 1979.

37. Yager, JD, Yager, R: Oral contraceptive steroids as promoters of hepatocarcinogenesis in female Sprague-Dawley rats. Cancer Res, 40:3680, 1980.

38. Cameron, R, Imaida, K, Ito, N: Promotive effects of ethinyl estradiol in hepatocarcinogenesis initiated by diethylnitrosamine in male rats. Gann, 72:339, 1981.

39. Wanless, IR, Medline, A: Role of estrogens as promoters of hepatic neoplasia. Lab Invest, 46:313, 1982.

40. Williams, GM: Sex hormones and liver cancer. Lab Invest, 46:352, 1982.

41. Schuppler, J, Schulte-Hermann, R, Timmerman-Trosiener, I, Gunzel, P: Proliferative liver lesions and sex steroids in rats. Toxicol Pathol, 10:132, 1982.

42. Kent, DR, Nissen, ED, Nissen, SE: Liver tumors and oral contraceptives. Int J Gynecol Obstet, 15:137, 1977.

43. Barrows, GH, Mays, ET, Christopherson, WM: Human liver neoplasia and steroid exposure. Toxicol Pathol, 10:145, 1982.

44. Ishak, KG, Rabin, L: Benign tumors of the liver. Med Clin N Am, 59:995, 1975.

45. Klatskin, G: Hepatic tumors: possible relationship to use of oral contraceptives. Gastroenterology, 73:386, 1977.

46. Ishak, KG: Hepatic neoplasms associated with contraceptive and anabolic steroids. Recent Results Cancer Res, 66:73, 1979.

47. Fechner, RE, Roehm, JOF: Angiographic and pathologic correlations of hepatic focal nodular hyperplasia. Am J Surg Pathol, 1:217, 1977.

48. Casarella, WJ, Knowles, DM, Wolff, M, Johnson, PM: Focal nodular hyperplasia and liver cell adenoma. Radiologic and pathologic differentiation. Am J Roentgenol, 131:393, 1978.

49. Knowles, DM, Casarella, WJ, Johnson, PM, Wolff, M: The clinical, radiologic, and pathologic characterization of benign hepatic neoplasms: alleged association with oral contraceptives. Medicine, 57:223, 1977.

50. Steinbrecher, UP, Lisbona, R, Huang, SN, Mishkin, S: Complete regression of hepatocellular adenoma after withdrawal of oral contraceptives. Dig Dis Sci, 26:1045, 1981.

51. Buhler, H, Pirovino, M, Akovbiantz, A, Altorfer, J, Weitzel, M, Maranta, E, Schmid, N: Regression of liver cell adenoma: a follow-up study of three consecutive patients after discontinuation of oral contraceptive use. Gastroenterology, 82:775, 1982.

52. Goldbarb, S: Sex hormones and hepatic neoplasia. Cancer Res, 36:2584, 1976.

53. Tesluk, H, Lawrie, J: Hepatocellular adenoma. Its transformation to carcinoma in a user of oral contraceptives. Arch Pathol, 105:296, 1981.

54. Pawlikowski, JR, Campbell, WJ, Campbell, TJ, Eden, M: A rationale for treating hepatic adenoma. Am Surg, 44:413, 1978.

55. Weil, R, Koep, LJ, Starzl, TE: Liver resection for hepatic adenoma. Arch Surg, 114:178, 1978.

56. Chan, CK, Detmer, DE: Proper management of hepatic adenoma associated

with oral contraceptives. Surg Gynecol Obstet, 144:703, 1977.

57. Fechner, RE: Benign hepatic lesions and orally administered contraceptives: a report of seven cases and critical analysis of the literature. Human Pathol, 8:255, 1977.

58. Stocker, JT, Ishak, KG: Focal nodular hyperplasia of the liver: a study of 21 pediatric cases. Cancer, 48:336, 1981.

59. Aldinger, K, Ben-Menachem, Y, Whalen, G: Focal nodular hyperplasia of the liver associated with high-dosage estrogens. Arch Int Med, 137:357, 1977.

60. Ross, D, Pina, J, Mirza, M, et al: Regression of focal nodular hyperplasia after discontinuation of oral contraceptives. Arch Intern Med, 85:203, 1976.

61. Stromeyer, FW, Ishak, KG: Nodular transformation (Nodular "regenerative" hyperplasia) of the liver: a clinicopathologic study of 30 cases. Hum Pathol, 12:60, 1981.

62. Wanless, IR, Godwin, TA, Allen, F, Feder, A: Nodular regenerative hyperplasia of the liver in hematologic disorders: à possible response to obliterative portal venopathy. A morphometric study of nine cases with an hypothesis on the pathogenesis. Medicine, 59:367, 1980.

63. Goodman, ZD, Ishak, KG: Hepatocellular carcinoma in women: probable lack of etiologic association with oral contraceptive steroids. Hepatology, 2:440, 1982.

64. Shar, SR, Kew, MC: Oral contraceptives and hepatocellular carcinoma. Cancer, 49:407, 1982.

65. Horii, K, Yasui, M, Adachi, Y, Yamamoto, T, Ishida, O, Itoh, H: An autopsy case of primary hepatoma associated with an oral contraceptive. Hepato-Gastroenterol, 29:187, 1982.

66. Dudley, AG, Sale, P: Hepatocellular carcinoma associated with oral contraceptive use and pregnancy. Diagnostic Gynecol Obst, 4:301, 1982.

67. Helling, TS, Wood, WG: Oral contraceptives and cancer of the liver: a review with two additional cases. Am J Gastroenterol, 77:504, 1982.

68. Mal, RA, Galdabini, JJ, Jeppsson, BW: Abnormal sex-steroid milieu in young adults with hepatocellular carcinoma. World J Surg, 7:247, 1953.

69. Gala, KV, Griffin, TW: Hepatomas in young women on oral contraceptives: report of two cases and review of the literature. J Surg Oncol, 22:11, 1983.

70. Vana, J, Murphy, GP: Primary malignant liver tumors. Association with oral contraceptives. NY State J Med, 79:321, 1979.

71. Piotrow, PT, Lee, CM: Oral contraceptives - 50 million users. Population Report, Series A, No. 1, Washington, D.C.: George Washington University Medical Center, Population Information Center, 1974.

72. Westoff, CF, Jones, EF: Patterns of aggregate and individual changes in contraceptive practice. United States 1965-1975 vital and health statistics. Series 3, No. 17, p 1, 1979.

73. MacCornack, FA, Nathan, JL, Covey, LS, Wynder, EL: Oral contraceptive use. Epidemiology NY State J Med, 77:200, 1977.

74. Hartz, SC, Shapiro, S, Kaufman, DW, et al: Factors associated with oral contraceptive use. Public Health Briefs, 70:1105, 1980.

75. Rinehart, W, Ravenholt, RT: U.S. Morbidity and mortality trends relative to oral contraceptive use, 1955-1975 and Danish morbidity trends 1953-1972. Population Report, Series A, No. 4, Washington, D.C.: George Washington University Medical Center, Population Information Center, p 105, 1977.

76. Higashi, S: Hepatocellular carcinoma induced by estrogen and progestogen: Development of hepatocellular carcinoma in rats following oral administration of synthetic estrogen and progestogen. Mie Med J, 30:295, 1981.

77. Ellis, EF, Gordon, PR, Gottlieb, LS: Oral contraceptives and cholangiocarcinoma. Lancet. 1:207, 1978.

78. Littlewood, ER, Barrison, IG, Murray-Lyon, I, Paradinas, FJ: Cholangiocarcinoma and oral contraceptives. Lancet, 1:310, 1980.

79. Caggiano, V, Chosney, B, Way, LW: Thrombotic thrombocytopenic purpura, cholangiocarcinoma, and oral contraceptives. Lancet, 2:365, 1980.

80. O'Sullivan, JP, Rosswick, RP: Oral contraceptives and malignant hepatic tumors. Lancet, 1:1125, 1976.

81. Meyer, P, LiVolsi, VA, Cornog, JL: Hepatoblastoma associated with an oral contraceptive. Lancet, 2:1387, 1974.

82. Ladaga, L, Kay, S, Melcher, M, King, JN: Combined epithelial and sarcomatous elements in a liver cancer associated with oral contraceptive use. Am J Surg Pathol, 3:185, 1979.

83. Monroe, PS, Riddell, RH, Siegler, M, Baker, AL: Hepatic angiosarcoma: possible relationship to long term oral contraceptive ingestion. JAMA, 246:64, 1981.

84. Shi, ECP, Fisher, A, Grouch, R, et al: Possible association of angiosarcoma with oral contraceptive agents. Med J Aust, 1:473, 1981.

85. Mowat, AP, Arias, IM: Liver function and oral contraceptives. J Reprod Med, 3:19, 1969.

86. Schinella, RA: Jaundice with Dubin-Johnson-Sprinz syndrome precipitated by oral contraceptives. NY State J Med, 72:2810, 1972.

87. Sherlock, S: Primary biliary cirrhosis. In: Weight, R, Alberti, KGMM, Karran, S, Millward-Sadler, GH (Eds): Liver and Biliary Disease, London-Philadelphia-Berlin, Saunders, 1979, p 715.

88. Schweitzer, IL, Werner, JM, McPeek, M, Thursby, MW: Oral contraceptives in acute viral hepatitis. JAMA, 233;979, 1975.

89. Jenny, S, Markoff, N: Oral contraceptives in liver disease. Schweitz Med Wochenschr, 97:1502, 1967.

90. Boston Collaborative Drug Surveillance Program. Surgically confirmed gallbladder disease, venous thromboembolism, and breast tumors in relation to postmenopausal estrogen therapy. N Engl J Med, 290:15, 1974.

91. Royal College of General Practitioners. Oral Contraceptives and Health. London, Pitman Medical, 1974.

92. Bennion, LG, Grundy, SM: Risk factors for the development of cholelithiasis in man. N Engl J Med, 299:1161, 1221, 1978.

93. Kern, F, Jr, Erfling, W, Simon, FR, Dahl, R, Mallory, A, Starzl, TE: Effect of estrogens on the liver. Gastroenterology, 75:512, 1978.

94. Friedman, GD, Kannel, WB, Dauber, TR: The epidemiology of gallbladder disease: observations in the Framingham study. J Chronic Dis, 19:273, 1966.

95. Everson, GT, McKinley, C, Lawson, M, Johnson, M, Kern, F: Gallbladder function in the human female: effect of the ovulatory cycle, pregnancy, and contraceptive steroids. Gastroenterology, 82:711, 1982.

96. Oral contraceptives and gallbladder disease: Royal College of General Practitioners' oral contraception study. Lancet, 2:957, 1982.

97. Mallory, A, Kern, F: Drug-induced pancreatitis. A critical review, Gastroenterology, 78:813, 1980.

98. Davidoff, F, Tishler, S, Rosoff, C: Marked hyperlipidemia and pancreatitis associated with oral contraceptive therapy. N Engl J Med, 289:552, 1973.

DISCUSSION

DR. DICZFALUSY: Thank you very much. I would like to invite questions.

DR. NASH: Relative to the adenomas, do you have an estimate of the risk or the incidence per 100,000 contraceptive users?

DR. ISHAK: About three or four per 100,000 users.

DR. NASH: Your survey of a large number of liver lesions indicated some association with contraceptive use. Which of these instances, beside the adenoma, do you feel convinced that there may be a causative association?

DR. ISHAK: We feel very confident that there is a relationship between hepatocellular adenomas and oral contraceptives; this is based on our large case control study with the CDC. Other associations are much less definite, particularly focal nodular hyperplasia. I mentioned that this tumor occurs in all ages, in both sexes, and while we acknowledge that it may grow slightly with the use of oral contraceptives, we feel it has no etiologic relationship to the pill.

We are not at all certain that there is a relationship at this time between nodular transformation or nodular regenerative hyperplasia and oral contraceptives.

DR. DICZFALUSY: In these epidemiological studies, do you find a difference between anabolic steroids and contraceptive combinations?

DR. ISHAK: There are no case control studies of anabolic steroids and hepatic tumors, but the reported cases of hepatocellular neoplasms that have been attributed to anabolic steroids have been generally called carcinomas. However, they rarely metastasize and, in fact, some have regressed after the anabolic steroid was discontinued.

DR. KNOPP: Our experience with the lipid research clinic program has provided us an opportunity to evaluate plasma bilirubin and SGOT concentrations among users of oral contraceptives across the board. We have also done this in pregnancy, and in contrast to what appears to be an idiosyncratic jaundice of pregnancy in oral contraceptive use, in fact, the bilirubin level is lower in ordinary users of oral contraceptive users. The same is true in pregnancy. SGOT in oral contraceptive users have not increased.

So I would think that the jaundice of pregnancy associated with oral contraceptive use would be an idiosyncratic effect rather than something that is to be expected over the dose range of the drug.

The other point that in response to hepatocellular proliferation is it appears that estrogen does have a stimulatory effect to cell growth and tissue culture, not when you add estrogen per se, but when you take the plasma from estrogen treated persons, there is a stimulatory effect which has led to the concept of estromedence, similar to that which mediates some of the effects of growth hormone, but not being the parent hormone.

DR. ISHAK: I am glad you mentioned those differences. I also thought there are underlying genetic factors. I already mentioned the high incidence in patients in Chile and in Scandinavia, and also the patients who develop the intrahepatic cholestasis of pregnancy and/or the steroid related jaundice. Relatives, sisters and mothers, have also had the same response to oral contraceptives. The exact inheritance pattern is not known.

DR. GOLDZIEHER: In respect to Dr. Nash's question, I think there are some data on incidence. The Royal College Study, the Oxford Study, the San Francisco Walnut Creek Study, the Puget Sound Study, and seven years of the Scottish National Disease Index, if taken collectively, represent approximately half a million women years of exposure. There is, as far as I know, only one case of hepatocellular adenoma.

DR. ISHAK: That is true. It might be pointed out that the effect is thought to be promotional rather than inductive. There must be a factor(s) that induces these lesions following oral contraceptive steroids which act as promoting agents. The relationship, as far as case control studies, is undoubtedly established in the U.S. The reason for the differences between the British and U.S. studies is unknown.

DR. VON EICKSTEDT: We are mainly concerned with animal studies, and I saw different morphological data in beagles and rats treated for long periods with progestational agents alone or in combination with estrogen. I saw some sinusoidal dilatation and cell proliferation. Do you think that the patient's history and the morphology which you saw is of importance, since the cases reported in the literature up to now are rare. On the other hand, the higher doses employed in animal toxicity studies don't cause any of these dramatic findings that you have shown.

DR. ISHAK: I must caution that these are all rare lesions considering the millions of women on the pill. I don't know why you are not seeing those lesions in animals.

DR. SCHUPPLER: I would just like to make one point concerning the androgen related or androgen associated tumors. These are very rare lesions, just like those seen in users of oral contraceptives. These androgens are given for aplastic anemia which is usually associated with either intoxication by organic solvents or microtoxins. We may have a case of classical promotion because the causative agents are cytotoxic and they may also be initiators. So we may have classical initiation and then promotion, a two-step mechanism of carcinogenesis.

I think we should consider such a mechanism if there is an association with oral contraceptives.

DR. EASTERLING: I believe I understood you to say that in cases of hepatocellular adenoma simply discontinuing the oral contraceptive was not enough, suggesting that ruptures had occurred in patients in whom the medication had already been terminated. Can you give us some idea about the frequency or number of cases in which that has happened?

DR. ISHAK: There have been a few cases reported in which that has occurred, either spontaneously or following a pregnancy after the patient had terminated oral contraceptive use.

We have had the opportunity of studying some patients who had been off the pill for as long as ten years and they still had adenomas. The patients underwent physical examinations, and adenomas detected by CAT scan or other radiographic techniques were subsequently removed. They don't completely disappear, the danger of possible rupture or other complications persists. If I had a wife who had an adenoma, I would want it surgically removed.

DR. BLYE: At this point, I am confused. We know, for example, that virtually any steroid will produce liver damage in the rat if given at a high enough dose for a long enough time. But, I'm not sure, as a result of all this discussion, whether anyone here believes that contraceptive steroids cause liver damage in women.

With respect to the androgens, are you referring to all androgenic hormones or to steroids such as methyltestosterone which, when taken orally, has well known hepatotoxicity.

Are the oral contraceptive steroids hepatotoxic in man?

DR. ISHAK: I didn't think there was any question about it, but I guess there is. Yes, they are hepatotoxic but not in every user. Intrahepatic cholestasis has been reported with the androgenic/anabolic steroids like methyltestosterone and other anabolic steroids as well as with the oral contraceptives, but the incidence is not very high. It can be reproduced by the natural estrogens during pregnancy.

As far as tumors are concerned there is only one which everyone agrees is related to oral contraceptive use, and that is hepatocellular adenoma, but its incidence is not very high, about three or four per 100,000 users. It does occur in these patients and there is no question that there is a dose effect, and that risk also increases with duration of use.

DR. BALAZS: Oral contraceptive steroids have two effects on the liver, one is a pure cholestasis, a dose-related decrease in bile flow that is reproducible in the rabbit and rat, and a familial relationship, perhaps a hypersensitivity reaction, maybe even HLA-type associated. A higher incidence has been reported in certain countries. The pruritis of pregnancy related to cholestasis is not necessarily a hypersensitivity reaction, but rather a toxic mechanism, with itching due to bile or degradation products. But cholestatic hepatitis might be considered as a hypersensitivity phenomenon, which never has been reproduced, to my knowledge, in experimental animals, in spite of the immense effort of all your colleagues.

DR. ISHAK: I did show vascular lesions. They are hyperplastic changes which occur in the intima of vessels throughout the body and have been definitely associated with oral contraceptives. Similar changes are seen in pregnancy. So the lesions can be caused by synthetic and natural estrogens. I illustrated the changes because they are frequent findings in patients with adenomas; they may also possibly explain some of the other vascular complications, such as the Budd-Chiari syndrome, in patients on oral contraceptives.

The other problems in pregnancy, pruritis and intrahepatic cholestasis, are a spectrum of one disease, because patients in one pregnancy may have pruritis and in another pregnancy many have intrahepatic cholestasis.

DR. McCONNELL: Dr. Ishak, can you classify these hepatocellular adenomas that you have seen as to their causative agent, whether they were in the 19-nortestosterone derivatives or the progesterone compounds? Do you have that data available?

DR. ISHAK: No, we couldn't do that. We did have the data, but we felt that the main effect was due to the estrogenic component of the oral contraceptive. There was no difference between ethinyl estradiol and mestranol, for example, but there was an effect of total potency of the estrogens in terms of greater risk. In other words, the higher potency preparations were associated with a greater risk of development of adenoma.

DR. McCONNELL: Do you feel that the estrogen component was more responsible than the progestin?

DR. ISHAK: Yes, I think so.

DR. DICZFALUSY: Thank you very much indeed for your presentation, Dr. Ishak.

NEW STEROIDAL CONTRACEPTIVES, IMPLICATIONS FOR TOXICOLOGICAL MODELS

Gerhard Zbinden

Institute of Toxicology
University of Zurich

HISTORICAL NOTES

When the first generation of steroidal contraceptives was introduced into clinical practice, toxicologists had to make their decisions under considerable pressure of time. Extensive clinical trials were going on in several countries and the compounds worked very well. It was easily predicted that this new method of contraception would rapidly be accepted by a large number of the female population. However, the biochemical mechanisms by which the compounds affected the endocrine equilibrium were not well understood and the analytical techniques to investigate them were in their infancy. As a consequence, clinical experience preceded ahead of experimental toxicology. The toxicologists' concern was mainly directed towards assurance of long-term safety rather than towards preparation of new compounds for Phase I and II clinical trials. Under these conditions, it was understandable that the conventional approach to drug safety testing was selected. Since many healthy women were exposed to these new drugs for a considerable length of time, it was believed prudent to demand long-term studies, not only in small rodents but also in beagle dogs and primates[1].

This great effort in safety testing yielded a mass of data which was difficult to understand. Never had so many animals been continously exposed to such large doses of hormonal drugs. No one was surprised by the organ changes which developed. However, it was not possible to extrapolate these findings to women who received these substances in much smaller doses in phase with their menstrual cycle. Over the past 15 years, much effort was spent to reconcile the toxicological findings in animals with the clinical and epidemiological experience in women taking steroidal contraceptives. It is fair to say that few valid correlations were found and that the tremendous toxicological effort had done little to further our understanding of the human risk created by these drugs.

This conclusion should not be viewed as a criticism of the original approach to safety testing of steroidal contraceptives. The methods selected at the time were the only ones known and the scientific basis for a more sophisticated concept was simply not available. However, it is clear that we cannot afford to test the steroidal contraceptives of the future with the toxicological methods of the past.

SCIENTIFIC BASIS OF THE NEW TOXICOLOGICAL APPROACH

For the better understanding of the toxicology of steroidal contraceptives it is useful to distinguish the following effects:

1. Changes related to hormonal activities
2. Changes related to metabolic activities
3. Toxicity related to the molecule as such and not mediated by hormonal or metabolic effects

Changes Related to Hormonal Activities

Most of the changes observed in standard toxicological experiments with steroidal contraceptives are a direct consequence of the hormonal effects of the drugs. They affect the stability of the hypothalamic, pituitary and gonadal functions, upset the intricate regulatory mechanisms, and through these effects alter the function and structure of organs such as mammary gland, urinary bladder and liver.

Experience has shown that effects of hormones and hormone-like drugs often differ among animal species. This is, at least in part, explained by the fact that the same reproductive functions are often regulated by different sex hormones and interactions with peptide hormones. The hormones important for the regulatory function are secreted in different amounts, and the sensitivity of target organs to these hormones differ considerably in various species.

Knowledge of these species differences is particularly important for dose selection. In the early phases of toxicological evaluation of steroidal contraceptives, dose selection was essentially based on the human contraceptive dose, expressed in mg per kg body weight. Owing to marked species different this practice led to controversial results. For example, many of the drugs studied were combinations of estrogens and progestogens in clincal ratios which were not optimal for the laboratory animals. Thus, if a combination which was optimal for women was tested in the rat, only the estrogenic component was expressed[2].

These species differences can greatly affect the outcome of toxicity studies. For example, in the rat, estrogens stimulate prolactin release an effect either enhanced or reduced by progestogens, depending on the compound and the dose. Thus, the resulting change in the mammary gland is a direct consequence of these hormonal interactions.

The best studied example is the difference between the response of beagle dog and man. It was shown that the effective dose of levonorgestrel in the beagle dog is 0.3 mg/kg. The human contraceptive dose of this drug is 0.005 mg/kg. If, for the animal studies, the human contraceptive dose is multiplied by 25, a test dose of 0.125 mg/kg is obtained and the ratio of this dose to the minimal effective progestational dose in the beagle is about 0.04. Cyproterone acetate, on the other hand, is a highly active progestational agent in the beagle, the minimal effective dose being 0.03 mg/kg. Since the human contraceptive dose is 0.04 mg/kg, the test dose (25 times the human contraceptive dose) is 1.0 mg/kg and the ratio between this dose and the minimal effective dose in the beagle is about 30. It is no wonder that, with such a large overdose, mammary gland nodules were induced. As a matter of fact, when levonorgestrel and similar compounds, including progesterone, were given to beagles in doses with equivalent relative progestational potencies, mammary nodules were also induced[2,3]. Moreover, it was found that progestogens produce an increase in growth hormone secretion in the beagle, leading to proliferation of the mammary gland and to the development of acromegaly. No such effect is observed in humans[4].

It was also demonstrated that various progestational agents used in oral contraceptives have a different hormonal spectrum in laboratory animals. For example, in the rat progesterone is an antiestrogen and a gestagen, but has no estrogenic and androgenic properties. Norethynodrel is a potent estrogen in the rat and thus can stimulate prolactin secretion. Norethisterone acetate on the other hand has estrogenic, antiestrogenic and androgenic properties while being a moderately potent progestational agent[4]. It is clear that such variations in the hormonal activities of individual compounds which usually do not correlate with the effects in man, greatly affect the outcome of toxicological studies, particularly those conducted at high doses.

From these examples it is seen that many changes observed in toxicological studies with steroidal contraceptives are a direct consequence of the hormonal functions of the test compounds. Since these effects predominate, the spectrum of changes seen in the toxicological studies usually represent the dose limiting characteristics and it is unlikely that potential toxic effects not due to the hormonal properties would be detected. Thus, the experimental model as it is currently used, is essentially reporting the reactions due to a derangement of hormonal balance and is poorly suited to detect inherent toxic effects of the molecules.

Changes related to metabolic activities

In clinical use the steroidal contraceptives have been associated with a variety of metabolic changes, affecting mainly lipid and carbohydrate metabolism and certain protein fractions. The routine animal toxicity studies of these agents have not reliably predicted these changes. Apart from certain fluctuations of lipoproteins and various protein fractions showing marked species variability, and occasional effects on bile flow, BSP extraction and bile acid excretion, no remarkable findings have been reported. It appears unlikely, that better animal models could be found and it is expected that human experience will, as in the past, be the main source of information for the exploration of metabolic effects of the new contraceptive steroids.

Toxicity related to the molecule

The hormonal effects of contraceptive steroids so dominate the spectrum of changes seen in routine toxicity experiments that other undesirable effects are usually masked. In some instances, particularly with compounds having estrogenic activity, mild to moderate anemia is found[5]. Occasionally an increase in fibrinogen concentration was mentioned as well as fluctuations in other coagulation factors. But a clear-cut thrombogenic effect does not emerge in routine toxicity studies.

CONCLUSIONS

The experience from extensive toxicology studies with many steroidal contraceptives has shown these compounds can lead to a great variety of endocrine effects particularly when they are given at high doses. The interpretation of these results is very difficult since clinical experience has yielded a totally different set of unwanted effects. In explaining this discrepancy one must consider the enormous species differences, the differences in dosing and in schedule of administration. Therefore, it is clear that routine long-term animal experiments conducted with arbitrarily selected multiples of the human contraceptive dose and without consideration of differences in hormonal efficacy, pharmacokinetics and metabolism, will be of very limited use.

Although the presently available steroidal contraceptives have a remarkable safety record, considering their widespread use by millions of women, it cannot be concluded that contraceptives of the next generation will be equally well tolerated. We must not only expect that they will have similar metabolic and hormonal side effects, but we must also consider that they could induce unexpected changes due to their novel chemical configuration. They might, for example, penetrate into the central nervous system and induce behavioral abnormalities. Their structural characteristics may lead to unexpected organ distribution and accumulation in certain tissues. Finally, they may profoundly alter reproductive function or exhibit serious teratogenic properties. For these reasons, toxicological assessment of future contraceptive steroids must continue, not necessarily along the conventional lines, but perhaps on the basis of a more scientific approach.

Before initiating a toxicity study, one should consider whether the new drug is an approved steroidal contraceptive which does not significantly differ chemically and pharmacologically from existing drugs. If its novel characteristics are mainly related to duration of action and potency it can be assumed that the side effects will be similar to those compounds presently marketed and the major effort to determine the drug's merits and drawbacks will be determined by the clinical pharmacologist.

If the compound has unusual structural features and clearly differs from the existing steroids with regard to its pharmacological and pharmacokinetic properties, it should be regarded as a new drug with unknown toxicological potential. The toxicological work-up should then proceed very carefully, and the clinical pharmacological evaluation must be conducted with great caution.

The major effort in the preclinical assessment of new steroidal contraceptives should be concerned with comparative hormonal activities in a variety of animal species. In these studies similarities and differences to known and established compounds should be determined. With a minimum of routine toxicology, i.e., a one to 3 month subchronic study in a rodent and a nonrodent (preferably a primate), the presence of unexpected toxic effects, unrelated to the hormonal activity, should be excluded. After this, human pharmacological studies should be initiated with the major goal of detecting pharmacokinetic characteristics and the basic effects on endocrine functions and hormone levels. If the general tolerance is acceptable, phase II studies designed to establish clinical efficacy can usually follow.

If a compound demonstrated good clinical efficacy and acceptable tolerance in humans, further extended clinical studies can be initiated. At the same time, long-term toxicity studies in animals must be started. In designing these studies an effort must be made to select a proper dose which takes into consideration the endocrinological spectrum in the test species as well as pharmacokinetic characteristics. In most instances a rodent and a primate should be used and a duration of two years appears appropriate. In the evaluation of the outcome of these investigations, the knowledge of species specific endocrinological activities must be considered.

This demand of chronic toxicity experiments with new contraceptive steroids may seem to be in contradiction to the conclusions reached in the first part of this paper. It is true, the record of routine chronic toxicological studies as a predictor of human tolerance of oral contraceptives has not been spectacular. On the contrary, many changes seen in animal toxicity studies have not only proven to be irrelevant, but were clearly erroneous. However, it is felt that much has been learned from these toxicological experiments and that better studies can be designed with the benefit of our accumulated knowledge of comparative endocrinology and pharmacokinetics. Moreover, we should not forget that the steroidal contraceptives of the future may differ fundamentally in certain respects from the drugs presently available. Thus, they may cause unknown, undesirable or even dangerous effects for which we have no appropriate and specific experimental models. Since we do not know what the new compounds have in store, it appears to be prudent to have recourse to the time honored procedure, the broad based chronic toxicity experiment. It may well be that it will disappoint us again and will burden us with many irrelevant, false positive effects. However, with the presently available knowledge we will be better prepared to deal with such events and will not reach the false conclusions drawn in the past. On the other hand, if any of the new generation steroidal contraceptives reach a worldwide distribution with millions of healthy women exposed for a substantial part of their lives, we will certainly not regret having solid experimental data on high dose, long-term administration to experimental animals, and to know that these studies would, at least, sound an alarm if the new agent differs significantly from the established contraceptives whose toxicological profile in animals and side effect liability in man are well established.

REFERENCES

1. Goldenthal, EI: Contraceptives, estrogens, and progestogens: A new FDA policy on animal studies. FDA Papers 3, November 1969, p 15.

2. Neumann, F and Graf, KJ: Some comparative endocrinepharmacological aspects and their relevance in the interpretation of adverse drug effects. Pharmac Ther. 5:271, 1979.

3. El Etreby, MF and Graf, KJ: Effect of contraceptive steroids on mammary gland of beagle dog and its relevance to human carcinogenicity. Pharmac Ther 5:369, 1979.

4. El Etreby, MF and Gunzel, P: Besonderheiten bei der Prufung von Sexualhormonen (am Beispiel der Gestagene) auf chronische Toxizitat. AMI-Berichte 1/80:127, 1980.

5. Kramer, M and Gunzel, P: The proof of drug effects on endocrine glands or endocrine target organs by means of toxicological investigations. Pharmac Ther 5:287, 1979.

DR. DICZFALUSY: Thank you very much, Professor Zbinden. I was pleased that you presented my summary. Perhaps we can wait for the Chairman's summary until Friday morning because it gives us a little bit more time for discussion now. I am sure that there are a number of questions. Who will start?

DR. SCHUPPLER: Did you imply that chronic toxicity studies should continue? Did you refer to 7-year dog and 10-year monkey studies as well, and if so, could you give your reason a bit more explicitly, especially in the sense for prediction of tumor formation?

DR. ZBINDEN: I indicated my personal interest in drug development is not limited just to oral contraceptives. My major concern is that clinical trials of new chemicals be done properly with a few patients. Once it is decided that the compound has major advantages, everything possible should be done and the type of toxicological study cannot, be based only on scientific considerations.

Once the drug is to be marketed, and has the desired therapeutic properties you must be prepared to study more human subjects. Under these conditions we are compelled to conduct additional chronic toxicity studies in animals.

We can debate the length of the chronic toxicity study. I certainly don't believe in seven or ten year chronic toxicity studies. However, every new drug that is taken for prolonged periods of time should also be given chronically to animals. If clinical untoward effects occur one has solid animal data available.

Based on present knowledge, you might be convinced that a long-term monkey study is not useful because it showed no undesirable effects.

However, in my opinion, the monkey study has reliably predicted the safety of the presently available contraceptives, and this, of course, is a very important toxicological finding.

I would think a two-year study in monkeys and rats should be mandatory once the drug enters extensive clinical trials and, if the compound were efficacious, I would even consider studying some monkeys indefinitely, just to have a continuous experience on which I could fall back, should that need arise.

DR. SCHAFFENBURG: By my previous remarks, I didn't mean to take toxicologists to task, particularly Professor Zbinden, because it is easy to make a diagnosis in retrospect. Toxicologists did what they were supposed to do at the time. What I was trying to recommend, and I think this is an inevitable conclusion here, deals more with chronic assessment. In acute studies, you identify, in 90 days in rats, dogs, or what have you, alerting symptoms or signs of toxicity, but you observe human adverse reactions in the clinic. I have never seen in animal studies those things that appear in the human in 15 or 20 years.

Let me give you an example. When the question of reserpine and mammary tumors came up, I was involved in the chronic toxicity of chlorpromazine in rats as well as a very potent prolactin inducer, sulfuride.

The rats were literally dragging mammary tumors around cages. They became ulcerated and died of these mammary tumors. I am not aware of a single mammary tumor found in women following 20 or 30 years of chlorpromazine use in various institutions.

Now, just imagine if the toxicity of chlorpromazine had been initially included because of different requirements such as a two-year toxicity in rats. I think probably we would have been looking for mammary tumors in women from the outset and spent a lot of money not finding them.

DR. ZBINDEN: Well, history is always interesting. I have been involved in developing similar compounds and at that time we used 90-day studies. We never looked at the mammary gland. If we had looked at the mammary gland we would have seen marked proliferation after two weeks. We may then have looked at prolactin synthesis and release. So I think it is certainly true that the way the studies are now being conducted, we observe more and more tumors which have no relevance for man.

A major reason for this is that we want to be on the safe side, and we utilize extremely high doses. Studies with 50 times, 100 times, or even higher multiples of the human dose of these extremely potent chemicals are bound to give irrelevant results.

DR. BARDIN: How would you react to a proposal similar to the way carcinogens are evaluated. There are some carcinogens, whether you want to call them inducers or promoters, that appear to cause tumors in a limited number of organs or species which are less of a concern than those that promote tumors in all species and in many organs. As long as there seems to be a hormone that causes tumors in a given species, perhaps related to some genetic susceptibility, be it an oncogene or whatever and could be predicted in a inherited way, would you be less concerned than about a chemical that caused multiple tumors in many species? Couldn't we arrive at some kind of evaluation scheme that would conclude that a tumor in this organ is of no concern because it occurs in only one species.

In other words is finding a tumor always of enormous concern from the toxicologist's point of view?

DR. ZBINDEN: No. In chronic animal studies, particularly when high doses are used, an increased tumor incidence is often observed. The evaluation of this finding requires that all available data be considered. I do not believe that if a tumor occurs only in one site, in a single species, it is a less dramatic situation than if it occurs in two species and three sites. You must consider its possible mechanism of action and other biological effects, such as the action as a mutagen in several in vivo or in vitro systems. You should consider covalent binding, the effect on repair, taking into a account comparative pharmacokinetics. There is a reasonable explanation why the animal model responds to most compounds by inducing tumor formation.

Sometimes this is a response which is also likely to occur in humans and in other cases there is biochemical and biological evidence to suggest that the animal response is most likely not relevant for man. The same is true for hormonal tumors. As long as there is no rational explanation, we cannot just disregard them and not worry about them. They may be relevant. Some estrogenic compounds are considered to be human carcinogens and long-term combination oral contraceptive use is associated with benign liver tumors. We cannot disregard them, and it is for that reason we must look at animal endocrine tumors and utilize all possible information to assess human risk.

DR. DICZFALUSY: The hour is late, but may I take the Chairman's privilege and ask the last question of Professor Zbinden. You rendered us a major service by putting the whole development of this field into perspective. As I mentioned earlier, after the thalidomide catastrophe, the methods employed in toxicological testing were the best possible ones at the time. Now it is less than 15 years since the first steroid radioimmunoassay was developed and it is only during the past ten years that we have been able to measure nanogram and picogram quantities.

My question is, and it is also a little philosophical, looking back at the beagle studies prior to the discovery that growth hormone was an important factor and considering carcinogenicity studies in different species, wouldn't it suggest that in addition to the steroids shouldn't we also examine pharmacodynamic effects? For instance, in terms of different hypophyseal hormones where the methods have not yet been developed for many species, i.e. we know little about the response of the hamster pituitary to steroids.

DR. ZBINDEN: I think that would be certainly more important than to have huge standard toxicity studies where you, like a blind date, just go into the unknown.

DR. DICZFALUSY: Then I thank very much Professor Zbinden for his presentation and his most stimulating remarks.

SUMMARY

Egon Diczfalusy

Reproductive Endocrinology Research Unit
Karolinska Sjukhuset (Swedish Research Medical Council)
Stockholm, Sweden

During the past two decades or so I have derived much comfort from a quotation from Max Gluckman: "A science is any discipline in which the fool of this generation can go beyond the point reached by the genius of the last generation."

Indeed, in a world rapidly and irreversibly changed by more and more sophisticated technology it is just not possible in any field to stop time in the hope that what we have done during the past 20 years is still the best possible approach.

In introducing my presentation during the first section, I recalled the historical background of safety testing saying that several of these regulations were formulated in the shadow of the thalidomide tragedy, which greatly strengthened the desire to adequately protect the public in the future by providing greater safety on the basis of animal studies. Indeed, the methods recommended were the best and most promising ones which could be devised at that time, some 20 years ago.

However, since then we have witnessed dramatic progress in analytical methods, which more or less revolutionized pharmacokinetic studies, especially those conducted in human subjects. As Professor Zbinden said, it would be simply wrong to continue the old-fashioned toxicology testing for another 15 years. The Sestri Levante meeting in 1976 (Europ. J. Clin. Pharmacol. 11, 233-238, 1977) rightly pointed out that, "Toxicity studies cannot be properly planned without knowledge of absorption, blood levels, half-life, excretion routes and plasma binding in the species used." Indeed the outstanding presentations amply confirmed and considerably expanded the conclusions reached by another group of scientists seven years ago.

There was a consensus among our speakers that meaningful toxicity studies cannot be based on predetermined arbitrarily chosen multiples of the human dose, but that the doses administered should be based on the assessment of the peripheral levels of the drug, using small multiples of the bioavailable dose in the human. This was emphasized by Drs. Humpel, Goebelsmann, Fotherby, Bardin, Edgren and Zbinden. Indeed, without adequate pharmacokinetic information one may reach wrong conclusions not only with regard to the true potency of the steroid, as emphasized by Dr. Clark, but also concerning its endocrine profile as elegantly demonstrated by Dr. Bardin, since a steroid administered in huge excess may occupy specific receptors for other steroids and thus produce misleading information. In addition to bioavailability in dose-dependency, we were repeatedly reminded of the importance of assessing the half-life of the active principle, and its possible accumulation in specific tissues. We were also reminded by Dr. Ishak of the importance of potential hepatotoxicity of some steroids.

A practical consequence of such a new approach is that pharmacokinetic properties of the new drug must be established as soon as possible in the human in order to initiate proper animal toxicological studies. For this, relatively little animal toxicology seems needed, provided we have established the broad endocrine profile of the drug, since only small doses will have to be administered to a few subjects for a short time. From here on there should be a shuttle between animal studies and clinical investigations.

From the various presentations we have heard, one might describe a scenario of a new and different drug development in the 80's and 90's characterized by a maximum of flexibility and if I may be somewhat provocative, it should be something like this. After conducting a large variety of studies on the hormonal profile and blood levels of the compound in two species, for instance rat and monkey, and the usual tests of acute toxicity, a more or less standard toxicology protocol would be undertaken in these two species for, say, four to six weeks with special attention to metabolic, cardiovascular, pulmonary and CNS effects after which one would immediately establish bioavailability in the early clinical pharmacokinetic study. On the basis of these data one would then design a subchronic toxicity study with graded doses of small multiples of the human blood levels say 1x and 5x but certainly not more than ten fold given for six months to the same two species. Since it is doubtful whether the absolute level of human safety can be increased by increasing the duration of administration of massive doses to experimental animals, the "overkill" principle with massive doses administered during many, many years should be abandoned. Rather, one might recommend the inclusion of a satellite group of animals in which a battery of hormonal and metabolic studies are carried out. With this information one would initiate Phase II clinical studies including a broad spectrum of hormonal and metabolic studies. The preclinical assessment of carcinogenicity is a problem because of the scarcity of animal models; a two year rat study was suggested.

As Dr. Sobel rightly pointed out, a good beginning could be made in this direction almost immediately by waiving the requirements for new formulations and delivery systems of well-known drugs, or when they are administered in such forms which are rapidly converted into steroids with adequate safety records provided the peripheral plasma levels are not exceeding those observed previously.

However, as Francis Bacon said, "hope is a good breakfast, but it is a bad supper", and I would hope that this will only be the very beginning.

SECTION 2

CONTRACEPTIVE STEROIDS AND CARCINOGENICITY

MODERATOR: MORTIMER B. LIPSETT

STEROIDS AND CARCINOGENESIS

Mortimer B. Lipsett*

National Institute of Arthritis, Diabetes, and Digestive and Kidney Diseases
National Institutes of Health
Bethesda, Maryland

This issue of the role of steroids in carcinogenesis is one of the hardest the FDA has to face. The definition of a carcinogen is in part at fault. The FDA can usually talk only about carcinogens, and isn't afforded the opportunity, at least in a variety of reports, of separating direct carcinogens from promoters of carcinogenesis. Once one is forced to lump these entities together, then the scientific aspects of the roles of steroids in carcinogenesis disappear. As biologists, we should, at least, have the luxury of thinking about types of carcinogens we are dealing with. It is now a reasonable and accepted assumption that steroids are not complete carcinogens.

With respect to direct carcinogens, I think we have to accept that animal models remain the cornerstone of carcinogenesis testing. Of the some 18 chemicals that have been identified as causing cancer in the human, 16 of them cause cancer in animal models; of the some 164 other chemicals that cause cancer in the animal, none of them has been shown to be safe in the human. So, for the direct acting carcinogens, the animal model is absolutely essential and I think it is going to remain with us.

Again, with respect to the differences between direct acting carcinogens, and promoters, such as steroids, a National Academy of Science study that was completed several years ago is pertinent. Let me just read one of their conclusions.

"In the absence of countervailing evidence for the specific chemical, it appears reasonable to assume that the lifetime cancer incidence induced by chronic exposure in man can be approximated by the lifetime incidence by similar exposure in laboratory animals at the same total dose per body weight." But such a statement just doesn't hold for the steroids acting as carcinogens in the very broad sense of the term that the FDA must use. If we consider their possible role as direct carcinogens, then we must admit to a paucity of evidence. The steroid hormones are not mutagens and reactive intermediates (epoxides) with the potential of binding to DNA have been shown only with large enough doses that permit metabolism to these rare species of metabolites[1]. The one human example that has been quoted on occasion is the effect of diethylstilbestrol

* Deceased

in the production of vaginal cancers in daughters of women who received this estrogen during pregnancy.

Perhaps this has been quoted because there were no obvious mechanisms to explain an indirect action. As a result of the work of Cunha and his collaborators[2] such mechanisms are now conceivable. He has shown, for example, that the relationships between the induction of epithelial changes by surrounding mesenchyme may be altered by hormone administration; presumably diethylstilbestrol could then have triggered inappropriate differentiation of the epithelial cells during a critical period. It is this effect that may be responsible for the changes that we see some 15 or 20 years later.

Most workers have agreed that steroids act as cocarcinogens or promoters of carcinogenesis. Berenblum[3] categorized the promoter effects as preparative, permissive and conditional. The preparative effect may be easily defined as preparing the cell for the carcinogen. All cells aren't equally susceptible to carcinogens; this has been shown experimentally for radiation, for viral carcinogens and for polycyclic hydrocarbons.

In each instance, the particular tissues have to be prepared, and this is particularly so for tissues that are induced to differentiate or grow by steroids. Radiation or dimethylbenzanthracene will induce a few mammary tumors in the ovariectomized rat. When the tissue is prepared by estrogen use, then the number of tumors increases dramatically.

In thinking of the permissive effect of steroids, we must look past the carcinogenic event. The putative role of steroids here is to permit the growth of the new cancer cell into a tumor capable of surviving in the host.

It is hard to show conditional effects in the experimental animal. There is one good human model for this, interestingly enough. It has been shown that latent prostate cancer, that is, nonclinical prostate cancer which the pathologist will identify as prostate cancer, has the same incidence in Japan as in the United States. On the other hand, the incidence of clinical prostate cancer is increased in Japanese men in Hawaii over Japanese men in Japan[4].

Now, there is no proof here that steroids are responsible. The diet and/or steroid hormones or unknown factors, may be causing this increase in clinical carcinoma. But this is an example, I think, of what might be called a conditional effect. Here we have a cancer which is microscopic but still it is many more than just a few cells, and something is conditioning this cancer so that in Japanese men in Hawaii it becomes clinical cancer more frequently than in Japanese men in Japan.

In an old, but relevant study, Doniach[5] showed the synergistic effects of TSH stimulation on the induction of thyroid cancer by irradiation (Table 1). Neither TSH nor radiation induced tumors; however, when the thyroid cells were placed in a growth phase by endogenous TSH, irradiation became a potent carcinogen.

Segaloff and Maxfield[6] have demonstrated that estrogens increase the rate of induction of the mammary tumor in the rat following radiation. It has subsequently been shown that in strains of rats susceptible to mammary cancer and in rats that are quite resistant to mammary cancer,

Table 1. Incidence of Thyroid Tumors in Rats After Irradiation of the Thyroid. From Doniach[5]. Reprinted by permission.

Treatment	Number of rats	Thyroid carcinoma
None	41	0
Methylthiouracil	50	0
30 μC^{131} (15,000 rads to the thyroid)	52	0
30 μC^{131} plus methylthiouracil	48	11
1,100 rads x rays to the thyroid	13	1
1,100 rads x rays to the thyroid plus methylthiouracil	22	7

estrogen sensitizes the mammary gland to the carcinogen, radiation. The timing of exposure to the promoter to the administration of carcinogen remains of interest and is pertinent to this discussion. If ovariectomy is done more than about a week before giving methylcholanthrene, it is very difficult to induce mammary tumor in the rat. If you give methylcholanthrene and do ovariectomy shortly thereafter, it is again very difficult to induce mammary tumor. If you do ovariectomy later, induction of mammary tumors is easier. Similarly, if estrogens are given to ovariectomized rats about a week after the methylcholanthrene, again there is induction of mammary tumors. The common theme here is that the ductal epithelium of the mammary gland has to be in the proliferative state under the influence of its growth hormone, estrogen, for a complete carcinogen to exert its maximal effect.

What does all of this imply? Well, if the direct carcinogens act randomly over time, that is, the chance of getting one hit or a certain number of gene rearrangements, or whatever the specific carcinogenic event(s) is, then the longer the promoter acts, the greater is the chance of these events occurring and the greater is the incidence of cancer.

The human data show that very nicely. For example, in breast cancer we know some of the important risk factors. An early menarche is an important risk factor for breast cancer. A late menopause is an important factor for risk of breast cancer. In each case the duration of time in which the ductal epithelium is stimulated by estrogen is increased. There are now additional data showing that if postmenopausal women take estrogen unopposed for up to 10 years, you can increase the risk of breast cancer by some twofold[7]. I should point out it is difficult to show small increases in the risk of breast cancer, because the disease is common; one of 11 women is going to have it. So, again, anything that extends the period of time that the tissue is being stimulated by its growth hormone, in this case estrogen, is going to increase the chance of developing a cancer.

It has been stated that promotion may be viewed as an epigenetic process which leads to aberrant expression of an otherwise blocked gene program for proliferation at the expense of maturation. This statement reiterates elegantly the idea that you must have proliferating tissue for carcinogenesis to occur.

It is curious that in the last decade, there has been much less interest in the steroid hormones as promoters of carcinogenesis, because the interest has shifted to much more specific compounds, the phorbol esters, where you can dissect the two-stage initiation of cancer in the skin and elsewhere. It seems that what you are doing with phorbol esters is blocking terminal differentiation in the skin. When terminal differentiation is blocked, then not as many cells leave the proliferative pool and go on or become keratinized. That is one of the reasons that the phorbol esters are acting as cocarcinogens. More cells remain vulnerable to the carcinogen for longer periods of time[8].

There is another class of compounds, the clastogens, compounds that cause aberrant changes in the chromosome, such as induction of chromosomal breaks or sister chromatid exchange that are pertinent to this discussion. Many of the clastogens are also carcinogens. Again the great majority of them have to be present during DNA replication to exert their effect.

Weinstein et al[8] have summarized the features of direct carcinogens and promoters (Table 2). The initiating agents are carcinogenic by themselves; promoting agents are not carcinogenic alone-and that applies to the steroids.

The concept of reversibility is important. The effects of a carcinogen are irreversible even though a tumor may not result. However, the promoter effect of steroids is certainly reversible. This can be nicely shown in the experimental mammary tumor system in the rat where estrogens can render the animal susceptible to carcinogenesis, and where you can show that reducing the estrogen stimulation will eventuate in a reduced incidence of cancer. Thus the promoter effect is reversible because what is happening in the tissue is reversible as a result of the effect of steroids.

The question of threshold is of interest. It has been discussed extensively for the carcinogens, but at low dose levels, it remains difficult to define. With respect to the steroids, I have looked through the literature to find good evidence that there are dose related effects of steroids as promoters of carcinogenesis.

This is difficult to find in the animal systems. In the human system, the only data that really suggest this are the studies relating the inci-

Table 2. A Comparison of Biologic Properties of Initiating Agents and Promoting Agents. From Weinstein et al[8]. Reprinted by permission.

Initiating agents	*Promoting agents*
1) Carcinogenic by themselves—"solitary carcinogens"	1) Not carcinogenic alone
2) Must be given *before* promoting agent	2) Must be given *after* the initiating agent
3) Single exposure is sufficient	3) Require prolonged exposure
4) Action is "irreversible" and additive	4) Action is reversible (at early stage) and not additive
5) No apparent threshold	5) Probable threshold
6) Yield electrophiles—bind covalently to cell macromolecules	6) No evidence of covalent binding
7) Mutagenic	7) Not mutagenic

dence of uterine cancer in postmenopausal women to the amount of estrogen that has been taken. Here there are only four studies, and the data are too poor to conclude that there is a dose related effect.

In general these studies have dealt with women receiving conjugated estrogens in the range of 0.6 to 1.25 milligrams. One would hypothecate that if enough estrogen is given to maximize the number of cells in a proliferative phase, that higher doses would not increase the incidence of cancer. To my knowledge, this hasn't been tested.

Now, let me just say a word or two about uterine cancer, because it has been a good model. The one thing that really shows up in studies of estrogen and uterine cancer is the effect of duration of use. That goes back to what I was talking about in breast cancer; that is, the longer the tissue is in a proliferative phase, the better the chance of a carcinogenic event. The incidence and the relative risk for postmenopausal endometrial cancer increases with the duration of estrogen use (reviewed in 7).

Now, just a few more words about uterine cancer. Although this conference is not directed at the risks of oral contraceptives, we need to bring the effects of progestins into perspective with respect both to endometrial cancer occurring before the menopause and after the menopause.

Risk factors for endometrial cancer before the menopause are obesity, polycystic ovarian disease and the estrogen-secreting tumors. The common denominator is anovulatory periods in which there is an unopposed estrogen effect. The tissue remains constantly stimulated by estrogen with resultant hyperplasia, adenomatous hyperplasia, and carcinoma. Epidemiologic studies have shown this clearly.

In postmenopausal women, what are the factors that predispose to endometrial cancer? Obesity and estrogen. What is the common denominator? Again, persistent estrogen stimulation. I would call to your attention the fact that almost all of the studies which have shown an increase in endometrial cancer after the menopause have been studies where progestational agents weren't given and where the dose was fairly continuous; again, an increased chance for expression of the carcinogenic event.

What are the progestins doing and why are the steroid contraceptives so different? Well, in fact, the progestins, you might say, "rest" the endometrium. They do it in several different ways.

They decrease the number of estrogen receptors thereby decreasing estrogen action. They increase sulfation of estrogens. When you increase sulfation, you are essentially removing them from reacting at the receptor site. They shift the equilibrium from estradiol to estrone and estrone is a less potent estrogen than estradiol.

And, recently, it has been shown that progestins accelerate the release of occupied estrogen receptors from the nucleus. So, in all of these ways, progestins are decreasing the effect of estrogens at the nuclear receptor sites. There is now some evidence that the incidence of endometrial cancer due to estrogen use after the menopause is decreased by intermittent use of progestins to induce withdrawal bleeding.

Well, of course, this is the reason why women and we as physicians have been so lucky with the oral contraceptives. I don't think any of this was appreciated or understood when the oral contraceptives were placed in use but we know now that we don't get endometrial hyperplasia. In fact, the endometrium is hypoplastic because of the progestational effect.

Now, with respect to breast cancer, Korenman[9] proposed an interesting idea in which he said that progesterone may be important for breast cancer as well; that period when there is unopposed estrogen in normal women is the period of greatest susceptibility of the breast to cancer.

He drew on studies of the survivors of the atom bombs in Hiroshima and Nagasaki. There is an excess incidence of breast cancer in these women, and there is some evidence that the excess incidence occurred either in women who were ages 10 to 15 at the time of the atom bomb, or who were in their perimenopausal periods.

Korenman[9] postulated that this is because those are the times when you have the greatest incidence of anovulatory cycles and unopposed estrogen effect. He also had some other data showing that during pregnancy they were less likely to develop breast cancers.

Although this is an attractive hypothesis, one would suspect that a larger number of prolonged anovulatory cycles would be necessary to demonstrate this. Further, there are a number of epidemiologists who have contested this rather vigorously. And recently Apter and Vihko[10] have shown that early menarche means early ovulatory cycles.

I would like to make one comment about uterine cancer in passing. Here is a cancer where the biologic, biochemical and epidemiologic data are in accord. This is relatively uncommon in epidemiology but when it does occur, considerable value can be placed on the findings.

Where does all this lead us in terms of the problems that the Food and Drug Administration has, or that we have as physicians with respect to the use of these steroids. I think it is pretty clear that if we give a steroid that promotes proliferation in a target tissue, we are going to increase the chance of cancer. Now, does that help us in our requirements for knowledge of toxicity, steroid kinetics, metabolism, steroid hormone action, and animal safety studies?

Well, the fact is, it really doesn't help us very much, because these steroids are really nontoxic at any sort of reasonable levels of use. We are unable to even talk about toxicity studies meaningfully unless something turns up in the future which is unique to some new steroid configuration.

That isn't to say we should not know about pharmacokinetics, because we should. But it doesn't help us with respect to this very difficult problem about carcinogenesis. And, again, the fact that there may not be any threshold for promoters makes it even harder to derive safe levels. The only safe level, in my opinion, would be one where there would be no stimulation of the tissue in question and of course no clinical usefulness.

Should the guidelines for preclinical animal safety studies be amended? The FDA must deal both with science and politics. For example, if they were forced to be consistent, oral contraceptives containing estrogens are carcinogens by any of the current definitions. They can be given to rats or mice and will increase the number, size and early recurrence of mammary tumors, and in hamsters you find other sorts of tumors. So, on that basis, one could call them carcinogens, the same as we now label the 17-acetoxy progestins as possible carcinogens. I find it very difficult to devise appropriate safety requirements for compounds such as steroid hormones that act as promoters of carcinogenesis if you assume that keeping the tissue in a proliferative state will increase the risk. Thus, if we find that there are reasons for the use of estrogens after the menopause, and those reasons are increasing all the time, the incidence of cancer in estrogen responsive tissues will increase. If progestins are given concurrently, the risk will be decreased. However, it will not be at the level seen in women not receiving estrogen.

Should the recommended dose levels be projected on the basis of an end organ's responsiveness? This is difficult to do because of our inability to define threshold effects. It is a lot easier if you are looking at discrete events such as thromboembolism and blood lipid changes.

I do think that we need more research to understand the mechanisms of cocarcinogenesis for steroid hormones and I am unable to offer suggestions on alternatives to long-term animal studies. We already know enough to say that a steroid hormone that causes growth of a tissue will, in fact, promote the chances of developing cancer in that tissue.

REFERENCES

1. Purdy, RH, Goldzieher, JN, LeQuesne, PW, Abdel-Baky, S, Durocher, KK, Moore, PH, Jr., and Rhim, JS: Active Intermediates and Carcinogenesis, In Merriam, GR, Lipsett, MB (eds): Catechol Estrogens, New York, Raven Press, p 123, 1983.

2. Cunha, GR, Chung, LWK, Shannon, JM, Taguchi, O, and Fujii, H: Hormone induced morphogenesis and growth: role of mesenchymal-epithelial interactions. Recent Prog Hormone Res, 39:559, 1983.

3. Berenblum, I: Established principles and unresolved problems in carcinogenesis. J Nat'l Cancer Inst, 60:723, 1978.

4. Akazaki, K, Stemmermann, GN: Comparative study of latent carcinoma of the prostate among Japanese in Japan and Hawaii. J Nat'l Cancer Inst, 50:1137 1973.

5. Doniach, I: Experimental induction of tumors of the thyroid by radiation. Brit Med Bull, 14:181, 1958.

6. Segaloff, A, Maxfield, WS: The synergism between radiation and estrogen in the production of mammary cancer in the rat. Cancer Res, 31:166, 1971.

7. Lipsett, MB: Hormones, medications and cancer. Cancer, 51:2426, 1983.

8. Weinstein, IB, Wigler, M, Fisher, P, Sisskin, E, Pietropaolo, C: Cell culture studies on the biologic effects of tumor promoters. In: Slaga, TJ, Sivak, A, Boutwell, RK (eds): Carcinogenesis, Vol. 2. (Mechanisms of Tumor Promotion and Cocarcinogenesis), New York, Raven Press, p 313, 1978.

9. Korenman, SG: The endocrinology of breast cancer. Cancer, 46:874, 1980.

10. Apter, D, Vihko, R: Early menarche, a risk factor for breast cancer, indicates early onset of ovulatory cycles. J Clin Endocrinol Metab, 57:2, 1983.

DISCUSSION

DR. PIKE: I would like to totally agree with Dr. Lipsett about what he said about proliferative effects but, in fact, if you accept that and you know the biology more initimately of breast cancer, in fact, the situation is extraordinarily encouraging.

I would like to draw a picture, because we tend to think that the breast is the uterus, and it certainly is not. If, in fact, you look at mitotic activity in the endometrium, which we all know from standard textbooks, in fact, the mitotic activity during the menstrual cycle behaves like this in the uterus.

There is a large proliferative phase until ovulation. Progestin comes around and mitotic activity decreases. In the breast, it is exactly the opposite. There is almost no mitotic activity in the breast in the follicular phase. You ovulate, and it is up here.

Now, this tells you all sorts of things. First of all, it tells you that, if you add progestins to postmenopausal estrogens, you might be doing a terrible thing if this is an effect of progesterone, so when we say that adding progestins to postmenopausal estrogen is going to be good, we ought to be very, very careful about which organ we are talking about.

I have no doubt that it is going to be true of endometrium. I am very frightened about what it will do in breast. This is exactly what the epidemiology would tell you. Postmenopausal estrogen, unopposed estrogens at the postmenopausal period will have a tremendously bad effect on the endometrium.

We get relative risks, as was shown by Dr. Lipsett and others, of the order of 8 and 10; in the breast, we can never get 2. Why is that? There is progesterone, possibly. Now, we keep on saying that the steroids might be carcinogens, but nobody has made the strong emphasis that we have wonderful evidence that oral contraceptives prevent cancer of the endometrium, right?

Now, this is quite easy to see in the proliferative phase. As Dr. Lipsett has mentioned, you look at women on oral contraceptives and there is mitotic activity, mitotic activity in the endometrium. Less mitotic activity, less cancer, exactly the biology as stated. Now, what happens when you look at mitotic activity in the breast on oral contraceptives?

It is not down here; it is up here. This tells you something that is really very, very interesting, because if oral contraceptives are up here, this is why the epidemiologists can't find any effect of oral contraceptives on breast cancer.

It tells you that on average we can't find anything. Oral contraceptives are not the same. If this is the average, which somehow the area under the curve is the same, we have the same mitotic activity, there are going to be some oral contraceptives up here and there are going to be some down here, and if you take these, it is going to protect you against breast cancer, and if you take those, it is going to give you breast cancer.

We have now quite convincing evidence that we can identify which these are. The point about it is that, in fact, if we are going to go on in this area, we need animal work now where we can measure mitotic activity in the right target organ. I think that is where I would like the FDA to put a lot of work.

What Dr. Lipsett said is absolutely, in my opinion, right on the ball. Mitotic activity is the name of the game. We must find the target organ in animals which is going to mimic the target organ in woman and, in fact, we might have the miracle drug for cancer -- not a carcinogenesis agent, but an anticarcinogenesis agent.

SPEAKER: Where did you get that evidence that there was increased activity in the breast?

DR. PIKE: There is a whole series of people who started work in Edinburgh, Dr. Kerr is now in Brisbane, Dr. Wiley, Dr. Anderson, Dr. Ferguson, it is all published in the British Journal of Cancer. They study the women who come in for reduction or augmentation mammoplasties, determine out what pills they are on, and obtain evidence from this group.

These are people who were not on the pill. This evidence is for people who were on the pill. In fact, you can do it from straightforward ordinary tissue blocks. You can even do it with stored tissue. But, they use a special technique, with light microscopy.

I am not a pathologist, but I think it is probably the most exciting thing that has happened in breast cancer in the last 10 years.

DR. LIPSETT: They certainly are very interesting data. Just two things. First, older data, both from England by Pohl and from Huggins and others in this country, have shown that progestins, under certain circumstances, can act as a promoter of carcinogenesis in the rat. It has not been shown, of course, in the human. The other is that Hoover and his colleagues at the National Cancer Institute have shown that with 10 years use of estrogen after the menopause there is about a doubling of the breast cancer risk. Ross had similar results.

DR. PIKE: My investigations are with Drs. Anderson and Ross from USC Medical School and, in fact, we have exactly the effect. There is a twofold increase in risk if you have long-term estrogen use postmenopausally.

DR. LIPSETT: Yes, it is a difficult problem. I remember two papers from the Los Angeles group ,one in which they said there was an increased risk with estrogens; and the second about a year or two later where the risk was denied. I think part of the problem is that there are so many variables and there are so many people with breast cancer.

DR. PIKE: We made a mistake.

(Laughter)

I don't deny we made lots of mistakes. The reason that the first paper showed -- I wasn't yet there, I was still in Oxford -- but when I arrived in LA the study was finished and I analyzed it. I knew no endocrinology, I am a mathematician. What we found was that, in fact, they did the study, they did a hospital-based case-controlled study, but because it was in Los Angeles, where everybody knows things are crazy, they in fact asked the physician who had been treating the breast cancer case to give us one of her other patients as a control.

Well, if you were a physician and you were in L.A. where people love going to the doctor, who would you send as your control? You would send someone, in fact, who was bugging you but had nothing the matter with them. Now, you know that in L A, again, if someone comes to you all the time bugs you and they have nothing the matter with them, you give them estrogens.

(Laughter)

So, you get the totally wrong answer and the first study is just rubbish.

DR. LIPSETT: That is a commentary on medicine in Los Angeles, I guess.

(Laughter)

DR. GOLDZIEHER: I would like to suggest to Dr. Pike that data from women who need reduction mammoplasties or augmentations gives you a U-shaped curve of the sensitivity of those tissues and it is a very unrepresentative population.

DR. PIKE: Well, Los Angeles might be crazy, but if in Texas you can do biopsies of normal women's breasts, I would love to know. It is the best data I'm aware of.

PROFESSOR VON EICKSTEDT: I would suggest you could simplify the problem by just counting mitoses in human breast biopsies.

The recommendation suggested should not forget that in some countries, we have already threephase pills which don't have a fixed content of progestogen. We have in many countries different kinds of progestogens combined with estrogens, and we must determine what the progestogen really is. Otherwise we return to the point where we were 20 years ago.

So, I think we have to find out where we are going in treating women with different kinds of progestogens, adding different doses of estrogens and then we come to quite another question. Dr. Lipsett, if you are discussing estrogens and endometrial cancer, what was the dosage?

In Germany, a lot of women have been treated with estrogens and no one could find an increase in endometrial cancer, but if you compare the population in Germany and over here, you find quite different dosages. So, the question is, how much is the dosage concerned?

Another question. How much is prolactin involved in the human? Prolactin is often measured and seems to play a role in breast cancer and we must differentiate between breast tissue concerning prolactin and the endometrium which reacts directly to estrogen.

DR. LIPSETT: The dosage phenomenon is really very hard to answer. As you point out, we are, for whatever the reasons, using conjugated estrogens, of which about 60 percent is estrone sulfate. But I am not sure it matters which estrogen we were using; what I guess matters is the degree to which we are stimulating the endometrium.

I suppose that in Germany you are using sufficient estrogen to get the desired clinical effects, and at that level there is probably some stimulation of the endometrium. Now, there must be some point at which you are just getting threshold effects with respect to carcinogenesis.

If that is the case, if you are at that level, the chances of developing cancer of the endometrium may be decreased as compared with women receiving higher doses of estrogens. My guess has been, and it is purely a guess, that in general if we get clinical effects with estrogens we are probably at threshold already. One of the reasons I say this is because in a number of studies of uterine cancer 0.3 milligram of conjugated estrogens, a fairly low dose, gives a clinical response and an increased carcinogenic effect. The progestin--we haven't answered that and we certainly need to.

DR. BRENT: You raised the question of the possibility that the DES model was evidence of a direct carcinogenic effect, although --

DR. LIPSETT: I don't subscribe to it, but it has been raised, right.

DR. BRENT: Don't you think the fact that high dosages of hormones can cause a change in differentiation of development, and that would probably fit in just as well with the whole area of displacement of tissue being susceptible to carcinogenesis in the pediatric age group? Because most hamartomas, most teratomas, most displaced tissue that is present at birth is more susceptible to carcinogenic breakdown --

DR. LIPSETT: That is certainly a reasonable alternative explanation.

DR. BARDIN: I would like to return to this interesting data that was just put up on the board, mitosis in the human mammary gland, and raise several issues. One, mitosis of the lobuloalveolar structure might mean something very different from ductal development, where the main part of carcinomas arise. That would be one comment.

Secondly, the comment seems to be a little at right angles to the idea that benign breast disease might in some way be related to the incidence of an increased risk, or might increase the risk for breast carcinoma. Is that an epidemiologic fact? Is that holding up?

Thirdly, progestins are used, certainly in Europe, to treat benign breast disease very successfully. In fact, there is a very large multi-center trial to see if they can reduce the incidence of breast cancer in women by treating benign breast disease with progestins. So, what are your reactions to these kinds of things? Are all these observations consistent, or are they yet to be explained?

DR. LIPSETT: Let me just make one comment, and ask Dr. Pike to comment, perhaps, and that is we have to be a little wary of benign breast disease. It is true that the most recent data show that there is an increased incidence of one-and-a-half to two-and-a-half-fold for breast cancer. But benign breast disease is about five or six different conditions.

If you look at specific types, such as a typical epithelial hyperplasia, the incidence is increased considerably. Now, which type is being successfully treated with progestin, I don't know, and maybe that will come out of this big study. Dr. Pike, would like to comment?

DR. PIKE: Oral contraceptives initially remarkably reduced fibrocystic disease of the breast and it was very confusing as to why we couldn't see something in epidemiologic studies on breast cancer because of the known relationship between the benign breast disease as a whole and breast cancer.

But as Dr. Lipsett just mentioned, in fact the relationship, as Black and others have shown, really is between a very small proportion, sort of hidden in these benign breast diseases, which in fact is related to cancer. There is a lot more work that needs doing.

Certainly progestins are effective agents for the overall majority of a lot of fibrocystic disease. So, I think that is an area which still needs work done.

Stanley Korenman, has an estrogen window hypothesis, which we never did like. The reason we didn't like it was because women whose menarche begins at 12 exhibit regular cycles very quickly, and have a much increased risk of breast cancer compared to those who at 12, have their first menses menses but doesn't go into regular cycling until three or four years later.

Dr. Korenman said exactly what you said, that somehow or other the mitotic activity is not in the right cells. Now, the right cells is really a difficult question. Cancer probably comes from stem cells and nobody knows which ones they are.

The other thing is, other pathologists are not at all convinced that those aren't the right cells. I am not a pathologist, but my feelings are that you can find pathologists who would tell you that the mitotic activity is in the right cells and not in the wrong cells. That is something that is obviously still open to debate.

DR. LIPSETT: Let me just emphasize one thing, and that is that 90 percent of breast cancer comes from the ductal epithelium.

DR. NASH: To try to take a lesson home from what you have said Dr. Lipsett, about the evaluations of candidate contraceptives that might be useful in predicting carcinogenic potential, as I interpret what has been said, the carcinogenic potential is a function of the hormonal activities, of estrogen activity, of the progestogenic activity, and so forth.

It would therefore seem logical that if one has an adequate endocrine profile, particularly in the human, that there is as good a basis as possible for predicting carcinogenic potential of contraceptive steroids.

DR. LIPSETT: Yes, I think that is essentially true, Dr. Nash, and I suppose we have to always have our minds open that there is going to be some new steroid structure that introduces a unique action and that, of course, has happened not with respect to cancer, but with respect to other effects.

But, in general, that is my feeling as well.

DR. BRENT: You didn't comment at all in developing the concept that this is an indirect effect. The work in the late sixties and seventies with regard to the possibility that these form toxic epoxides, the work of Waters, when you reviewed that and your experience in this area, do you feel that that supports the fact that this is not a direct mutagen-carcinogen?

DR. LIPSETT: I didn't do that because Dr. Clark reviewed it very well, yesterday and I agree with him. Both Dr. Purdy in San Antonio and McLaughlin at NIEHS have shown that epoxide formation occurs. Epoxides are very reactive compounds and can covalently bind to DNA. Whether that is a significant at the levels of estrogens that we are all dealing with has not really been proved.

The other point is one I made yesterday, and I think it is just an indication of a terribly good debating point. You do have clear-cut dosage effects with direct carcinogens, and it has been very hard to demonstrate this with steroids.

DR. BLYE: If reproductive tract and gonadal cancers are related to mitotic activity and steroid hormone levels, why is there an increasing incidence of them as a woman ages, particularly in the postmenopause when these tissues are not proliferating and circulating sex hormones are reduced.

DR. LIPSETT: Of course, there is much we don't know. We don't know latency periods or how many half-lives are involved, and there are many half-lives involved in the time of the one to two cell stage to the diagnosis of a clinical cancer.

You can say the same thing about carcinoma of the prostate. Carcinoma of the prostate occurs in older men when testosterone is certainly not increasing; if anything, perhaps decreasing a little bit. On the other hand, you have had exposure, the cells have been exposed to testosterone for a long period of time.

There has never been, that I am aware of, a cancer of the prostate occurring in a eunuch, for example. So, that is a clear-cut example of a permissive effect, of testosterone acting how, we don't know. Well, what is the latent period of carcinoma of the prostate until it becomes cancer? These are the sorts of very difficult questions that I think we can answer in the future.

DR. PIKE: It is sort of a well-known problem for epidemiologists. If you look at it in the normal way that an epidemiologist would look at it. The effects that you say, occur more often when mitotic activity is decreasing, is not true.

It is that if you plot something which is not related, like cancer of the lung or cancer of the colon or cancer of the stomach, and you plot the logarithm of the probability of getting it that year against the logarithm of age for most epithelial tissue, you get, in fact, a straight line. So, in fact, all cancers of epithelial tissue simply increase with age in this way, if they are not hormone-dependent or mitotic activity-dependent, which will change with age.

But if you plot endometrium, breast, or ovary, the rate of increase always decreases as the mitotic rate decreases, so that the epidemiology is, in fact, what you would expect, except for prostate where, in fact, the turnover seems to be much, much later.

DR. LIPSETT: Concerning this concept of phase and mitotic activity, so many carcinogens and so many clastogens have been shown to work only during the S phase, the time of DNA replication. That is very important.

MR. HALL. I was looking for Dr. Stadel. He referred yesterday to the ongoing WHO studies in about 11 centers throughout the world in which we are looking at five cancer sites, breast, cervix, endometrium, ovary, and liver, and the association with hormonal contraception.

We have already collected a large number of cases, but at this time we have only one or two preliminary analyses in this case-controlled study. It might be worth just proposing at this moment on the very preliminary analyses on DMPA users that, in fact, from this particular study one is seeing, say, with cervical cancer, where there are sufficient cases to be able to estimate a relative risk of 1.6, that this is not being achieved.

So, the relative risk is considerable lower than that, and with breast cancer there appears to be a protective effect. I think this just backs up some of the other knowledge from epidemiological studies that we have at the present time. I hope within the next year we will have some concrete data and, of course, one of the things that must be done, and we have planned to do, is to continue surveillance studies.

Because, as just mentioned one is always concerned about the latency period, and the duration of drug use. So, we are intending, particularly with the progestin-only therapy, to continue surveillance for a long period into the future.

DR. LIPSETT: Yes, I think we will look for the results of those studies with interest. It does remind me that the recent CDC-NICHD study on effects of oral contraceptives showing that ovarian cancer is decreased, again, is further evidence of this effect. I assume and, of course, I have no way of knowing if it is correct, that what we are doing is inhibiting gonadotropic stimulation of a variety of several ovarian cells by oral contraceptives.

DR. KRAUSS: This may be an obvious point, but I would just like to raise it for discussion. There is, certainly, some variation in the estrogen receptor levels in mammary carcinomas from individuals undergoing surgery. Wouldn't this play a role, that, plus possible differences in progesterone receptors in the individual susceptibility to the effects that you were discussing? Isn't this a factor to be considered which might be a confounding one?

DR. LIPSETT: Well, of course, I don't know what the relationship is of both estrogen and progesterone receptors in carcinoma to what existed in the tissue previously. What we do know is that the presence of progesterone receptors is necessary for a response to progestational agents. But other than that, I couldn't answer.

DR. KATZENELLENBOGEN: I just had a comment to your question. I think there is certainly evidence in the human as well as with animal models that some breast cancers have reasonable levels of hormone receptors. Probably in these cases physiologic levels of estrogen, in fact, serve as growth factors or maintenance factors for these tumors, and some of these patients certainly respond well to endocrine manipulation or antiestrogen therapy.

I think there are many aspects related to what these stored hormones may be doing and, in addition to acting at the phase of initiation, in a sense, the promotion aspect, they also may be growth regulators in already overt tumors.

AN ASSESSMENT OF THE TOXICOLOGICAL AND CARCINOGENIC HAZARDS OF CONTRACEPTIVE STEROIDS

Ralph Heywood

Huntingdon Research Centre
Huntingdon Cambs., England

INTRODUCTION

With the world's population due to reach five billion in seven years, population growth must be slowed humanely through foresight and leadership, otherwise there will be severe economic hardship amd famine. Against this background, those of us concerned with the safety evaluation of contraceptive methods must ensure that the advice we give is relevant to the balance of hazards and benefits. Toxicologists have made assumptions that have nothing to do with the real world and, on the basis of these premises, have perpetuated theories and animal models that have resulted in some degree of confusion. This Workshop will attempt to resolve some of the issues.

It is now generally accepted that oral contraceptives are associated with deep vein thrombosis, pulmonary embolism and certain types of acute cerebrovascular disease. They may cause myocardial infarction and can lead to hypertension. An important non-cardiovascular adverse effect is cholelithiasis. Minor side effects include cervical erosion, nausea, breast tenderness and temporary impairment of fertility after cessation of dosing[1]. Tumors, both benign and malignant (hamartoma), have been caused by contraceptive use[2].

The first alerts of adverse effects of the oral contraceptives (OCs) were anecdotal reports, which were later verified by prospective and case-control studies[3]. The OCs were first marketed in 1958, the first alert for pulmonary embolism was in 1961 and this was later verified in 1967[4]. Myocardial infarction was alerted in 1963, and verified in 1970[5].

The question we have to answer is, what role have animal studies played in predicting adverse drug reactions? Here, an empirical review of data generated from studies in animals receiving progestogens or oestrogens, or a combination of both, could be a starting point for discussion on better systems for assessing safety. The open literature on the toxicity of oral contraceptive steroids in animals is sparse, and what is available has been reviewed[6].

CARDIOVASCULAR EFFECTS

a. Thrombotic complications. Oestrogens cause depression in

erythrocyte and white cell counts in mice. In the rat, there is a slight reaction in haemoglobin and haematocrit values[6]. Rats given 0.5 mg/kg of ethinyloestradiol show significant increases in the prothrombin index and thrombotest time but there was no effect on the activated partial thromboplastin time following 2 weeks of drug administration[7]. These changes were shown to be reversible. Oestrogens have profound effects on the haemopoietic system of dogs: neutrophil leucocytosis, anemia and thrombocytopoenia resulting in haemorrhagic diathesis have been recorded[8]. Bone marrow samples showed myeloid hyperplasia and depression of the megakaryocytes. In the female rhesus monkey, a slight progressive dose dependent decrease in haemoglobin and haematocrit has been recorded following oestrogen administration[9].

Progestogens in the rat can cause a slight depression in values relating to the red blood cells. In the dog the haematocrit and haemoglobin values are lowered, and the white blood cell count is increased. The data for clotting factors show great variation and prothrombin time may be affected; with massive doses, it is usually prolonged. Activated partial thromboplastin time shows inconsistent differences, but values from treated dogs tend to be lower than those of the controls. Fibrinogen concentration is generally higher in the higher dose groups. The platelet counts tend to increase with time. Higher serum cholesterol levels are associated with progesterone treatments[10]. Little or no effect has been recorded in monkey species, although norethindrone has been found to elevate plasma fibrinogen levels[11].

Naturally occurring thromboembolic disease is rarely recorded in laboratory animals and, from the published studies in rodents, dogs and monkeys with contraceptive steroids, there is no real evidence that progestogens induce vascular and/or thrombotic disease. The one exception is a study on Depo-Provera and injections of progesterone, in which dogs receiving the median (10 times) and the high (25 times) doses of Depo-Provera died from multiple thrombosis and metastatic carcinoma by the end of the sixth year[12]. The three basic causes of thrombosis, hypercoagulability of the blood, injury to or pathological lesions of the blood vessel wall, and stasis of blood flow through the blood vessels, were investigated but no satisfactory explanation was found for the thrombi. Amyloidosis was found in the majority of animals and many of the pathological changes seen may have been related to the amyloidosis. It is known that in cases of spontaneous amyloidosis in the dog thrombosis is a frequent complication[13].

This study on Depo-Provera and progesterone was by injection and the evidence suggests that chronic inflammation and repeated immunoreactions occurred at the injection sites and it was because of the dosage form that amyloidosis was seen. It was the injection site reaction which was the major factor in inducing thrombosis and not the progestogens.

b. <u>Myocardial infarction</u>. This has not been reported in any of the animal studies.

c. Hypertension. Changes in blood pressure are difficult to record in an experimental animal, but there is no substantive evidence that OCs induce hypertension in laboratory animals.

EFFECTS ON THE GALL BLADDER

Cystic mucinous hyperplasia of the gall bladder has been recorded by all pathologists examining dogs that have received progestogens. The gall bladder wall is thickened, and accumulation of mucoid material may completely occlude the lumen. The pathogenesis of this condition in the dog is uncertain, and is probably unrelated to gall bladder disease in women. The Boston Collaborative Drug Surveillance Program[14] suggests that the oestrogenic component of the Pill is an important factor. In a study in which ethinyloestradiol was administered to rhesus monkeys with intact enterohepatic circulation, a fall in bile acid concentration with accompanying decreases in cholesterol, phospholipid, cholesterol saturation index, and a significant rise in daily bile volume were observed[15]. These results in rhesus monkeys are consistent with those found in the baboon by Morrissey and co-workers[16] and conflict with the data from women[17], which suggest that the cholesterol saturation of the gall bladder and reduction in chenodeoxycholic acid occurs in oral contraceptive use.

CARCINOGENIC RISK

a. Liver. A report by the Committee on Safety of Medicines[18] concluded that there was no evidence of increased incidence of liver cell tumors in mice given oestrogens or progestogens. Examination of the data suggests that this is not strictly true, for animals receiving some progestogens did show a slight increase in benign neoplasia. Rats given ethinyloestradiol show increased serum alkaline phosphatase (SAP) levels, which is attributed to new synthesis by the liver[19]. With some progestogens, there may be minor elevation of serum glutamate pyruvic transaminase (SGPT) values, particularly in the early stages, of the study, and elevation of serum protein values is a common finding. There is an increase of proliferative changes in the liver and, at high dose levels, progestogens, particularly in combination with oestrogens, bring about a slightly increased incidence of liver tumors. These are generally benign, but may be malignant with some progestogens (megestrol acetate and norethynodrel)[18].

Ethinyloestradiol does not affect liver enzyme or liver morphology in the dog. In this species, administration of progestogens causes an increase in SGPT values. With some progestogens given over a 7-year period (lynestrenol) there is an increased incidence of areas of hyperplasia, which is considered to be compensatory hyperplasia[6]. Hansel and co-workers have reported liver cell adenomata in dogs receiving parenteral doses of medroxyprogesterone acetate or progesterone, but similar lesions have not been found by other pathologists[20]. In the monkey, liver enzyme values, notably SGPT and leucine amino peptidase (LAP), are increased with the administration of ethinyloestradiol, but morphological change can be identified with electron microscopy (EM) only[21]. The administration of progestogens to monkeys appears to have little effect, if any, on liver enzymes, although ultrastructural changes have been induced with norethindrone in baboons[22].

Adenomata and focal nodular hyperplasia have been described in the livers of OC users; associated increased vascularity of the tumors carries the risk of ruptures[2]. Some correlations of liver findings can be made between the laboratory animal species and women.

b. Mammary Tumors. There is no increase in mammary tumors following steroid administration to the rodent species. There is, however, no doubt that the long-term administration of progesterone and some progestogens (both the 17-hydroxyprogesterone and 19-nortestosterone derivatives) cause the development of mammary nodules in the beagle dog, and that some of these nodules can progress to become malignant[6]. The administration of progestogens to the dog induces a variety of changes indicative of considerable endocrine disturbance.

In the beagle dog there is evidence of the stimulation of growth hormone by progestogens[23]. The other factor that may be of importance is that mammary hyperplasia can be induced with progesterone The data on mammary nodules and tumors in beagle dogs suggest that the mechanisms operating in the beagle dogs differ from those in women, and that the findings cannot be extrapolated across species boundaries[24]. I am of the opinion that if all available progestogens were investigated at equal progestational potency in the dog, they would be equally tumorigenic.

There is only one case in which an oral contraceptive (Enovid) has been associated with infiltrating duct carcinoma in the rhesus monkey, although there is a possibility that a spontaneous occurrence cannot be excluded[25]. Mammary nodular hyperplasia in the monkey has provoked some controversy. This is a condition occurring spontaneously in the rhesus monkey[26]. In my experience, these nodules are often transient and there is no evidence that they are progressive.

The WHO report on steroid contraceptives and the risk of neoplasia[27] concludes that there is no clear evidence to suggest either an adverse or a beneficial effect of OC use on breast cancer. The data now suggest strongly that the use of OCs lowers the risk of fibrocystic breast disease.

c. Tumors of the Reproductive Tract. A low incidence of uterine tumors was recorded in mice which received a number of progestogens[18]. These tumors were found particularly to involve the cervical epithelium and were more prevalent in the groups given a high dose levels of ethinyloestradiol. There was no increase in the incidence of endometrial tumors in rats[18].

In the dog the effect of progestogens on the reproductive tract is well known, causing cystic endometrial hyperplasia, as also does administration of oestrogens[6]. Long term administration of oestrogens to the dog induces proliferative serosal changes and these proliferative lesions are indistinguishable from mesotheliomas and are hormone dependent. Oestrogens can induce uterine mesotheliomas in the New World monkey, particularly the squirrel monkey, but this effect has not been shown in the rhesus monkey[7]. The administration of progesterone and synthetic progestogens to the non-human primate induces a degree of atrophy of the endometrial, glandular and mucosal epithelium and decidualisation of the endometrial stroma[28,11]. In two monkeys receiving high dose-levels of Depo-Provera, and in one monkey receiving norethisterone enantate, endometrial carcinomas were found. These tumors were poorly differentiated carcinomas. The histogenesis of these tumors is not known, although there is some resemblance to the epithelial plaque cells of the rhesus monkey. It is generally considered that these tumors are unique to the monkey[29].

There is no epidemiological evidence of a correlation between the use of OCs and carcinoma of the vulva and vagina, or ovarian tumors, nor is there any evidence of increased incidence of endometrial cancer in women using combined OCs or long-acting injectable progestogens.

TOXICOLOGICAL PREDICTIONS

Testing for Toxicity. The purpose of toxicity testing is to define doses that can be given with reasonable safety to man. The studies are designed to elucidate target organ effects, to characterize the type of toxicity and, from this information, to deduce the dose that causes no adverse effect. It is unlikely that no-effect levels can be established with any steroid given at greater than physiological levels. Biotransformation and pharmacokinetic studies should be the basis for the selection of dosages and selection of the appropriate species. Unfortunately, this information is frequently not available early in drug studies. Biotransformation, protein binding and excretion are compound limited procedures: deviations from linear (dose dependent) pharmacokinetics preclude extrapolation from high to low dosages. All the available evidence indicates that toxicity can be defined within a six-month period. A standard toxicity study at three dosage levels, in an appropriate species and at proper dosage levels, would be sufficient to establish safe doses for clinical investigation of any steroid in women: firstly, the traditional safety factor approach, which sets arbitrarily chosen limits of safety; secondly, mathematical modeling to predict from observed response to the zero dose. At the moment, the best approach to low dose extrapolation is to rely on simple linear extrapolation.

I would like to suggest that for toxicity testing of contraceptive steroids, the low dose could be set at that dose which just suppresses ovulation; the high dosage should be selected on the basis of pharmacokinetics and should be near the upper limit of linearity; and, as I do not feel that there is a need for massive safety factors with this type of compound, I think that the intermediate dosage levels should be no more than 5 to 10 times the low dose.

Testing for Carcinogenicity. There is no doubt that the long-term treatment of laboratory animals with high doses of contraceptive steroids increases the incidence of a variety of neoplasia. The question is, what is the relevance of these findings to the risk of neoplasia in women? The animal bioassay is the accepted definitive test for carcinogens. The basis for this test is the assumption that chemicals that cause tumors in animals may cause tumors in man. These studies are normally performed in rodent species; only with steroids is there a requirement for primate and dog carcinogenicity studies. Rodent carcinogenicity studies are being continually questioned, for some would argue that these studies have have not been properly validated and, on reviewing published literature, it would appear that they lack sensitivity and specificity[30].

Carcinogenicity testing of steroids poses further problems because overdosing with steroids induces general endocrine disturbances. The dog is undoubtedly the most sensitive of the laboratory species to female sex steroids.

The animal model required for carcinogenicity testing of steroids should exhibit anovulation with a cyclic endometrium. Such as animal model does not exist, and we therefore have to compromise by using the species that are available to us. The monkey is the best with respect to reproductive cycles.

The greatest improvement we can make to the design of these studies is in the selection of appropriate dosages. The current practice of selecting dose-levels as multiples of the human dose level on a mg/kg body weight basis is too simplistic. This practice has given rise to our present position of selecting as a high dose level for rodents 200 times the human dose, for monkey studies 50 times the human dose, and for the dog, 25 times the human dose. Findings at very high dose levels are of significance in the context of dose and duration of exposure in a particular species, and cannot be extrapolated to other species, including man.

I would suggest for the carcinogenicity study that the low dosage be selected as that which just suppresses ovulation. I see no need for a three dose study, and the second test group could be investigated at 10 times this level.

I appreciate that by selecting the ovary as the end organ I am making a major compromise, for I know that steroids have different potencies for different end organs. Binding affinities to receptor sites differ between species[24]; for example, chlormadinone acetate has greater progestational activity with respect to the uterus of the bitch, as measured by the Clauberg type assay, than in women, whereas norgesterol is less progestational in the bitch than in women using the same endpoint. Norethisterone is known to be a weak progestogen in the dog, but potent in women[31]. Recent studies have shown low affinity for levongesterol and norethisterone for the receptors of dog tissue as compared with those of woman[24]. Treatment with progesterone may significantly increase progesterone receptor concentrations in cytosols of end organs. This has been shown in the uterus and in the mammary tissue of the dog, but there is no evidence that this occurs in the rat. In the dog, the matter is further complicated by the fact that altered tissues, such as spontaneous benign mammary tumours, have concentrations of progesterone receptors almost twice as great as those seen in mammary tissues after progesterone stimulation. Any study for carcinogenicity must take into consideration receptor binding and the possibility of receptor proliferation in the main target end organs, for the proper interpretation of the data.

There is now so much evidence against the use of the dog as a model for carcinogenicity of steroids that I would hope that the regulatory agencies would reject this model. If this is not possible, I would hope that they would seek some compromise with respect to the length of the study and with respect to dosage levels. In this species, it is known that growth hormone is stimulated by progestogen and I would suggest that, if progestogens are given at dosages which cause elevation of growth hormones, the model is invalid.

It is easy to generate animal toxicological data. It is important that we should be able to interpret these data properly. There is always uncertainty about the shape of the dose-response relationship at the levels of actual human exposure. Some regulatory authorities assume that a carcinogen has a no-zero risk of cancer, however small the dose. This assumption is not accepted by everyone, but I think there are thresholds of a real and practical nature. With steroids, carcinogenic thresholds can be established.

In the final analysis, I conclude that animal studies have not been predictive of the main effects of contraceptive steroids, with the possible exception of liver toxicity. The animal models for carcinogenicity are of dubious value, but if we use them, then I must plead for realistic dosage levels.

REFERENCES

1. Vessey, MP, Doll R: Evaluation of existing techniques: Is "the Pill" safe enough to continue using? Proc R. Soc Lond (Biol), 195:69, 1976.

2. Ishak, KG: Hepatic neoplasms associated with contraceptives and anabolic steroids. In Lingeman, CH (ed): Carcinogenic Hormones. Recent Results in Cancer Research. Berlin, Heidelberg, New York, Springer-Verlag, p 73, 1979.

3. Venning, GR: Identification of adverse reactions to new drugs. I: What have been the important adverse reactions since thalidomide? Br Med J, 286:199, 1983.

4. Medical Research Council: Risk of thromboembolic disease in women taking oral contraceptives. A preliminary communication. Br Med J, 2:355, 1967.

5. Inman, WHW, Vessey, MP, Westerholm, B, Engelund, A: Thromboembolic disease and the steroidal content of oral contraceptives: a report to the Committee on Safety of Drugs. Br Med J, 2:203, 1970.

6. Heywood, R: The experimental toxicity of systemic fertility regulatory agents in laboratory animals. In: Serio, M, Martini, L, (eds): Animal Models in Human Reproduction, New York, Raven Press, p 433, 1980.

7. Heywood, R, Wadsworth, PF: The experimental toxicolgy of oestrogens. In: Chaudhury, RR (ed): Pharmacology of Oestrogens, Pergamon Press, p 63, 1981.

8. Capel-Edwards, K, Hall, DE, Sansom, AG: Hematological changes observed in female Beagle dogs given ethynyloestradiol. Toxicol Appl Pharmacol, 20:319, 1971.

9. Geil, RG Lamar, JK: FDA studies of estrogen, progestogens and

estrogen/progestogen combinations in the dog and monkey, J Toxicol Environ Hlth, 3:179, 1977.

10. Heywood, R: Unpublished results, 1983.

11. Wadsworth, PF, Heywood, R, Allen, DG, Hossack, DJN, Sortwell, RJ, Walton, RM: Treatment of rhesus monkeys (Macaca mulatta) with intra-vaginal rings impregnated with either progesterone of norethisterone. Contraception, 20:339, 1979.

12. Carlson, RG: Long-term Depo-Provera study in dogs. Dawson Research Corporation, Final Report (DRC No. 6205).

13. Slauson, DO, Gribble, DH, Russell, SW: A clinicopathological study of renal amyloidosis in dogs. J Comp Pathol, 80:335, 1970.

14. Boston Collaborative Drug Surveillance Programme: Oral contraceptives and venous thromboembolic disease, surgically confirmed gallbladder disease, and breast tumors. Lancet, 1:1399, 1973

15. McMaster, P, McLeish, RN, Medd, RK, Heywood, R: The studies of bile kinetics in the rhesus monkey after ethinyloestradiol. IRCS Med Sci, 6:127, 1978.

16. Morrissey, K, Panveliwalla, D, McSherry, C, Deitrick, J, Niemann, W, Gupta, G: Effects of contraceptive steroids and pregnancy on bile composition and kinetics in the baboon. J Surg Res, 22:598, 1977.

17. Bennion, LJ, Ginsberg, RL, Garnick, MB, Bennett, PH: Effects of oral contraceptives on the gallbladder bile of normal women. N Eng J Med, 294:189, 1976.

18. Committee on Safety of Medicines: Carcinogenicity Tests of Oral Contraceptives. H.M. Stationary Office, London, 1972.

19. Gopinath, C, Rombout, PJA, Van Versendaal, RG: Serum alkaline phosphatase elevation in female rats treated with ethinyl estradiol. Toxicology, 10:91, 1978.

20. Hansel, W, Concannon, PW, McEntee, K: Plasma hormone profiles and pathological observations in medroxyprogesterone acetate treated Beagle bitches. In: Garattini, S, Berendes, HW (eds): Pharmacology of Steroid Contraceptive Drugs. New York, Raven Press, p 145, 1977.

21. Wadsworth, PF, Heywood, R, Toxicology of ethinyl oestradiol in rhesus monkeys. In: Chivers, DJ, Ford, EHR (eds): Recent Advances in Primatology, Vol. 4- Medicine. London, Academic Press, p 179, 1978

22. Chai, LS, Colson, JG, Kirdani, RY, Sandberg, AA: Ultrastructural study of hepatic effects of a contraceptive steroid in baboon. Contraception, 10:79, 1974.

23. Concannon, P, Atlszuler, N, Hampshire, J, Butler, WR, Hansel, W: Growth hormone, prolactin, and cortisol in dogs developing mammary nodules and an acromegaly-like appearance during treatment with

medroxyprogesterone acetate. Endocrinology, 106:1173, 1980.

24. Briggs, MH: Progestogens and mammary tumors in the Beagle bitch. Res Vet Sci, 28:199, 1980.

25. Kirchstein, RL, Rabson, AS, Rusten, GW: Infiltrating duct carcinoma of the mammary gland of a rhesus monkey after administration of an oral contraceptive: a preliminary report. J Natl Cancer Inst, 48:551, 1972.

26. Squire, RA, Goodman, DG, Valerio, MG: Tumors. In: Benirschke, K, Garner, FM, Jones, TC (eds): Pathology of Laboratory Animals, New York, Springer Verlag, p 1204, 1978.

27. WHO Technical Report Series No. 619: (Steroid contraception and the risk of neoplasia: Report of a WHO scientific group), 1978.

28. Scommegna, A, Pandya, GN, Christ, M, Lee, AW, Cohen, MR: Intrauterine administration of progesterone by a slow releasing device. Fertil Steril, 21:201, 1970.

29. Salsburg, D: The lifetime feeding study in mice and rats - an examination of its validity as a bioassay for human carcinogens. Fund Appl Toxicol, 3:63, 1983.

30. WHO Special Programme of Research, Development and Research Training in Human Reproduction: facts about injectable contraceptives. Bulletin of the World Health Organization, 60:199, 1982.

31. Briggs, MH: Animal models and the carcinogenicity of contraceptive steroids. In: Animal Models in Human Reproduction, Serio M, Martin, L, eds., Raven Press, New York, pp 423-431, 1980

DISCUSSION

DR. LIPSETT: Dr. Heywood, do you agree continuing with the use of the three animal models?

DR. HEYWOOD: I am not enthusiastic about the beagle dog as a model for contraceptive steroids for reasons I have listed. It is endocrinologically different in that progestogens stimulate growth hormone. The beagle mammary gland has been shown to be susceptible to progesterone alone but, more importantly, receptor affinities vary with different progestogens. With respect to mammary cancer, the presence of nests of foci of preneoplastic lesions in the normal beagle dog has been suggested. For these reasons, I would hope that the FDA would review its position on the beagle dog. I am not for discarding the rodent and the monkey model.

DR. LIPSETT: Dr. McConnell?

DR. McCONNELL: Any model system must have a long range of uniquely susceptible individuals, ones that are in the intermediate stage, and those at the low end of the spectrum. I don't agree with the dosages that have been set for dogs in the past, and I think that we have produced some very unusual lesions which are in no way correlated with the human experience with OCs.

I think that if we can rearrange our dosage schedules so as to not overstimulate the pituitary and induce exaggerated responses in the beagle, that model system will be better than we think. We have years of experience with the beagle, we know how it overreacts, and certainly if we were able to use that system in a more thoroughly scientific way to get better dosage levels, it may still be a useful model. Then, hopefully, those data can be used in a better way.

If it overreacts at the dosage levels we think are appropriate levels, then, perhaps, we should suspect the compound.

PROFESSOR VON EICKSTEDT: Concerning the beagle, we know that it overreacts if you compare human and beagle endometrium, but this doesn't say it all. May I show a slide to explain.

It doesn't only overreact, it also acts in a different manner, when you compare the rate of growth of the breast tissue in normal animals with animals dosed with a C-21 progestogen. We are concerned with this progestogen, especially in our country, since it has been licensed as an oral contraceptive with special indications concerning hirsutism and, therefore, we always are seeking new data.

Here you see hypophysectomized dogs on the right side and normal dogs on the left side treated with the steroid. I think this is not a question of oversensitivity; this is a question of difference of reaction of rebound effects of hormones where the hypophysis is involved, when you see such a big difference between hypophysectomized and nonhypophysectomized animals.

DR. DICZFALUSY: I have two questions for Dr. Heywood. I understand you suggest subchronic toxicity testing in two species, a rodent and a non-rodent, but not canine; probably rat and monkey.

Do I also understand that for carcinogenicity testing you suggest the same, you don't even recommend the lifetime two year study? The other question which I feel is important is you mentioned that one of the stumbling blocks in this whole field is the paucity of published information, that toxicological studies were sponsored mostly by industry and those studies never get published.

Could you recommend a mechanism by which one could reverse this state of affairs? I think it is very important that toxicological data which have been obtained should be published; otherwise, we could not have all this hassle we have today, that we are trying to draw sufficient conclusions from insufficient data.

DR. HEYWOOD: There is a paucity of published toxicological data on the contraceptive steroids and I feel that these could be made available. The published summaries are insufficient.

Steroid testing has posed considerable problems for toxicology, but this does not mean that we discard the current-day philosophy of toxicity testing. I am suggesting that we take a more reasoned approach to steroids, looking to end organ toxicity and, in particular, using pharmacokinetic data.

DR. McCONNELL: If I could also add to that. There are many times we observe lesions of extrememly low incidence which are not considered compound related. I wonder how many of these lesions may have some relationship to drug exposure.

For example, I have seen leiomyomas and benign tumors in the floor of the vagina, cervix, and uterus in rhesus and beagles. I have also had an opportunity to observe at necropsy some small lesions in the liver of dogs on a 19-nortestosterone. Maybe those are related to the human experience, I don't know. The granular cell myoblastoma has been cited in the literature as being associated with estrogens.

I would like to review completed studies to glean from them all those low incidence lesions and make them available to other pathologists.

DR. LIPSETT: I must just say the International Agency for Research on Cancer (IARC) in Lyons has the responsibility at least for the carcinogenicity testing and should be apprised of this. The National Toxicology Program decided the National Institute of Environmental Health Sciences has responsibility for pulling together a variety of the other effects. One of the recommendations from this meeting might be that the FDA and/or CHT contact the National Toxicology Program.

DR. BRENT: Since both Drs. Heywood and McConnell were directing discussions towards the use of animal models, I was surprised that they didn't examine the question of threshold. Dr. Lipsett introduced that as the morning topic, since the crucial element in protecting the public (utilizing animal studies) is to answer that question.

When you consider a direct carcinogen like irradiation, we conclude that it is a stochastic phenomenon, the risk goes all the way down to zero. But Dr. Lipsett presented a vast amount of data that would indicate that many effects of the sex steroids are threshold effects and neither of you addressed the use of animal models for examining that particular question. It should be very important to a regulatory agency. In your discussions you didn't mention in any of the pathological discussions the differences in the various progestational agents. I got the feeling they are endocrinologically similar, and yet the endocrinologist tells us about differences in their metabolism and function.

At least if we didn't know anything else, we would get the feeling that all those tissue sections that you showed us could be produced by any progestational agent.

But is the dogs' uniqueness so different from the metabolism in man that makes it inapplicable to the human? The field that I happen to be in is particularly interested in teratogenesis. We throw out animal models if the basic science of the animal model, like the chick embryo, is so far from the human situation that we can't use it.

I don't know what the answer is with the beagle dog, but I think the question comes down to not that it is uniquely sensitive, but how appropriate it is for the human model.

DR. HEYWOOD: In animal safety studies we fulfill government requirements for toxicity testing. These are not necessary scientific, the precepts were established some 20-25 years ago, and there has been little change over the years.

From these data, one would hope to be able to detect the threshold levels for several carcinogens. I have pointed out the problems of threshold levels with respect to end organ sensitivity in laboratory animal species.

DR. BRENT: You did, but I got the feeling that this conference was to look toward the future, and since you had the podium and the obligation and the right to make suggestions and since threshold is a key issue here what do you look for in the future.

DR. HEYWOOD: Well, it obviously can be done. The ED01 study that was commissioned in this country some years ago generated a certain amount of controversy but did show that you can demonstrate threshold values for a known carcinogen.

In that case they used 2-acetylaminoflourene, which is a known carcinogen.

They demonstrated real threshold with respect to bladder and hepatic carcinogenicity. If you look at the time to tumor formation, you could demonstrate real threshold levels, It is an expensive study and logistically a difficult experiment to undertake.

To suggest this for the steroids in our current state of knowledge would be another complicating factor to an already very difficult situation.

DR. LIPSETT: Would you like to address the question about the differences in progestational agents?

DR. McCONNELL: I would like to speak on that. You heard the comment yesterday that an estrogen is an estrogen is an estrogen. For the most part, that may be true. There are some differences, but it is very difficult to distinguish between EE and MEE, or between stilbestrol and any one of the other nonsteroidal estrogens that I have looked at. They do essentially the same thing. They stimulate the same end organs, the same tissues. There is a difference between the progestational compounds and you have to know the response in each species, because they react differently in each species.

The 19-nortestosterones act more like an estrogen in the bitch than as a progestin, while the progesterone derivatives act typically as a progestin. You detect the formation of mammary nodules and so on and the effect on the mammary glands is different.

Then you should know whether the drug inhibits ovulation. If it doesn't, you have endogenous progesterone levels to deal with, which produces a combination effect. So, it depends upon the animal species, the dose level, and a number of factors. That is what makes it so difficult to get an accurate assessment of just exactly what is happening in these model systems.

DR. LIPSETT: I think we talked a bit around the question. I don't think it is all so difficult to determine threshold effects if one sets out properly.

DR. McKENZIE: I tend to support Dr. Heywood's statement that the dog should be negated as a model in the testing of oral contraceptives. But, more importantly, it is not so much the fact that the dog is very sensitive, but the fact that the dog is inappropriate. Reference was made to the cystic endometrial hyperplasia complex which we see in the dog and, incidentally, Dr. Heywood has stated that it is due to oral contraceptives. I think it is not induced but rather enhanced by oral contraceptives. It is a progesterone phenomenon in the dog. In man cystic endometrial hyperplasia is more an estrogen phenomenon. So, I think this is a case in point of the fact that the dog is certainly not an appropriate model.

DR. BLYE: I have two points. The first is that the Freedom of Information Act was written and is interpreted by lawyers and the present legal interpretation is that if you release some data, it jeopardizes the proprietary nature of the rest of it.

Secondly, I don't think the dog is more sensitive to sex hormones that other species; I think it is uniquely responsive. For example, a daily dose of one milligram of stilbestrol can kill a dog in a month. It develops thrombocytopenia. I don't know of another species in which you can do that. I don't know of another species that develops pyometra spontaneously or following progestin treatment.

I think the trouble with the dog is that it is unique, period. It isn't uniquely sensitive; it is uniquely responsive.

DR. PERLMUTTER: As a clinician, and in reviewing the literature, I have seen nothing to indicate that long term use of oral contraceptives is harmful. It is a woman's decision as to what she is going to use. What detrimental effect can occur from long term use.

I don't know if there is a risk of liver tumors, since they comprise only a couple of hundred cases in the literature worldwide.

DR. LIPSETT: Dr. Perlmutter has opened a very difficult problem and I am going to just permit one comment.

DR. McCONNELL: I think in any animal population, human included, that you have subsets who are uniquely susceptible to these types of products. If they are closely monitored some will be identified with hepatocellular adenomas or thromboembolism and these are the ones that suffer from prolonged usage.

DR. PERLMUTTER: But interrupted usage may do the same thing. We don't know that, because your animal models have not shown us that.

DR. BARDIN: There has been a recommendation that we continue to use the monkey as a test for carcinogencity. In how many of the studies testing contraceptives were sufficient monkeys used to allow proper statistical assessment of whether there was indeed a carcinogenic effect? I know of none.

DR. HEYWOOD: I must make it clear that I did not recommend proceeding with monkey carcinogencity studies. I said that if the FDA demanded carcinogenicity studies in non-rodent species, the only model that might be appropriate is the monkey. I do not think you can carry out studies in group sizes which are sufficiently large for the performance of appropriate statistical analysis. I do not think that 10 years is the life span of a monkey, and I feel that if one is performing a carcinogenicity study, it is essential to look at the life span of the animal species one uses.

DR. LIPSETT: Do you agree, Dr. McConnell?

DR. McCONNELL: Yes

DR. McKENZIE: I want to comment on the multistudies. Those studies were really not intended to be carcinogenesis studies. For sure, we have not considered the monkey studies carcinogenic studies; the number of animals would be inadequate and the duration would not be appropriate.

So, that is why I think the question was raised as to whether we should continue with the two year rat studies. Those would be carcinogenic studies, not the monkey studies.

DR. HEYWOOD: The monkeys studies were initiated at FDA's request and they were designated carcinogenicity studies. In my opinion, the dosage levels selected were wrong and the experimental periods inadequate.

DR. McKENZIE: Dr. Heywood referred to the tumors in the rat as being due to oral contraceptives. What we have seen is an increased incidence of nodular hyperplasia and I have no evidence that nodular hyperplasia is transformed to adenoma or carcinoma and don't know if there is any available evidence to show that. Furthermore, even in the epidemiological studies in man it is clear that the incidence (of these lesions) is relatively low. Last year at the Liver Symposium in Reston, Virginia, Dr. Burroughs from the Kentucky Medical Center, where there is a registry for oral contraceptive studies and are studying the liver, indicated that the incidence was less than one percent.

DR. GABELNICK: Dr. Heywood, you alluded to the problem that the ten year monkey studies really do not represent their lifetime. Is there any value in starting with older animals and looking at them for a shorter period of time?

DR. HEYWOOD: We are dependent on wild caught monkeys and do not know the age of these animals at the onset of our studies.

DR. GABELNICK: But now there are more colony bred animals available.

DR. HEYWOOD: The cost of breeding laboratory primates is very high. To breed them in sufficient numbers to the point of sexual maturity for the purpose of testing contraceptive steroids would impose phenomenal costs on industry.

DR. LIPSETT: I think we are going to have to move on. I would like to thank Dr. Heywood. Obviously there are many problems in this area and we haven't covered all of them.

ESTROGENS AND CARCINOGENICITY: AN OVERVIEW OF INFORMATION FROM STUDIES IN EXPERIMENTAL ANIMAL SYSTEMS

Benita S. Katzenellenbogen

Department of Physiology, Biophysics and Biochemistry
University of Illinois
Urbana, Illinois

INTRODUCTION

It has long been known that sex steroid hormones regulate the growth and differentiation of many normal reproductive tissues. This review will focus on the role of estrogen in several animal tumor systems. Information will be presented on the role of estrogenic hormones in tumor induction as well as their role as regulators of tumor growth and maintenance in a variety of relatively well characterized experimental animal tumor systems. In particular, an attempt is made to relate these effects on tumor induction and tumor maintenance to the general growth stimulatory effects of estrogenic hormones. The systems described include dimethylbenz(a)anthracene (DMBA)-induced mammary tumors in Sprague-Dawley rats, several other experimental mammary tumor systems that differ in their responsiveness to hormones, estrogen induced pituitary tumors in Fischer rats, estrogen induced Leydig cell tumors in Balb/C mice, and estrogen induced renal tumors in hamsters.

Estrogens are not easily categorized as standard inducers, cocarcinogens or promoters. Further, structure-activity relationships for estrogenic hormones suggest a good correlation between estrogenic potency measured as growth stimulation, and tumorigenicity. Hence if one compares the potencies of potent estrogens such as diethylstilbestrol and estradiol versus a weak estrogen such as estriol, there is a good correlation between the potency of these different estrogens in stimulating tissue growth, for example uterine weight gain, and the ability of these compounds to stimulate tumor development in various animal model systems.

ESTROGEN EFFECTS IN EXPERIMENTAL MAMMARY TUMOR SYSTEMS

The tumor system studied most intensively in analysis of estrogen and carcinogen interrelationships in induction of mammary tumors has been the dimethylbenz(a)anthracene-induced mammary tumor system in Sprague-Dawley rats, a system that was detailed initially by Charles Huggins and coworkers[1,2]. In this system, Sprague-Dawley female rats are treated at 45 to 50 days of age with the carcinogen dimethylbenz(a)anthracene (DMBA).

Usually over 90 percent of the animals will develop mammary tumors following carcinogen treatment and in most cases there will be multiple mammary tumors per rat.

It is of note that there are marked strain and species differences in susceptibility to mammary tumorigenesis by this carcinogen. Hence Sprague-Dawley rats, for example, are the most susceptible of various rat strains to the carcinogenic action of DMBA. In addition, the developmental stage of the mammary gland is critical for tumor induction. The mammary gland is most susceptible to carcinogenesis by DMBA when animals are approximately 45 to 50 days of age, that is, approximately two weeks after the animals have reached puberty and the mammary gland is undergoing extensive proliferation[1,2]. This proliferation very much depends on the hormonal status of the animal and it is quite clear that estrogenic and progestogenic hormones alter the mammary gland cells. The sensitivity to initiators such as DMBA appears to be related to the rate of proliferatio of these mammary gland cells[3]. It is clear that the ability of hormones to alter the mammary cell sensitivity to DMBA is not due to an effect of

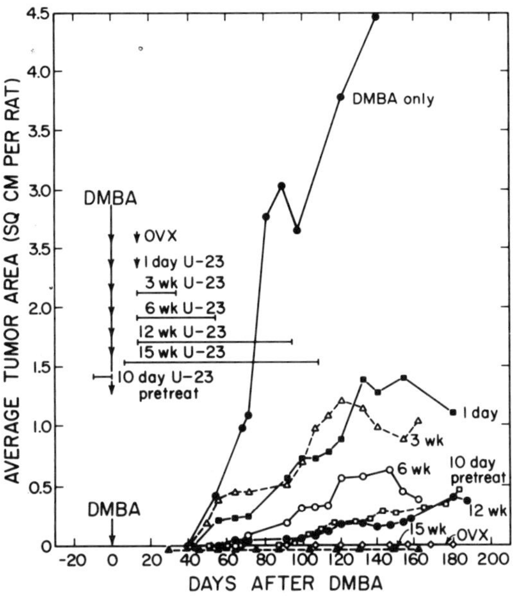

Figure 1. The influence of treatments on the development and growth of DMBA induced rat mammary tumors. Female Sprague-Dawley rats received DMBA at 47 to 50 days of age, and then following a two-week period, groups of rats were ovariectomized (OVX) or they received the antiestrogen U23,469 (U-23) injections of 250 μg/day either for one day or for 3, 6, or 12 weeks. Another group was pretreated with U23,469 for ten days before DMBA administration and another group received 15 weeks of U23,469 exposure starting at only one week after DMBA. There were 8-13 rats per treatment group and 58 rats in the control group. Values represent the average tumor area per rat of animals in these different treatment groups. (From reference 6).

hormones on altering the effectiveness of carcinogen activation. Rather, the effect appears to be one of changing the state of proliferation and the sensitivity of the mammary epithelial cells to the carcinogen.

In this mammary tumor system, carcinogen as well as endogenous estrogen is essential for tumor development. Neither carcinogen nor estrogen alone is effective in initiation of tumors[1-3]. Hence, estrogen is co-carcinogen-like in this tumor system: it appears to alter the effectiveness of the carcinogen. This may be by influencing the rate of mammary cell proliferation or possibly by reducing the efficiency of DNA repair, or by increasing error prone repair as related to the rapid proliferation of these cells. A similar situation is seen in carcinogen induced uterine endometrial tumors in rabbits where both carcinogen and the proper hormonal milieu are essential for tumorigenesis[4,5].

As mentioned above, the state of the mammary gland is critical for successful induction of mammary tumors with the carcinogen DMBA. Hence, if animals are ovariectomized shortly after DMBA exposure, essentially no tumors appear[1-3]. Likewise, if animals are pretreated with an antiestrogen prior to carcinogen administration, or if antiestrogen is given beginning shortly after carcinogen, tumorigenesis is suppressed markedly[6] (Figure 1).

The circulating estrogen concentration is also very important in induction of tumors in this DMBA-induced mammary tumor system. Hence when estrogen levels are very low due to ovariectomy, or if the effectiveness of circulating endogenous estrogen levels is antagonized by giving

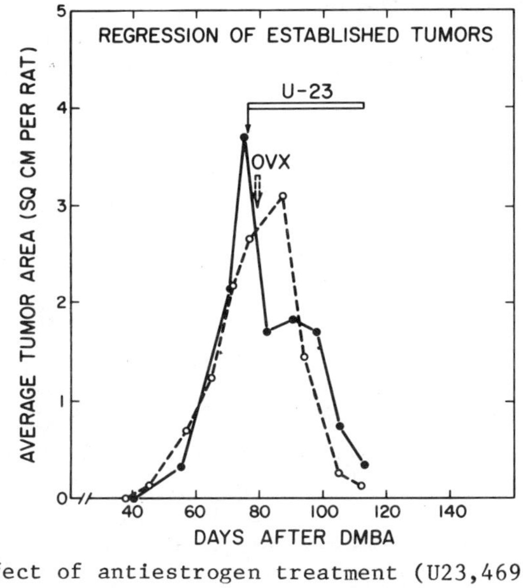

Figure 2. The effect of antiestrogen treatment (U23,469) or ovariectomy (OVX) on the regression of established tumors. At the time indicated (arrows) after DMBA treatment, animals (15 per group) received U23-469 injection (250 μg/day, 6 days per week) for 36 days or were ovariectomized and followed for 34 days. Values represent the average tumor area per rat for each group of 15 rats. (From reference 6).

antiestrogen, there is an extremely low incidence of tumor development. Physiologic estrogen concentrations are optimal for tumor development and when estrogen levels are in the physiologically normal range, i.e., those of mature cycling females, approximately 90 percent of animals will develop tumors. The effects of estrogen on tumor induction in this system appear to be mediated via the estrogen receptor system[7-11].

Another aspect of interest related to this DMBA mammary tumor system concerns the conditions required for maintenance of tumors after they develop. Approximately 90 percent of the tumors that appear in this system are hormone dependent for their growth. Animals require the presence of the ovaries as well as the pituitary (as a source of prolactin) for maintenance of tumor growth[7,12]. Hence one sees the effects of estrogens in this system at times far after carcinogen exposure. Estrogens are "growth regulators" here and the tumors require continuous estrogen not just one exposure for this maintenance. A similar situation is seen in some human breast cancers that are hormone dependent and, in these cases, removal of the estrogen source such as by ovariectomy or effective elimination of the estrogen effects by treatment with antiestrogen can very effectively extinguish these hormone dependent breast cancers[7,13].

Once tumors have become established in this DMBA mammary tumor system, regression of these tumors can be evoked by ovariectomy or by treatment with antiestrogen (Figure 2). In addition, and interestingly, regression of established tumors can also be evoked by treatment with very high, pharmacologic concentrations of estrogen[14]. Again, pharmacologic

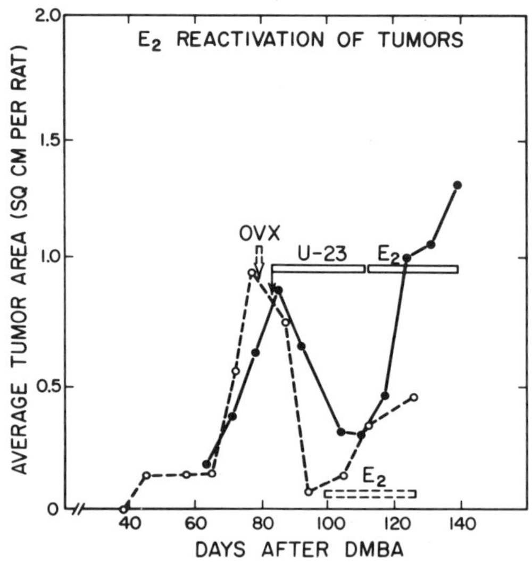

Figure 3. The ability of estradiol (E_2) to elicit regrowth of tumors caused to regress by antiestrogen treatment or ovariectomy. Animals received DMBA at 47 days of age, and at the time indicated (arrows) rats (6 per group) were ovariectomized or received U23,469 injections (250 μg/day) for 28 days, prior to administration of estradiol (5 μg/day) for 27 days. Values represent the average tumor area per rat for the six rats in each group. (From reference 6).

concentrations of estrogen also extinguish the growth of endocrine responsive human breast cancers[7,13]. Hence, using physiologic concentrations of estradiol, one can reactivate the growth of DMBA mammary tumors that had been caused to regress by ovariectomy or antiestrogen treatment (Figure 3).

It is important to note that there are significant interrelationships between estrogens and prolactin in this rodent mammary tumor system[7,10,12,14-18] Estrogens increase blood levels of prolactin and elevated prolactin levels are stimulatory to tumorigenesis in the DMBA mammary system[19]. Prolactin also increases the concentration of estrogen receptors in these tumors[20] and in the normal rodent mammary gland[21] thereby probably increasing the sensitivity of the mammary epithelium to estrogens. However, the role of prolactin in the etiology and growth regulation of human breast cancer is much less clear. Although many human breast cancers do contain prolactin receptors[18], the data at this time suggest a limited role, if any, for prolactin in human breast cancer[22,23].

A variety of experimental mammary tumor systems have been studied with interest because they differ in their extent of hormonal dependence (Table 1). Hence DMBA mammary tumors and nitrosomethylurea (NMU)-induced mammary tumors in rats show substantial dependence on the ovary for their growth and these tumors contain high levels of estrogen receptors[6,7,24] In the middle of this spectrum of hormone dependence is the R3230AC mammary tumor system in rats in which low levels of estrogen receptors are present[10,25]. In this tumor system, ovariectomy has no effect on the rate of tumor growth but high doses of estrogen as well as treatment with antiestrogens reduce but do not extinguish tumor growth (Figure 4). Estrogens and antiestrogens also modulate the activities of several enzymes in R3230AC mammary tumors[26,27]. At the opposite end of the spectrum are ovarian autonomous mammary tumors which have very low levels of estrogen receptor and which are totally autonomous of the ovary for their growth[12,28].

This spectrum of hormonal dependence in experimental mammary tumor systems is mirrored by that seen in the human situation. Human breast cancer also covers a spectrum from high estrogen receptor content and strong ovarian dependence to hormone responsive tumors which have low to intermediate levels of estrogen receptor, to totally hormonally independent tumors with low or nondetectable estrogen receptor content in which endocrine therapy has absolutely no effect on tumor growth[13]. Several adenocarcinoma cell lines derived from human breast cancers have been found to serve as good models for the spectrum of hormonal sensitivity

Table 1. Hormone-dependence in experimental mammary tumor systems.

DMBA rat	NMU rat	R3230AC rat	13762 rat	C_3H mouse
Ovarian Dependent	⟵		⟶	Ovarian Autonomous
High Estrogen Receptor				Low Estrogen Receptor

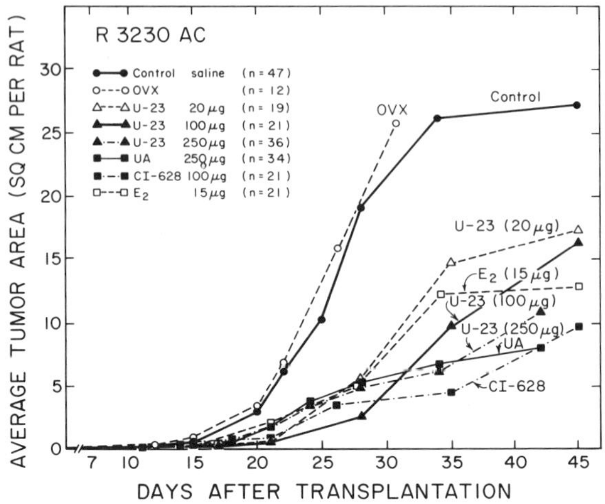

Figure 4. The influence of treatment with antiestrogens or estrogen on the growth of R3230AC mammary tumors. Tumors were transplanted into intact female Fischer 344 host rats, and, beginning on the day after tumor transplantation, rats received the indicated daily doses of antiestrogen or estradiol (E_2). In one group, tumors were transplanted into host rats that had been ovariectomized five days prior to the time of tumor transplantation (OVX). The antiestrogens utilized were U23,469 (U-23), U11,100A (UA), and CI-628. (From reference 10).

seen in human breast cancer. MCF-7 breast cancer cells have high levels of estrogen receptors and their growth is inhibited by antiestrogens such as tamoxifen; T47D cells have low levels of estrogen receptor and their growth is suppressed only slightly by antiestrogens; while MDA-MB-231 human breast cancer cells do not contain estrogen receptors and the growth of these cells is not altered by antiestrogen treatment[29] (Figure 5).

ESTROGEN EFFECTS ON TUMORS IN TISSUES OUTSIDE OF THE MAMMARY GLAND

There are several tumors arising in estrogen target tissues other than the mammary gland that have been extensively studied in experimental animal systems. One of the most interesting is the estrogen induced pituitary tumors that develop in certain strains of rats. Again, as seen in the DMBA-mammary tumor system, various strains of rats differ substantially in their sensitivity to carcinogenesis. Hence, Fischer 344 rats show a high incidence of pituitary tumors induced by estrogen administration while Sprague-Dawley Holtzman rats have a very low incidence of pituitary tumors even when estrogen is administered at high concentrations for a prolonged period of time[30-32]. It is of interest that these animals do not develop tumors in other estrogen target tissues such as the uterus or the mammary gland but that tumors appear exclusively in the pituitary gland. It is also of interest that, in Fischer 344 rats, estrogen appears to bring on at an early time susceptibility to pituitary tumors that normally develop spontaneously at a later stage in the life of these animals. Hence, Fischer 344 rats normally have a high spontaneous incidence of pituitary tumors later in life, while Sprague-Dawley Holtzman rats show a very low incidence of spontaneous onset of

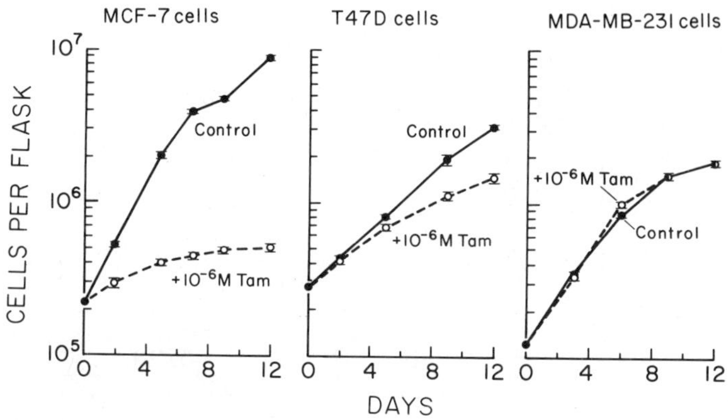

Figure 5. The effect of the antiestrogen tamoxifen (Tam; 10^{-6}M) on the growth of three different human breast cancer cell lines, MCF-7 cells, T47D cells, and MDA-MB-231 cells. Cells were grown in the continuous presence of the antiestrogen tamoxifen, and media with fresh tamoxifen were renewed every other day. On the days indicated, triplicate flasks of cells were counted. Values are the means of the triplicate determinations $\pm$ SEM. (From reference 29).

pituitary tumors throughout life. As documented by interesting studies of Wiklund and coworkers[30], when estrogen is administered to weanling Fischer 344 rats (Figure 6), the animals are very susceptible to the development of pituitary tumors. In these Fischer 344 rats, estradiol and diethylstilbestrol are equally effective in inducing pituitary tumors and tumors develop equally well in male and female animals. One may question in this system whether estrogens are indeed acting alone to induce pituitary tumors, whether the estrogen receptors in the pituitary tumors are somehow different from those in other estrogen target tissues, or whether the estrogen receptor system or pituitary-estrogen interaction may differ among different strains of rats and among animal species.

Another interesting system involves estrogen-induced Leydig cell tumors in inbred Balb/C mice. Implantation of pellets containing diethylstilbestrol results in the appearance of tumors at seven to 10 months after exposure to the estrogen. Transplantable tumor cell lines have been developed from these Leydig cell tumors, and interestingly, these transplantable tumor lines differ in terms of their responsiveness to estrogen although all were initially estrogen-induced[33-35]. Estrogens also induce renal tumors in hamsters[36-39]. Again, animal strains and species differ markedly in their susceptibility to tumorigenesis by estrogens. Adult castrated male Syrian hamsters given implants of diethylstilbestrol which release approximately 100 micrograms of DES per day, develop renal tumors after six to 12 months. Tumorigenesis can be inhibited by antiestrogens or by androgens[37].

Progestin enhanced development of mammary nodules and mammary tumors is documented in beagles[40]. Again, it is of note that beagles have a high spontaneous incidence of mammary nodules and dysplasias[40] and progestins appear to bring on at an earlier time, and at a higher incidence, mammary hyperplasia and tumorigenesis that would occur normally in many

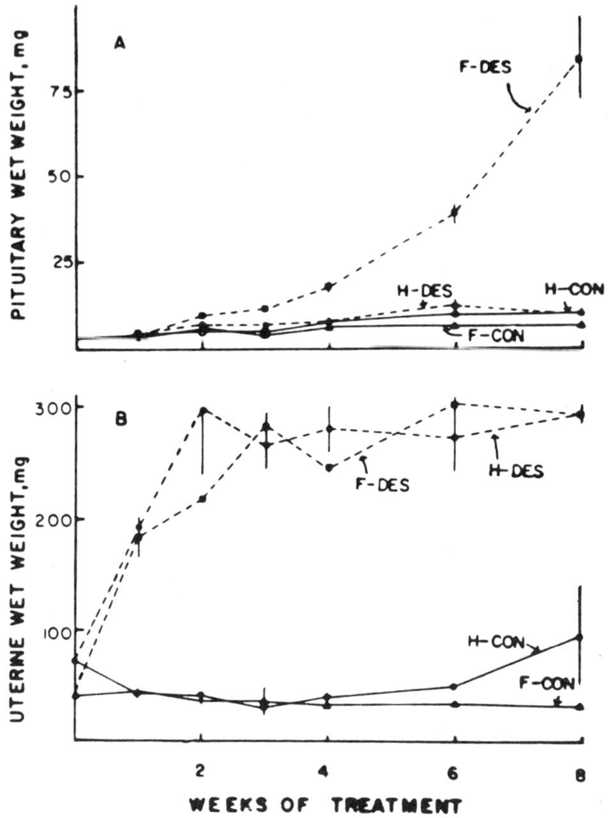

Figure 6. The influence of chronic diethylstilbestrol (DES) treatment on pituitary weight and uterine weight of Fischer 344 rats and Holtzman Sprague-Dawley rats. At zero time, weanling females were ovariectomized and given silastic tubing implants containing 5 mg. DES. At the indicated times, pituitaries and uteri were removed and weighed. Values represent the mean ± SEM of four animals. (From reference 30).

of these animals at a later stage of life.

CONCLUDING COMMENTS

It is clear that estrogens regulate the growth of some established tumors. This appears to be the case for both some experimental tumor systems as well as some human breast cancers which require estrogens for their growth and maintenance. In these tumors then, elimination of estrogen or overcoming the effects of estrogen by competition from administered antiestrogens can very effectively suppress further growth of the tumors and, in many cases, result in tumor regression or total disappearance of the tumor.

The mechanisms by which estrogens regulate the growth of established tumors are not completely understood but appear to involve the estrogen receptor system. Hence, tumors that contain high concentrations of estrogen receptors are the most responsive to treatment by endocrine therapy and it is only in these tumors that substantial benefits can be achieved by antiestrogen administration or other endocrine manipulations[13]. Exactly how estrogen normally stimulates growth of these tumors is not clear. Many of the effects of estrogen are likely mediated via the estrogen receptor system, and there is increasing evidence that estrogens may stimulate the production of critical growth factors termed estromedins[41,42] or conditioning factors[43]. It is possible that these factors may function as essential protein products stimulated by estrogens in rapidly proliferating cells.

In addition to regulating the growth of established tumors, estrogens play an important role in tumor reduction, at least in experimental animals. The role of estrogens in tumor induction in humans is much less clear (see refs. 23 and 44 for reviews). Of especial note, is the observation from animal studies of marked differences among strains and species of animals in susceptibility to hormone modulated carcinogenesis. It seems quite likely that a similar situation may exist among humans, with human subpopulations also differing considerably in their sensitivity to problems that may result from excessive hormonal exposure. In experimental tumor systems, the growth promoting effects of estrogens appear to alter the sensitivity of estrogen target cells to carcinogens. Hence endogenous estrogen appears to sensitize the mammary tissue to carcinogens such as DMBA. Likewise, exogenous estrogen may increase sensitivity to environmental carcinogens or viruses. Estrogen, in these systems, probably acts as a co-carcinogen; that is, it enhances the potency of a carcinogen, rather than acting as a classical carcinogen that reacts via activated metabolites with DNA. Although in *in vitro* systems, estrogen metabolites can be found attached covalently to DNA, the significance of this in terms of the quantity of reaction and the extent to which it occurs in the *in vivo* situation with stilbene and non-stilbene estrogens still needs careful evaluation[44]. The general parallelism that is observed between the growth promoting and "co-carcinogenic" effects of estrogens suggests a common mechanism via the estrogen receptor system of target cells.

ACKNOWLEDGEMENTS

Some of the studies described in this chapter were supported by United States National Institutes of Health Grants HD06726, CA18119 and CA31870.

REFERENCES

1. Huggins, C, Grand, LC, and Brillantes, FP: Mammary cancer induced by a single feeding of polynuclear hydrocarbons and its suppression. *Nature (London)*, 189:294, 1961.

2. Huggins, C, and Yang, NC: Induction and extinction of mammary cancer. *Science*, 137:257, 1962.

3. Dao, TL: The role of ovarian hormones in initiating the induction of mammary cancer in rats by polynuclear hydrocarbons. *Cancer Res*, 22:973, 1962.

4. Meissner, WA, Sommers, SC, Sherman, G: Endometrial hyperplasia, endometrial carcinoma, and endometriosis produced experimentally by estrogen. Cancer (Phila), 10:500, 1957.

5. Papadaki, L, Beilby, JOW, Chowaniec, J, Coulson, WF, Darby, AJ, Newman, J, O'Shea, A, and Wykes, JR: Hormonal replacement therapy in the menopause: a suitable animal model. J Endocrinol, 83:67, 1979.

6. Tasi, TL, Katzenellenbogen, BS: Antagonism of development and growth of 7,12-dimethylbenz(a)anthracene-induced rat mammary tumors by the antiestrogen U23,469 and effects on estrogen and progesterone receptors. Cancer Res, 37:1537, 1977.

7. McGuire, AL, Chamness, GC, Horwitz, KB, Zava, DT: Hormones and their receptors in breast cancer. In O'Malley, BW, Birnbaumer, L (Eds.): Receptors and Hormone Action, Academic Press, 1978, vol. 2, p 401.

8. Katzenellenbogen, BS, Bhakoo, HS, Ferguson, ER, Lan, NC, Tatee, T, Tsai, TL, Katzenellenbogen, JA: Estrogen and antiestrogen action in reproductive tissues and tumors. Recent Prog Horm Res, 35:259, 1979.

9. Katzenellenbogen, BS, Rorke, EA, Eckert, RL: Mechanisms of estrogen and anti-estrogen action in mammary cancer. J Steroid Biochem, 15:219, 1981.

10. Tsai, TS, Rutlege, S, Katzenellenbogen, BS: Antiestrogen modulation of the growth and properties of ovarian-autonomous and ovarian-dependent mammary tumors in rats. Cancer Res, 39:5043, 1979.

11. Horwitz, KB, McGuire, WL: Antiestrogens: mechanism of action and effects in breast cancer. Biological activities of antiestrogens. In McGuire, WL (Ed): Breast Cancer: Advances in Research and Treatment, New York, Plenum Publishing Corporation, 1978, vol. 2, p 155.

12. Segaloff, A: Hormones and mammary carcinogenesis. In McGuire, WL (Ed): Breast Cancer: Advances in Research and Treatment, New York, Plenum Publishing Corporation, 1978, vol. 2, p 1.

13. McGuire, WL: Steroid receptor sites in cancer therapy. Adv Internal Med, 24:127, 1979.

14. Kledzik, GS, Bradley, CJ, Marshall, S, Campbell, GA, Meites, J: Effects of high doses of estrogen on prolactin-binding activity and growth of carcinogen-induced mammary cancers in rats. Cancer Res, 35:621, 1975.

15. Leung, BS, Sasaki, GH, Leung, JS: Estrogen-prolactin dependence in 7,12-dimethylbenz(a)anthracene-induced tumors. Cancer Res, 35:621, 1975.

16. Heuson, JC, Waelbroeck, C, Legros, N, Gallez, G, Robyn, C, L'Hermite, M: Inhibition of DMBA-induced mammary carcinogenesis in the rat by 2 alpha-Br-ergocryptine (CB 154), an inhibitor of prolactin secretion, and by nafoxidine (U11,100A), an estrogen antagonist. Gynecol Invest, 2:130, 1971.

17. Manni, A, Trujillo, JE, Pearson, OH: Predominant role of prolactin in stimulating the growth of 7,12-dimethylbenz(a)anthracene-induced rat mammary tumor. Cancer Res, 37:1216, 1977.

18. Kelly, PA, Djiane, J, Gandilhon, P, Rosa, AAM, St-Arnaud, R: Prolactin and prolactin receptors in tumor development, growth and cellular functions. In Leung, BS (Ed): Hormonal Regulation of Mammary Tumors, Montreal, Eden Press, 1982, vol. 2, p 25.

19. Welsch, CW, Nagasawa, H: Prolactin and murine mammary tumorigenesis: a review. Cancer Res, 37:951, 1977.

20. Vignon, F, Rochefort, H: Regulation of estrogen receptors in ovarian dependent rat mammary tumors: effects of castration and prolactin. Endocrinology, 98:722, 1976.

21. Muldoon, TG: Interplay between estradiol and prolactin in the regulation of steroid hormone receptor levels, nature, and functionality in normal mouse mammary tissue. Endocrinology, 109:1339, 1981.

22. MacMahon, B, Cole, P, Brown, J: Etiology of human breast cancer: a review. J Natl Cancer Inst, 50:21, 1973.

23. Henderson, BE, Ross, RK, Pike, MC, Casagrande, JT: Endogenous hormones as a major factor in human cancer. Cancer Res, 42:3232, 1982.

24. Turcot-Lemay, L, Kelly, PA: Characterization of estradiol, progesterone, and prolactin receptors in nitrosomethylurea induced mammary tumors and effect of antiestrogen treatment on the development and growth of these tumors. Cancer Res, 40:3232, 1980.

25. Hilf, R, Michel, I, Bell, C, Freeman, JJ, and Borman, A: Biochemical and morphologic properties of new lactating mammary tumor line in the rat. Cancer Res, 25:286, 1965.

26. Hilf, R: The effect of the anti-estrogen, MER-25, on the estrogen-induced responses in growth and enzyme activities in the R3230AC mammary carcinoma of Fischer rats. Enzyme, 14:318, 1973.

27. Rorke, EA, Katzenellenbogen, BS: Comparative effects of estrogen and antiestrogen on enzyme activities in R3230AC rat mammary tumors and uteri of tumor-bearing animals. Cancer Res, 40:3158, 1980.

28. Bogden, AE: Therapy in experimental breast cancer models. In McGuire, WL (Ed): Breast Cancer: Advances in Research and Treatment, New York, Plenum Publishing Corporation, 1978, vol. 2, p 283.

29. Miller MA, Katzenellenbogen, BS: Characterization and quantitation of anti-estrogen binding sites in estrogen receptor-positive and -negative human breast cancer cell lines. Cancer Res, 43:3094, 1983.

30. Wiklund, J, Wertz, N, Gorski, J: A comparison of estrogen effects on uterine and pituitary growth and prolactin synthesis in F344 and Holtzman rats. Endocrinology, 109:1700, 1981.

31. Wiklund, J, Rutledge, J, Gorski, J: A genetic model for the inheritance of pituitary tumor susceptibility in F344 rats. Endocrinology, 109:1708, 1981.

32. Wiklund, JA, Gorski, J: Genetic differences in estrogen-induced deoxyribonucleic acid synthesis in the rat pituitary: correlations with pituitary tumor susceptibility. Endocrinology, 111:1140, 1982.

33. Sato, B, Huseby, RA, Samuels, LT: Characterization of estrogen receptors in various mouse Leydig cell tumor lines. Cancer Res, 38:2842, 1978.

34. Sato, B, Spomer, W, Huseby, RA, Samuels, LT: The testicular estrogen receptor system in two strains of mice differing in susceptibility to estrogen-induced Leydig cell tumors. Endocrinology, 104:822, 1979.

35. Sato, B, Maeda, Y, Noma, K, Matsumoto, K, Yamamura, Y: Estrogen binding component of mouse Leydig cell tumor: an in vitro conversion from nonreceptor to receptor-like molecule. Endocrinology, 108:612, 1981.

36. Kirkman, H, Bacon, RL: Malignant renal tumors in male hamsters (Cricetus auratus) treated with estrogens. Cancer Res, 10:122, 1950.

37. Li, JJ, Cuthbertson, TL, Li, SA: Inhibition of estrogen tumorigenesis in the Syrian golden hamster kidney by antiestrogens. J Natl Cancer Inst, 64:795, 1980.

38. Reznik-Schuller, H: Carcinogenic effects of diethylstilbestrol in male Syrian golden hamsters and European hamsters. J Natl Cancer Inst, 62:1083, 1979.

39. El-Etreby, MF, Graf, KJ: Effect of contraceptive steroids on mammary gland of beagle dog and its relevance to human carcinogenicity. Pharmac Ther, 5:369, 1979.

40. Sirbasku, DA, Benson, RH: Estrogen-inducible growth factors that may act as mediators (estromedins) of estrogen-promoted tumor cell growth. In Sato, G. Ross, D (Eds): Hormones and Cell Culture, New York, Cold Spring Harbor Laboratory Press, 1979, p 477.

41. Sirbasku, DA, Leland, FE: Growth factors for hormone-sensitive tumor cells. In Leung, BS (Ed): Hormonal Regulation of Mammary Tumors, Montreal, Eden Press, 1982, p 88.

42. Vignon, F, Derocq, D, Chambon, M, Rochefort, H: Les proteines oestrogenoinduites secretees par les cellules mammaires cancereuses humaines MCF7 stimulent leur proliferation. C R Acad Sci Paris, 296:151, 1983.

43. Hoover, R: Association of exogenous estrogens and cancer in humans. In McLachlan, J (Ed): Estrogens in the Environment, New York, Elsevier/North Holland Publishers, 1980, p 353.

44. Metzler, M, Gottschlich, R, McLachlan, JA: Oxidative metabolism of stilbene estrogens. In McLachlan, J (ED): Estrogens in the Environment, New York, Elsevier/North Holland Publishers, 1980, p 293.

DISCUSSION

DR. DAS GUPTA: Dr. Katzenellenbogen, your second slide was slightly perplexing because as the number one conclusion you said that hormone does not alter the effectiveness of carcinogens.

DR. KATZENELLENBOGEN: Do you mean the effectiveness of carcinogen activation?

DR. DAS GUPTA: And the next one you said that they altered effectiveness. Would you clarify?

DR. KATZENELLENBOGEN: Yes, I am sorry. The slide indicated that hormones do not act by altering the effectiveness of carcinogen activation to the DNA reactive form. Many carcinogens need to be activated to be biologically effective in reacting with DNA.

Hormones clearly alter the effectiveness of the carcinogen, which is why I consider them in many cases to be co-carcinogens, which enhance tumor production when a carcinogen is present. That this is by affecting the target cell and its state of proliferation or differentiation, and not by an effect on the DMBA itself in terms of whether the carcinogen is in a reactive or nonreactive form.

DR. DAS GUPTA: My second question is, do you feel that when promoted, estrogen is estrogen is estrogen, and when you say that probably certain actions are not being explained, that we relate it to the different responsiveness of estrogen receptors? Is it because we have less or inadequate knowledge of estrogen receptors? What is your view? Or would you like to generalize that estrogen is estrogen for biological effectiveness?

DR. KATZENELLENBOGEN: Your question has several aspects. I think that as far as we know, the estrogen receptors in different tissues are quite similar. The effect of the receptor interaction, in other words what end point is stimulated as a result of hormone binding to this receptor, can differ between species.

I believe it is modulated by the genetic susceptibility of that cell to appropriate or inappropriate DNA synthesis. In Fischer rats, for example, though the uterus grows very well in response to estrogen, it stops growing, whereas in the pituitary of those animals, the pituitary just keeps growing.

In both cases, the receptor system is active and has a similar affinity for estrogen. In fact, in Holtzman rats that do not get DES-induced pituitary tumors, estrogen stimulates prolactin production very well, so that having the cell respond to estrogen gives it, in a sense, the potential, perhaps to respond to other carcinogenic agents as well. But it is not alone, perhaps, sufficient.

DR. LIPSETT: I wonder if Jim Clark would agree, when we say an estrogen is an estrogen is an estrogen, this is somewhat of a simplification. We are really talking about strong estrogens because, as Dr. Clark showed, you get a variety of other factors that come into play in terms of receptor occupancy, the nucleus and receptor regeneration.

DR. KATZENELLENBOGEN: What I mean by an estrogen is an estrogen, which is similar to what Jim Clark means, is that biologically there is a spectrum of responses that will be evoked which is similar providing one has a biologically equivalent amount of compound. So, with estriol, for example, you may need 10 times as much, because it is cleared rapidly and has a lower affinity for receptor, but if you give 10 or 20 times as much estriol, it will evoke the same sequence of events that estradiol will.

DR. CLARK: I was just going to echo Dr. Katzenellenbogen's comments. The pharmacokinetic properties are just for receptor occupancy. Not only are the response profiles very similar, but the pathological profile is also very similar.

DR. SCHAFFENBURG: I think, since we are talking about animal models, it is very important to raise the question of prolactin in rats. If you induce prolactin elevation and then give a direct carcinogen, you inhibit the cancer, and the other way around. If the direct carcinogen is there first, and then you induce prolactin elevation by any number of means, you enhance the appearance of tumors.

The important thing is that prolactin is a luteotropic hormone in rats and works through the ovary, while in humans it is mostly not luteotrophic and such effects are probably not seen.

DR. KATZENELLENBOGEN: Yes, I agree with you completely. The prolactin effect in the human in terms of breast cancer is highly debatable.

DR. LIPSETT: The interesting thing about prolactin is that it is not a proliferative hormone as far as ductal epithelium is concerned.

DR. DICZFALUSY: Dr. Katzenellenbogen, in the DMBA-induced tumors, you stated that the pituitary is needed, so that pituitary function must be expressed in certain hormonal secretions or alterations. Do you have information on the role of prolactin or growth hormone in that species?

DR. KATZENELLENBOGEN: People consider prolactin to be very important in this tumor system and, again, estrogen and prolactin interact and modulate each other's level, so I think that prolactin probably is of importance here here in the DMBA system. The relevance of this model per se in terms of the prolactin component to the human situation, I think, is debatable, because in the human it is not clear that prolactin has a role.

Is this what you are asking?

DR. DICZFALUSY: Not exactly. You said that in the absence of the pituitary, DMBA did not induce mammary tumors, so that estrogen must have an effect on the pituitary. My question was, have you or anyone else measured relevant pituitary hormones and how they are changed when you administer the estrogen?

And I have kind of a second question in mind, if you answer the first one.

DR. KATZENELLENBOGEN: I guess what I should say is that in the absence of the pituitary, you can in fact induce tumors with the ovary alone. The tumors are not maintained as well without the pituitary.

It has been suggested that prolactin is the important agent and not growth hormone in this system. There have been interesting studies recently of human breast tumor cells transplanted into nude mice. The results suggest that estrogen as well as some pituitary factor is important in the stimulation of growth of these breast cancer cells. In this case it is clear that it is neither growth hormone nor prolactin which is important, but perhaps some as yet undescribed pituitary factor.

DR. LIPSETT: About 15 years ago Olaf Pearson demonstrated that hypophysectomy and subsequent administration of a prolactin antiserum could markedly diminish the effect of DMBA. That has been reported not only in the Sprague-Dawley rat, but also with the nitrosomethylurea-induced rat mammary cancer.

So, there is no question that prolactin is a very important hormone in the rodent with respect to the induction of mammary tumors. And, by the way, estrogen does increase prolactin in the rodent.

DR. DICZFALUSY: Does it also in the mouse?

DR. KATZENELLENBOGEN: Does estrogen increase prolactin?

DR. DICZFALUSY: In the mouse.

DR. KATZENELLENBOGEN: Yes. It does in humans, also.

DR. SCHUPPLER: I noticed you were very careful about the way you discussed the role of active metabolites and DNA. Have you any evidence that estrogens or, in particular, estrogen in any test system, really can classify as a genotoxic agent?

I have never heard estrogens to be mutagenic and they don't transform hepatocellular cells in culture. They are also negative in the Farber system and this applies to progesterone as well. So, I was wondering why you were so careful, or that was my impression any way, about that prospect.

DR. KATZENELLENBOGEN: Well, I have to say that I have not done any of these studies myself in terms of reactive metabolites of estrogens and their possibility in terms of DNA interaction. All I can say is what I understand of the literature.

I think Jim Clark had a slide with DES and all the various forms that can be generated.

Epoxides and other forms of estrogens associated with DNA in cultured cells under in vitro conditions have been identified. Now, whether these metabolites ever accumulate in significant levels in vivo, or when appropriately low levels of hormones are utilized, is unknown.

I think that many have the impression that estrogens very likely act directly by inflicting damage on DNA. My view is that this is highly unlikely. We can explain most of estrogens' actions on promotion and co-carcinogenesis by acting through the estrogen receptor system to modulate the physiology of that cell.

PROFESSOR VON EICKSTEDT: You demonstrated a good correlation between estrogenicity and tumor promoting effects. Since yesterday we heard that estrogens are estrogens, I would like to ask you, on which model, on which tissue, did you measure estrogenicity?

DR. KATZENELLENBOGEN: The estrogenic assay that I referred to is the uterotropic test, i.e., uterine weight gain in rats, and while one can argue with that, I think it is reasonably reliable.

PROFESSOR VON EICKSTEDT: You stated that receptors probably are important in these tumor-promoting effects. Shouldn't we then measure dose dependent estrogen effect on the receptors and not in any other organ?

DR. KATZENELLENBOGEN: I think that if one correlates receptor occupancy with uterotropic activity, the correspondence is really quite good. Compounds that interact with a receptor well and that occupy the receptor for a prolonged period of time evoke very good uterine weight gains.

PROFESSOR VON EICKSTEDT: Then, from my understanding, estriol should be either a weak or non tumor promoting estrogen.

DR. KATZENELLENBOGEN: Well, if you give it as just one injection every three days, it doesn't do very well. You see, again, the pharmacokinetic aspects that Dr. Clark mentioned and which both of us have studied, are of great importance. What you need to know is the biologically effective blood concentration.

PROFESSOR VON EICKSTEDT: Yes, but you remember we heard yesterday from Dr. Zbinden that you must give it all day to have steady state levels in the tissue.

DR. KATZENELLENBOGEN: Yes, but if you do that with estriol, it is very effective in tumor induction.

DR. CLARK: I would like to speak to the lack of specificity of the uterotropic assay which you just mentioned. I think that is an overstatement, because, as a matter of fact, androgens induce uterine growth and they are clearly not estrogens. You have to give enough androgen to the point that it illicitly occupies the estrogen receptor. When the estrogen receptor is occupied by an androgen, the uterus thinks it is an estrogen.

So, an androgen becomes an estrogen. In fact, the uterotropic assay is more specific than you might imagine and it does correlate very well with vaginal cornification, which we have also tested.

DR. GLOCKLIN: Perhaps you addressed this and I may have missed it, but I am concerned about sources of endogenous estrogen. Exogenous estrogens are likely to be at pharmacologic levels rather than physiologic, and DMBA is, after all, an environmental carcinogen.

DR. KATZENELLENBOGEN: I am sorry if I confused you. Looking at the growth promoting effect, we have to consider both the situation of both endogenous and exogenous estrogens, and from what we know of studies on endogenous estrogens physiologic levels are optimal perhaps, for sensitizing mammary tissue to various carcinogens.

In the case of exogenous estrogens, as one might see in menopausal replacement therapy, which has nothing to do with the DMBA system, it is just my impression that one would very likely expect this to increase the sensitivity of target tissues to other agents.

DR. PIKE: I just wanted to make a few comments about reactive metabolites. Of course, the most reactive metabolites in blood are those that come from cigarettes and you are absolutely riddled with them if you are a cigarette smoker. There is no question that cigarette smoking has nothing to do with breast cancer, except that it might reduce it by reducing your weight.

DR. KATZENELLENBOGEN: If I can just make a comment. I think that many of these reactive metabolites are very readily conjugated and excreted.

DR. PIKE: They are still reactive in the urine.

DR. LIPSETT: We will accept that they are all mutagens in the Ames test.

DR. PIKE: The other thing I would like to say is that all the evidence about prolactin in man is in not negative. It is just very complicated. You can quite easily show that young girls whose mothers have breast cancer have higher prolactin levels than normal girls, but that would appear to be because they cycle more regularly.

There are lots of case-controlled studies that show that premenopausal breast cancer cases have higher prolactin levels than normal women, although we are not exactly sure whether that isn't because of the actual disease.

But in postmenopausal women you can never find that and it would appear that this is an explanation for something that was raised yesterday about reserpine. Prolactin is not important in postmenopausal women, possibly because of the absence of progesterone. Studies on reserpine in postmenopausal women were just slightly positive and they were all just a bit above one.

We shouldn't ignore prolactin in that area. Thus far prolactin is only one criteria that might be responsible for the protection afforded by the first birth against breast cancer. Prolactin is the only hormone that we have found which is actually changed by having a baby.

After first birth, prolactin levels are permanently reduced. Estrogen or binding globulin levels are not reduced however, prolactin is reduced about a third and it seems to last for 10 years.

DR. KATZENELLENBOGEN: I would just comment, though, that I think people also believe that the high levels of estrogen during pregnancy may have a permanent effect on the morphologic and physiologic state of the breast, so that it may then reduce its sensitivity to other harmful agents as they come along later in life.

But both of these may be important.

DR. LIPSETT: I think we have to move on. I don't want to argue with Dr. Pike, because he is too adroit, but it has always interested me why so many epidemiologists interested in prolactin tend to ignore all the results on the phenothiazine derivatives, where we know that thousands of women have had higher prolactin levels and nobody has been able to demonstrate any sort of an increased risk.

A TWENTY YEAR SUMMARY OF FDA ANIMAL SAFETY TESTING OF CONTRACEPTIVE STEROIDS

Solomon Sobel

Center for Drugs and Biologics
Food and Drug Administration
Rockville, Maryland

I think it is useful to present a little history. In 1962, the Kefauver-Harris Amendments were enacted and a new approach to the drug approval process was implemented. That approach included a formalized investigational new drug application. As part of that program there were suggestions made that certain preclinical tests be performed before the Phase I studies of the IND could be initiated.

The manufacturers came to the FDA and said we are working under new stringencies. Please help us in telling us what you will consider as adequate preclinical tests. The Agency attempted to help but I don't know how grateful they have been for our assistance in this matter.

In general, while all drugs were provided with guidelines, the guidelines for steroidal contraceptives were unique.

I think we can all agree that steroidal contraceptives deserved a particular degree of stringency in evaluation. They are drugs given to healthy women for long periods of time to prevent a non-pathological condition.

The studies that we requested, which would be applied even to marketed steroidal contraceptives at that time, were the seven-year beagle studies, and the 10-year rhesus monkey studies. It was neither accidental nor arbitrary that the beagle was chosen as there was some history that influenced the decision. A study by one drug company had revealed a carcinogenic effect on the mammary glands in beagle dogs with a chloroethynyl derivative of norethindrone.

The beagle seemed to be a sensitive model, and we were looking for sensitive models. As far as the duration of testing, one may ask why did we choose seven years study in beagles and 10-years in monkeys.

This too was not arbitrary. Since the reproductive life of a woman spans approximately half of her life time, the Agency decided that it would be appropriate to choose half the life span for those test species.

We have developed a point of reference in these models. We have a 16 year experience in beagles. Before we discard them, we should consider modifying the studies and try to make them better models, but I don't think starting with an entirely new species is a good idea at this time.

We bracket the range of sensitivities with our models. In regard to carcinogenesis, we have a sensitive model in the beagle on the one hand, and a resistant model in the rhesus monkey on the other. The monkeys are known to be quite resistant to the development of reproductive tissue carcinomas; spontaneous endometrial and mammary carcinomas are rare.

Some of the speakers made a plea for more liberal release of information that we have in our files from drug companies. That, of course, is a legal question. It has become involved in the issue of new drug applications that are based on published studies. Companies are reluctant to release information that would jeopardize their proprietary interests in a drug and one of the means of maintaining this, is having information that is available only to the company, and not in the published literature.

So, the position of the pharmaceutical companies in the face of our system of drug approval is understandable from a strictly commercial standpoint.

I agree that it would probably serve the scientific community well to have free exchanges of ideas and information in all areas. I can assure you that if a serious safety issue should develop, we do have regulations that permit us to release otherwise privileged information.

Committee members who were present at our previous meeting know we had some specific problems which lead to this workshop. We anticipated the introduction of new contraceptives using old molecular entities in new delivery systems. For example, how does one consider a progestin in a silastic implant that gives certain levels in the blood that we have already studied quite well in animal models for years.

Does one require standard beagle and monkey testing, or does one consider the pharmacokinetics and apply previously obtained data from animal studies of the same molecular entity?

We have new esters of various progestins that are metabolized to drugs whose parent compounds we know very well. Does one mandate 7 and 10-year studies in this situation? One would think not.

Some of the Committee members asked what it takes to begin the various phases of clinical testing and perhaps it would be worthwhile to outline the requirements.

I don't think they are particularly stringent. For Phase I studies, that is the initial introduction into man usually limited to a few subjects for up to about 10 days of administration, we require 90-day studies in rats, dogs and monkeys. For Phase II studies, which is a limited introduction for actual clinical use in about 50 subjects for three menstrual cycles, we require the completion of one year studies in rats, dogs and monkeys. If one wishes to administer the drug for a single menstrual cycle, we require only a six month study in two species.

For Phase III, that is large-scale clinical trials, we require completion of two year studies in rats, dogs, and monkeys and, in addition, initiation of the seven year dog and ten year monkey studies.

Are there alternatives to the long range animal studies that the FDA can rely on for the preclinical assessment of safety of steroidal contraceptives? Certainly there are ancillary tests that would be helpful, but I don't think the complete animal model is likely to be displaced.

DISCUSSION

DR. ANDREWS: Dr. Sobel, thank you very much. Dr. Lipsett asked me if I would close. Are there any questions to be directed to Dr. Sobel?

DR. EDGREN: Just a practical consideration that I think the Committee will eventually have to cope with, and that is that a field trial of a new drug requires two year toxicological information in three species. From a practical consideration, these two-year studies would require at least a year to initiate, two years of treatment and somewhere between a year and two years to analyze the data and assemble an IND supplement. I think we are actually talking about four to five years from conception to final testing at that level.

DR. STADEL: Within a year or two we should have some data on Depo-Provera and cancer. If it doesn't confirm the anticipation of a large breast cancer increase, do you think the Agency would be prepared to abandon the dog?

DR. SOBEL: No, I don't think that would be a compelling reason. The dog model stands on its own in many areas besides primary tumor induction.

DR. STADEL: I was referring specifically to breast cancer.

DR. SOBEL: To breast cancer? I don't know. That certainly is a very sensitive model and I really can't say. We will just have to wait and see. As high quality epidemiological data come in on depo-medroxyprogesterone acetate, we certainly may reevaluate our interpretation of the model to some degree.

DR. KUZMA: I have been asked what will happen after the workshop. I think the intent of the question was what recommendations are we going to make and, more specifically, what is the FDA going to do with the recommendations. Underlying that question was, what is the attitude for willingness to change the perhaps old rules and guidelines. I wonder if you can say something about the attitude of willingness to change these, based on the information presented here.

DR. SOBEL: The Division looks favorably upon implementing modifications. I don't think one has to have a major change in policy on current testing to deal with some of the questions. We can keep our current animal testing system and yet make modifications on a case by case basis that permit us to facilitate development.

DR. ANDREWS: Thank you very much.

SECTION 3

EFFECTS OF CONTRACEPTIVE STEROIDS ON COAGULATION AND LIPID METABOLISM

Moderator: Heinz Berendes

INTRODUCTION

Heinz Berendes

Epidemiology and Biometry Research Program
National Institute of Child Health and Human Development
National Institutes of Health

Adverse health effects of contraceptive steroids resulting in an increased risk of several cardiovascular diseases are well documented and have been the subject of intensive investigation. Diseases of the cardiovascular system which have been linked to the use of contraceptive steroids include venous thrombosis, pulmonary embolism, thrombotic and hemorrhagic stroke, hypertension, subarachnoid hemorrhage and myocardial infarction. There is evidence that the relative risks of venous thrombosis, pulmonary embolism, and thrombotic stroke increase with the amount of estrogen in oral contraceptive formulations. This observation has led to a change of formulations containing 100 micrograms of estrogen to those with lower doses of estrogen like 50 or 35 micrograms. One study has reported that the relative risk of hypertension may depend upon the progestin dose.

Considerable attention has been focused on the design of studies to develop a better understanding of the pathogenetic mechanisms underlying the increased risks for certain diseases of the cardiovascular system associated with the use of contraceptive steroids. Such knowledge of the pathogenesis of these effects should be useful in developing new formulations of combination contraceptive steroids which may carry lower risks of adverse cardiovascular effects. We now know that combination contraceptive steroids effect blood coagulability by decreasing antithrombin III and also fibrinolytic activity. The resultant increased blood coagulability may underlie the known increased risk of venous thromboembolism among certain contraceptive steroid users. There is a good deal of evidence that oral contraceptives affect a number of factors associated with the process of atherogenesis. Combination oral contraceptives are associated with an increase in mean systolic and diastolic blood pressure, they have been shown to decrease glucose tolerance and, more recently, several investigators have reported a decrease in HDL cholesterol associated with the use of certain formulations of oral contraceptives, with some progestins in oral contraceptives in use producing a greater decrease than others.

How can we then improve the screening for possible adverse cardiovascular effects of new formulations of steroid contraceptives? Can a demonstrated effect of a given formulation of contraceptive steroids on one or more of these possible pathogenetic factors be used as a screen to identify formulations associated with a possible increased risk of adverse effects on the cardiovascular system? Do we know enough to say that formulations which decrease antithrombin III, decrease fibrinolytic activity, or which affect an increase in mean systolic and diastolic blood pressure and/or a decrease in HDL cholesterol are more likely associated with an increased risk of cardiovascular disease? If the evidence for the predictive value of these effects were compelling, and I'm not sure that it is, given our current state of knowledge, then effects on these various parameters of coagulation or on HDL fraction may be used as markers to identify contraceptive formulations which are potentially safer than those currently in use. Work currently in progress, some of which to be reported in this session, is addressing this question in a nonhuman primate model by testing different formulations of contraceptive steroids in terms of their effects on various lipoprotein fractions as well as on atherogenesis. It appears that this type of work is of paramount importance to identify animal models for screening of new formulations of contraceptive steroids to ascertain potential hazards to the cardiovascular system associated with their use. This should help settle the question as to whether effects on the cardiovascular system can be predicted by observing effects on lipoprotein fractions or other factors in the pathogenetic chain of events which would permit one to use such effects as markers for screening purposes both in animal models as well as in phase II studies.

It is a pleasure for me to preside over a session which brings together four distinguished investigators who will talk on the effects of contraceptive steroids on coagulation and lipid metabolism, addressing the question of atherogenesis in animal models, and also of the use of markers for screening of new formulations of contraceptive steroids.

CONTRACEPTIVE STEROIDS AND THROMBOSIS

Stanford Wessler

Department of Medicine
New York University School of Medicine
New York, New York

INTRODUCTION

This presentation will discuss two issues relevant to thrombosis and oral contraceptives. First, a definition of hypercoagulability and the evidence that compounds preventing ovulation induce an hypercoagulable rather than a thrombotic state, together with the laboratory and clinical implications of this distinction. Second, the demonstration of how an animal model has provided insights into an understanding of the relationships between thrombosis and oral contraceptives.

ESTROGENS, PROGESTINS, MIXED STEROIDS AND THROMBOSIS IN MAN

Most of the linkage of atherosclerosis and thrombosis with estrogens is epidemiologic in origin. The initial connection, based on the higher incidence of coronary heart disease in men, led to the thesis that endogenous estrogenic hormones in some manner protected women against atheroscelerosis, in the genesis of which the hemostatic process plays a role[1]. This inferred hormonal protective effect, coupled with the favorable results on coronary artery disease of exogenous estrogens administered to some experimental animals, suggested the use of these estrogens to prevent coronary heart disease in men. But exogenous estrogens given to men with prior myocardial infarction increased rather than decreased the risk of thromboembolism[2]. Similarily, exogenous estrogens in the treatment of advanced prostatic cancer resulted in increased arterial and venous thromboembolic phenomena and mortality[3]. Also to be noted was the high incidence of venous thromboembolism among women given diethylstibestrol to prevent postpartum lactation[4]. Not the least disturbing connection between sex hormones and thrombosis followed epidemiologic evaluation of the side effects of oral contraception.

Epidemiologic data can at best demonstrate an association and suggest a causal relation between a drug and disease[5]. In addition to this inherent limitation, epidemiologists were hampered, in examining the data on contraceptive use, by factors beyond their control: most importantly by low event rates, but also by soft clinical endpoints, meager autopsy data and frequent changes in the concentration and nature of the various steroids. Nevertheless, a clear association was established between oral contraceptive use and an increased incidence of venous thromboembolism[6,7], stroke[7-9] and acute myocardial infarction[10,11]. In addition, the data indicated that the frequency of these thrombotic episodes was increased for all categories by age[12], for venous thrombosis by surgery[13,14], and for arterial disease by cigarettes[11]. Less definitively, venous thromboembolism has been related, in a dose dependent manner, to the estrogen component of the drug[15-20]. More fragile is the intriguing suggestion that arterial thrombosis is a reflection of the progestin content of the mixed steroid[15,19,20], with its presumed facilitation of arterial thrombosis possibly related to the compound's capacity to decrease high density lipoprotein cholesterol[21,22].

No tissue is free from the influence of contraceptive steroids. These effects are manifest in carbohydrate, lipid and protein metabolism and involve liver, lung, bone, electrolytes, nerve and the cardiovascular system including hypertension and the mechanism of hemostasis[23]. It is to the effects of the hemostatic system that one turns for an interpretation of the connection between oral contraceptives and thrombosis.

THE HEMOSTATIC MECHANISM AND ORAL CONTRACEPTIVES

Vascular patency depends upon the balance of at least seven subtly interrelated systems, each by itself exceedingly complex: the endothelium and its subjacent structures including local and regional vascular differences, the platelets, the deformation and flow characteristics of blood within the circulation, vascular tone, the coagulation and fibrinolytic systems, and their plasma inhibitors. Alterations in the intricate interplay of these various parameters can result in either hemorrhage or thromboembolism.

Endothelium

The meager autopsy data concerning the coronary and cerebral arteries among women taking oral contraceptives indicate that these steroids increase the risk of occlusive vascular disease primarily by precipitating thrombosis rather than augmenting atherosclerosis. Proliferative intimal arterial lesions in autopsied women who received oral contraceptives have been described[24,25]. Since these changes were mainly in the pulmonary arteries, and since most of the cases also had pulmonary artery thrombi, the proliferative changes may have been secondary to thrombosis. Thus, any primary effect of oral contraceptives on endothelial morphology remains to be established.

Platelets

Early studies suggested that platelets of women taking oral contraceptives were more reactive than controls to a number of stimuli[26] but these findings have not been substantiated[27,28]. Nor has helpful data been derived from platelet survival experiments. New techniques including circulating platelet aggregates, radioimmunoassays for β-thromboglobulin and assays for platelet factor 4 are of great interest. A major limitation of the immunoassays is the uncertainty as to whether the rise in plasma levels is a primary or secondary event, as well as whether the rise truly occurs in vivo.

Vascular Tone and Rheology

Dilatation of peripheral veins is associated with oral contraceptive use diminishing vascular tone and contributing to venous stasis[29]. Retarded blood flow, itself unable to induce intravascular coagulation, does, however, facilitate the thrombotic process once initiated[30]. In areas of retarded flow thrombus formation is favoured in the plasma phase within the static red cell network because of at least six phenomena: 1) serine clotting proteases, including thrombin, are protected from dilution to subcritical concentrations, 2) nascent fibrin is prevented from premature dispersion, 3) liver clearance of activated species, is delayed, 4) the inflow of protease inhibitors is retarded, 5) the prostaglandin, PGI_2, is locally decreased, and 6) stasis profoundly alters the physical properties of a column of blood so as to predispose to fibrin formation. The only factors opposing thrombosis are fibrinolysis and the impaired influx of clotting procoagulants or zymogens. Stasis, therefore, can be viewed as a facilitator of thrombosis, once intravascular coagulation has been initiated.

There remains, then, in addition to stasis, the question of whether abnormalities among any of the plasma proteins and their cofactors involved in coagulation, fibrinolysis or the inhibition of either system can identify individuals who, before or after contraceptive use, are at risk of thrombosis.

Hypercoagulability

Since the articulation more than 300 years ago by the English physician Richard Wiseman[31], the concept of hypercoagulation has led a phantom like existence until recent times. For the recognition of hypercoagulation requires that a critical distinction be made; namely, between a perturbed, but partially contained system in which intravascular coagulation is occurring but has not yet progressed to actual thrombus deposition such as may be reflected by a rise in fibrinopeptide A or an increase in β-thromboglobulin on the one hand and an unperturbed system on the other hand in which the threshold resistance to thrombogenesis has been decreased, but intravascular coagulation has been initiated, such as occurs in congenital antithrombin III deficiency or impaired fibrinolysis. Some investigators would label all four examples as reflecting prethrombotic states and equate each with hypercoagulability. It can be suggested, however, that only the latter two be given such a designation. This view, moreover, leads to an operational and experimentally verifiable definition which claims that hypercoagulability represents a state of circulating blood in which intravascular coagulation has <u>not</u> been initiated, but requires a smaller quantity of clot promoting substance to induce intravascular coagulation than is required to produce comparable thrombosis in a normal subject. This definition has the additional advantage of categorizing retarded blood flow itself as an hypercoagulable state that operates not only on the venous side, where stasis is readily appreciated, but also in arterial circuits at normal bends and bifurcations as well as at areas of pathologic narrowing.

Stasis, therefore is not a unique mechanism for thrombus formation, as Virchow originally suggested in 1856[32] but is, itself, an example of a hypercoagulable state. It is no ordinary form of hypercoagulability, but rather the example par excellence because of the ubiquity with which retarded flow complicates so many of the thrombosis prone states, including those in users of oral contraceptives.

Coagulation

There is no clear evidence that anovulatory compounds are inducers of thrombotic states. Observation in three areas, coagulation, fibrinolysis and the serine protease inhibitors have suggested, however, that these steroids may function as facilitators of intravascular coagulation. In one study, by Gordon and colleagues, a marked elevation in Hageman Factor, functionally and immunologically associated with the modest increase in C1 inhibitor, was found in the menstrual cycle[33]. These data suggest that the increase in Hageman Factor may enhance in vitro fibrinolysis possibly abetted by diminished inhibitory control of C1 inhibitor. As the investigators themselves noted, however, the linkage of these findings to thrombosis, as with a host of other relevant clotting abnormalities[34-36], remains to be determined.

Fibrinolysis

Dryer et al knew from prior studies that in some women there was a preexisting state of impaired fibrinolysis[37]. Based on these observations they carried out studies suggesting that when such women received oral contraceptives, thrombosis might occur because the pretreatment defect was enhanced by anovulatory compounds through an as yet undefined abnormality attributable to the contraceptives[38].

Protease Inhibitors

In the third area, plasma inhibitors of coagulation, Gitel and associates[39] demonstrated a change in the coagulation inhibitory reaction rate associated with the use of contraceptive compounds. I should like to describe some of Gitel's findings, for they led to the demonstration, by animal model, that oral contraceptives do, in that fact, cause an hypercoagulable state.

Of the several known plasma inhibitors of coagulation, antithrombin III is, by far, the most effective in protecting against thrombosis. Antithrombin III, an α_2 globulin of 62000 daltons, present in human plasma at a concentration of 20 mg/dl, neutralizes most clotting protease at a 1:1 molar ratio of enzyme active site to inhibitor.

Since it is known that patients with congenital deficiencies in antithrombin III are highly susceptible to thrombosis, Gitel chose to determine, by separate coagulation assays, whether women taking oral contraceptives had either a diminished quantity of antithrombin III or a retardation of the rate at which this inhibitor neutralizes clotting proteases.

Plasma samples were obtained at Bellevue Hospital from 57 women receiving oral contraceptives all containing 50μg of ethinyl estradiol, and from 48 women who were using intrauterine devices. There was no difference in the quantity of antithrombin III between the two groups. In contrast, the mean reaction rate between the plasma and the clotting protease, activated Factor X (for which the term Xa inhibitory activity will be used hereafter) was significantly decreased ($p \leq 0.001$) among women taking oral contraceptives compared to their controls[39].

So far, so good. But really neither very far nor very good, for what is the evidence that a depression in Xa inhibitory activity reflects an increased risk of thrombosis? None of the 57 Bellevue women on oral contraceptives had experienced clinical thrombosis moreover the majority had normal Xa inhibitory activities. And since the event rate of clinical thrombosis in this population would be expected to be low, it would be an Herculean task to mount a clinical trial to establish a positive relationship.

THE ANIMAL MODEL AND Xa INHIBITORY ACTIVITY

Accordingly, our laboratory decided it would be more practical to address the question in an animal model with which we had previously obtained correlations between drugs and thrombosis. Our model can be defined as a living animal in which an artificial pathologic process is induced that in one or more respects closely resembles the same phenomenon occurring in man. Such a model can never provide final answers, but can offer only approximations for no single animal model can ever duplicate a disease in man. Thus, while it should not be expected to be ideal and suitable for all foreseeable purposes, to be useful at all, it must provide a new insight, have relevance to a particular problem and respond predictably[40].

Technique

Granted these constraints, let me briefly describe the method[41]. A rabbit jugular vein is freed from its surrounding structures, and if a thrombogenic substance such as a clotting protease is injected into a contralateral ear vein, there forms a thrombotic cast of the isolated segment. That this cast resembles a typical red thrombus is confirmed by scanning electron micrography to be morphologically indistinguishable from a human venous thrombus, where are seen erythrocytes enmeshed in a network of spaghetti-like fibrin strands with only an occasional platelet visualized.

This type of thrombus can also be produced in arteries and atrial appendages[42] and embolized, fresh or aged in predetermined lengths, from leg veins to pulmonary arteries[43,44] or from central sites to peripheral systemic arteries[42]. In addition to rabbits, the model has been sucessfully employed (though not for studies of oral contraceptives) in mice, rats, guinea pigs, hamsters, cats, dogs, birds, rhesus monkeys and baboons. In regard to the relative quantities of clotting zymogens, the baboon most resembles man among the non human primates. The model has also been employed in human volunteers[45].

Various sizes of thrombi can be produced in the model. If one injects lesser amounts of protease than the quantity necessary to induce the thrombus that forms a cast of the isolated segment (a score 4 thrombus), score 3, 2, or 1 thrombi can be obtained, and if the quantity of infusate is sufficiently reduced, no thrombus will form. Despite its apparent crudity, quantitative relationships can be realized. Thus, a linear plot of the log purified thrombin infused, in µg quantities, against the resulting average thrombotic score indicates that a 100 percent increase in the amount of thrombin infused is required to raise a score 1 to a score 2 thrombus. To raise a score 2 to a score 3 thrombus, an additional 40 percent increase in thrombin is required[46].

Oral Contraceptives

To apply this model to oral contraceptives, rabbits were fed either of two doses of a mixture of 0.5 mg norgestrel and 50 µg ethinyl estradiol. Bloods were obtained for determinations of thrombin times and both the quantity and reactivity of antithrombin III. The amount of thrombin was so selected that infusates would result in a score 2 thrombus in untreated animals. Thus, if oral contraceptives had no effect on thrombus formation, treated animals would also yield a score 2 thrombus; if the compounds had an anticoagulant effect, score 1 or score 0 thrombi would result, but, if score 3 or 4 thrombi were produced, it would indicate that the contraceptives caused an enhancement in thrombogenicity.

Three groups of rabbits were tested over a seven week period: controls, a low dose group (0.8 μg estrogen/kg), and a high dose cohort (2.5 μg estrogen/kg). There was no difference between the thrombin times of the control rabbits and those given either dose of oral contraceptives throughout the experiment. This indicated that the compounds neither accelerated nor inhibited the thrombinfibrinogen reaction. For all three groups the quantity of antithrombin III also remained unchanged. However, Xa inhibitory activity was depressed by contraceptives in dose dependent manner. In the low dose group there was a slight, but nevertheless significant, decrease in Xa inhibitory activity, whereas in the high dose group this decrease was more marked[47].

Correlations were also obtained between Xa inhibitory activity and the average thrombotic score for the three groups. The control group exhibited 100 percent Xa inhibitory activity and score 2 thrombi, the low-dose group a significantly but slightly depressed Xa inhibitory activity and a higher thrombotic score than the control group; whereas the high-dose cohort revealed an even more marked depression of Xa inhibitory activity and still higher thrombotic score[47].

One additional finding of clinical relevance was obtained. In still another group of rabbits, on a higher dose estrogen regimen, that was given five units of heparin/kg immediately prior to thrombin infusion, Xa inhibitory activities and thrombotic scores after heparinization were indistinguishable from the controls[47].

Additionally, four rabbits on high dose contraceptives, all with significant decreases in Xa inhibitory activity and four control rabbits with normal Xa inhibitory activity were subjected to the stasis assay in which saline was substituted for thrombin as the infusate. In none of the eight animals was a stasis thrombus formed[47]. These control experiments demonstrate the contraceptive treated rabbits, despite a marked decrease in Xa inhibitory activity, do not form thrombi in the absence of a thrombogenic stimulus, an observation consistent with the fact that the vast majority of women on oral contraceptives and without other risk factors for thrombosis, rarely develop intravascular coagulation.

Tobacco

The exploitation of the animal model was taken one step further by examining, in preliminary experiments, the connection between smoking and oral contraceptives. Becker, et al had isolated, from cured tobacco leaves and tobacco smoke condensate, a glycoprotein with the capacity in vitro to activate the clotting zymogen, Hageman Factor[48]. In the model, infusates of this glycoprotein produced a low grade thrombogenicity (score 1-2). If, however, female rabbits on oral contraceptives were infused with tobacco glycoprotein, the average thrombotic score was doubled[49].

RELEVANCE OF Xa INHIBITORY ACTIVITY TO THROMBOSIS IN MAN

We had asked two further questions, answers to which were only forthcoming after the experiments just summarized were undertaken: 1) is there any evidence in man that a normal quantity of antithrombin III with a depressed Xa inhibitory activity represents a hypercoagulable state, and 2) do estrogens alone depress Xa inhibitory activity?

Congenital

In one report, a Danish family was described in which four of seven members studied developed venous thromboembolism. All seven had normal quantities of antithrombin III, but marked decreases in Xa inhibitory activity without other associated hemostatic abnormalities[50]. The values in the Danish subjects were comparable to the depressed levels of Xa inhibitory activity noted among some of the Bellevue women on oral contraceptives.

Premenopausal

In a report from Great Britain, 37 young women subjected to relatively minor abdominal surgery, such as appendectomy, were followed postoperatively by ^{125}I limb scanning. Six of 22 on oral contraceptives developed deep venous thrombosis by scan though not clinically, and all six had preoperative Xa inhibitory activities at or below 60 percent by our assay method. Deep venous thrombosis did not develop in the 16 remaining women on contraceptives nor in any of the 15 matched controls, and all 31 of these two latter groups had normal Xa inhibitory activities[51].

Postmenopausal

The second question was addressed in our laboratory by measuring Xa inhibitory activity in three groups of postmenopausal women: one receiving no estrogen, another on low doses of conjugated estrogens (0.625 - 1.25 mg/day) and the third receiving high doses of conjugated estrogens (2.5 mg/day). Xa inhibitory activity was depressed in both of the latter two groups in a dose dependent manner[52].

CONCLUSIONS FROM MODEL RELEVANT TO ORAL CONTRACEPTIVES

The hazards involved in transferring to man inferences from the data obtained in the animal studies just reviewed is epitomized by the English novelist Samuel Butler's 1912 statement: "Life is the art of drawing sufficient conclusions from insufficient premises"[53]. With this epigramatic message in mind, allow me to suggest that the animal model data support the following four conclusions.

(1) The estrogenic content of oral contraceptives, while not itself thrombogenic, aggravates the thrombotic process once intravascular coagulation has been initiated. This statement is consonant with the definition of hypercoagulability stated earlier. In short, oral contraceptives, like retarded blood flow, alter the normal hemostatic balance such that after a thrombotic challenge, as from surgery or cigarette smoking, intravascular coagulation is favored.

(2) The extent to which hypercoagulability is augmented by oral contraceptives is reflected in the extent to which Xa inhibitory activity is depressed.

(3) Heparin's primary anticoagulant action is to accelerate the rate of reaction between antithrombin III and clotting proteases. When the drug is injected in trace quantities into high dose oral contraceptive treated rabbits, both Xa inhibitory activity and thrombotic scores return to control levels even though the whole blood clotting times and the partial thromboplastin times remain within the normal range. This finding is in accord with the clinical observation that patients on oral contraceptives, whose risk of venous thromboembolism is increased six fold over controls when subjected to surgery[14], have that portion of their increased risk of post operative thrombosis attributable to the anovulatory agent, eliminated by a regimen of low dose heparin[51]. In fact, it provides further justification for the prophylactic use of low dose heparin regimens in women on oral contraceptives who are subjected to abdominal or thoracic surgical procedures.

(4) Aside from supporting the epidemiologic data indicating that older premenopausal women on oral contraceptives are at increased risk of acute myocardial infarction if they are also cigarette smokers, the data further suggest a mechanism whereby this untoward result may be precipitated. For, while the tobacco protein is activating Hageman Factor, thereby initiating a low grade state of intravascular coagulation, the contraceptives are simultaneously inducing a hypercoagulable state that, by decreasing the reactivity of antithrombin III, enhances the thrombogenicity caused by the tobacco glycoprotein.

Clotting abnormalities other than Xa inhibitory activity may also reflect a hypercoagulable state among women on oral contraceptives. Proof of such a relationship, however, will require studies in man or in animals correlating the abnormality in the clotting system with the development of thrombosis. The major difficulty of obtaining this proof in man, in the absence of other risk factors, is the low event rate of thrombosis among oral contraceptive users, necessitating large scale clinical trials, reason enough to utilize this or another animal model, aside from the issue of feasibility, rights of individuals and cost effectiveness.

Sensitivity and Specificity

The model can recognize, by the intravenous or oral route, inciters, inhibitors or facilitators of thrombosis. Its sensitivity is reflected in the finding that infusions of as little as 0.04 nmols of activated Factor X or 2 picomols of activated Factor IX are thrombogenic[46]. Specificity is demonstrated by the fact that the duration of hypercoagulability induced by infusions of phospholipids depends on their lipid composition and surface potential. Thus, phosphatidylserine is active alone or when mixed with phosphatidylcholine, phosphatidylethanolamine or cetyltrimethylammonium bromide with the optimal proportion of phosphatidylserine being 35 percent of the total lipid corresponding to a surface potential of -80 millivolts. In contrast, no thrombotic potentiation was noted with infusions of mixtures of phosphatic acid with either phosphatidylethanolamine or phosphatidylcholine[54].

Effects of Other Substance in the Model

Several other agents have been found to be positive in the model. These include serum[41], tissue thromboplastin[55], tryspin[56], ellagic acid[57], activated clotting factors XII, XI, IX, X and II[46], saturated and unsaturated long chain fatty acids (C_{14}-C_{22})[58], endotoxin[59], Factor IX concentrates[60], and 6-azauridine[61].

Substances failing to initiate or facilitate thrombosis include saline[47], plasma[42], clotting zymogens[62], short chain fatty acids (C_6-C_{12})[58] and activated Factor VII[55]. This activated species (VIIa), even though it is a serine protease, does not fool the model because to initiate coagulation VIIa requires a co-factor, tissue thromboplastin, that does not normally enter the circulation and hence infusions of VIIa are inert. To date there have been no known false positives or false negatives.

SUGGESTIONS FOR FUTURE STUDIES

Three separate investigations can be suggested that may have different interests for investigators in hemostasis, regulatory agencies, population study groups and the pharmaceutical industry.

The first is directed towards elucidating the mechanism whereby oral contraceptives depress Xa inhibitory activity, determining why it is depressed in only some women and, as a corollary, automating the assay procedure and employing it in conjuction with studies involving plasma levels of steroid metabolites and cholesterol related lipids.

The second type of study is suggested by the likelihood that the versatility of the model would be further enhanced by examining with light and electron microscopy, histopathologic sections of vessels from within and without the occluded arteries and veins of treated and control animals. The third, and perhaps the most immediately relevant experiment relates to the fact that the ability of the current model to detect minor change in thrombosis is limited by the nonparametric nature of the scoring procedure. Since a given score, except for 0 or 4, can cover a range of thrombus sizes, it becomes a judgmental decision, when assigning a size to a thrombus that is between any two scores. The only method presently of overcoming this inherent limitation is by blinding the observer responsible for scoring and employing a large number of animals. This presents a particularly difficult situation with thrombogenic substances that initiate only small thrombi, even when large quantities of clot initiator are employed, yet scores greater than 1 cannot be obtained.

This limitation can be resolved, however, by altering the model so that the endpoint is determined isotopically rather than by gross visual inspection. In this manner, the extent of thrombus formation would be measured by the ratio of thrombus weight to segment volume using ^{125}I labelled fibrinogen and obtaining thrombotic dose response curves providing a broader and more discrete scale of thrombotic potential.

If this latter goal were to be achieved, and mice or rats were substituted for rabbits, an extremely effective, rapid and inexpensive screen would be available to test minor modifications on either the dose or clinical structure of steroid sex hormones for their thrombotic potential prior to their entry into clinical trials. On the basis of available data, this proposed modification would provide a better predictor of thrombogenicity than any assay currently available to predict mutagencity or carcinogenicity with regard either to sensitivity or specificity.

SUMMARY

An animal model has demonstrated that oral contraceptives induce a dose dependent, hypercoagulable, rather than a thrombotic, state that is reflected in a depression of the reaction rate between the plasma inhibitor, antithrombin III, and the clotting protease, activated factor X. This model mimics many of the findings in man induced by oral contraceptives. With minor modifications, the model could become an effective screen for the recognition of the potential thrombotic hazard, or lack therof, of newly developed steroid contraceptives.

REFERENCES

1. Chandler, AB, Eurenius, K, McMillan, GC, Nelson, CB, Schwartz, CJ, Wessler, S (Eds): The Thrombotic Process in Atherogenesis. New York, Plenum, 1978.

2. The Coronary Drug Project Research Group: The coronary drug project. Findings leading to discontinuation of the 2.5 mg/day estrogen group. JAMA, 226:652, 1973.

3. The Veterans Administration Co-operative Urological Research Group: Treatment and survival of patients with cancer of the prostate. Surg. Gynec Obstet, 124:1011, 1967.

4. Daniel, DG, Campbell, H, Turnbull, AC: Puerperal thromboembolism and suppression of lactation. Lancet, 2:287, 1967.

5. MacMahon, B: Strengths and limitations of epidemiology. In: The National Research Council in 1979: Current Issues and Studies. Washington, D.C. National Academy of Sciences, p 91, 1979.

6. Vessey, MP, Doll, R: Investigation of relation between use of oral contraceptives and thromboembolic disease. A further report. Brit Med J, 2:651, 1969.

7. Sartwell, PE, Masi, A, Arthes, FG, Greene, GR, Smith, HE: Thromboembolism and oral contraceptives: an epidemiologic case-control study. Am J Epidemiology, 90:365, 1969.

8. Bickerstaff, ER: Neurological complications of oral contraceptives. Oxford, Clarendon Press, 1975.

9. Jick, H, Porter, J, Rothman, KJ: Oral contraceptives and nonfatal stroke in healthy young women. Ann Int Med, 89:58, 1978.

10. Inman, WHW, Vessey, MP: Investigation of deaths from pulmonary coronary, and cerebral thrombosis and emobolism in women of child-bearing age. Brit Med J, 2:193, 1968.

11. Mann, JI, Vessey, MP, Thorogood, M, Doll, R: Myocardial infarction in young women with special reference to oral contraceptive practice. Brit Med J, 2:241, 1975.

12. Tietze, C, Lewit, S: Mortality and fertility control. Internat J Gynec Obstet, 15:100, 1977.

13. Vessey, MP, Doll, R, Fairbairn, AS, Glober, G: Postoperative thromboembolism and the use of oral contraceptives. Brit Med J, 3:123, 1970.

14. Greene, GR, Sartwell, PE: Oral contraceptive use in patients with thromboembolism following surgery, trauma or infection. Am J. Pub Health, 62:680, 1972.

15. Inman, WHW, Vessey, MP, Westerholm, B, Engelund, A: Thromboembolic disease and the steroidal content of oral contraceptives: a report to the Committee on Safety of Drugs. Brit Med J, 2:203, 1970.

16. Royal College of General Practitioners: Oral Contraceptives and Health. An interim report from the oral contraceptive study of the Royal College of General Practitioners, London, Pitman, 1974.

17. Stolley, PD, Tonascia, JA, Tockman, MS, Sartwell, PE, Ruttledge, AH, Jacobs, MP: Thrombosis with low-estrogen oral contraceptives. Am J Epidemiology, 102:197, 1975.

18. Meade, TW, Greenberg, G, Thompson, SG: Progestogens and cardiovascular reactions associated with oral contraceptives and a comparison of the safety of 50 and 30μg estrogen preparations. Brit Med J, 280:1157, 1980.

19. Bottiger, LE, Boman, G, Eklund, G, Westerholm, B: Oral Contraceptives and thromboembolic disease: effects of lowering oestrogen content. Lancet, 1:1097, 1980.

20. Kay, CR: The happiness pill? J Royal Coll Gen Pract, 30:8, 1980.

21. Bradley, DD, Wingerd, J, Petitti, DB, Kraus, RM, Ramcharan, S: Serum high-density-lipoprotein cholesterol in women using oral contracepives, estrogens and progestins. New Engl J Med, 299:17, 1978.

22. Wahl, P, Walden, C, Knopp, R, Hoover, J, Wallace, R, Heiss, G, Rifkind, B: Effect of estrogen/progestin potency on lipid/lipoprotein cholesterol. New Engl J Med, 308:862, 1983.

23. Salhanick, HA, Kipnis, DM, Vande Wiele, RL (Eds): Metabolic Effects of Gonadal Hormones and Contraceptive Steroids, New York, Plenum Press, 1969, p 1.

24. Irey, NS, Manion, WC, Taylor, HB: Vascular lesions on women taking oral contraceptives. Arch Path, 89:1, 1970.

25. Irey, NS, Morris, HJ, Intimal vascular lesions associated with female reproductive steroids. Arch Path, 96:227, 1973.

26. Johnson, M, Ramey, E, Ramwell, PW: Sex and age differences in human platelet aggregation. Nature 253:355, 1975.

27. Tsao, CH, Lo, R, Raymond, J: Critical importance of citrate-blood ratio in platelet aggregation studies. Am J Clin Path, 65:518, 1976.

28. Kelton, JG, Powers, P, Julian, J, Boland, V, Carter, CJ, Gent, M, Hirsh, J: Sex-related differences in platelet aggregation: influence of the hematocrit. Blood, 56:38, 1980

29. Goodrich, SM, Wood, JE: Peripheral venous distensibility and velocity of venous blood flow during pregnancy or during oral contraceptive therapy. Am J Obstet Gynec, 90:740, 1964.

30. Wessler, S: The role of stasis in thrombosis. In: Sherry, S, Brinkhous, KM, Genton, E, Stengle, J, (Eds): Thrombosis, Washington, D.C., National Academy of Sciences, 1969, p 461.

31. Wiseman, R: Several Chirurgical Treaties, 2nd edition, London, Norton and Macock, 1686, p 64.

32. Virchow, R: Gesammelte Abhandlungen zur Wissenchaftlichen Medicin, Frankfurt, Meidinger, Sohn, 1856, p 219.

33. Gordon, EM, Ratnoff, OD, Saito, H, Donaldson, VH, Pensky, J, Jones, PK: Rapid fibrinolysis, augmented Hageman Factor (factor XII) titers, and decreased C1 esterase inhibitor titers in women taking oral contraceptives. J Lab Clin Med, 96:762, 1980.

34. Ambrus, JL, Mink, IB, Courey, NG, Niswander, K, Moore, RH, Ambrus, CM, Lillie, MA: Thromboembolic complications of oral contraceptive therapy. Res Comm Chem Pharm Path Pharm, 10:197, 1975.

35. Carvalho, ACA, Vaillancourt, RA, Cabral, RB, Lees, RS, Colman, RW: Coagulation abnormalities in women taking oral contraceptives. JAMA, 237:875, 1977.

36. Poller, L: Oral contraceptives, blood clotting and thrombosis. Brit Med Bull, 34:151, 1978.

37. Williams, RS, Logue, EE, Lewis, JL, Barton, T, Stead, MW, Wallace, AG, Pizzo, SA: Physical conditioning augments the fibrinolytic response to venous occlusion in healthy adults. New Eng J Med, 302:987, 1980.

38. Dreyer, NA, Pizzo, SV: Blood coagulation and idiopathic thromboembolism among fertile women. Contraception, 22:123, 1980.

39. Wessler, S, Gitel SN, Wan, LS, Pasternack, BS: Estrogen-containing oral contraceptive agents; a basis for their thrombogenicity. JAMA, 236:2179, 1976.

40. Frenkel, JK: Choice of animal models for the study of disease processes in man. Fed Proc, 28:160, 1969.

41. Wessler S, Reimer, SM, Sheps, MD: Biologic assay of a thrombosis inducing activity in human serum. J Appl physiol, 14:943, 1960.

42. Wessler, S, Reiner, L, Freiman, DG, Reimer, SM, Lertzman, M: Serum-induced thrombosis. Studies of its induction and evolution under controlled conditions in vivo. Circulation, 20:864, 1959.

43. Wessler, S, Freiman, DG, Ballon, JD, Katz, JH, Wolff, R, Wolf, E: Experimental pulmonary embolism with serum-induced thrombi. Am J Path, 38:89, 1961.

44. Frieman, DG, Wessler, S, Lertzman, M: Experimental pulmonary embolism with serum-induced thrombi aged in vivo. Am J Path, 39:95, 1961.

45. Johnson, A: Personal communication.

46. Gitel, SN, Stephenson, RC, Wessler, S: In vitro and in vivo correlation of clotting protease activity: effect of heparin. Proc Natl Acad Sci, 74:3028, 1977.

47. Gitel, SN, Stephenson, RC, Wessler, S: The Activated Factor X-antithrombin III reaction rate: a measure of the increased thrombotic tendency induced by estrogen-containing oral contraceptives in rabbits. Haemostasis, 7:10, 1978.

48. Becker, CG, Dubin, T: Activation of Factor XII by tobacco glycoprotein. J. Exper Med, 146:457, 1977.

49. Wessler, S: Atherothrombology. In: Chandler, AB, Eurenuis, K, McMillan, GC, et al (Eds): The Thrombotic Process in Atherogenesis, New York, Plenum Press, 1978, p 409.

50. Sorenson, PJ, Dyerberg, J, Stofferson, E, Jensen, MK: Familial functional antithrombin III deficiency. Scand J Haemat, 24:105, 1980.

51. Sager, S, Thomas, DP, Stamatakis, JD, Kakkar, VV: Oral contraceptives, antithrombin III activity, and postoperative deep-vein thrombosis. Lancet, 1:509, 1976.

52. Gitel, SN, Wessler, S: Do natural estrogens pose an increased risk of thrombosis in post-menopausal women? Throm Res, 13:279, 1978.

53. Butler, S: The note-books of Samuel Butler, London, AC Fifield, 1912, p 11.

54. Barton, PG, Yin, ET, Wessler, S: Reactions of activiated factor X-phosphatide mixtures in vitro and in vivo. J Lipid Res, 11:87, 1970.

55. Gitel, SN, Wessler, S: the antithrombotic effects of warfarin and heparin following infusions of tissue thromboplastin in rabbits: clinical implications. J Lab Clin Med, 94:481, 1979.

56. Wessler, S, Reiner, SM, Freiman, DG, et al: Factors involved in the initiation of thrombosis. In: Anticoagulants and Fibrinolysis, Toronto, MacMillan, 1961, p 108.

57. Botti, RE, Ratnoff, OD: Studies on the pathogenesis of thrombosis: an experimental "hypercoagulable state" induced by the intravenous injection of ellagic acid. J Lab Clin Med, 64:385, 1964.

58. Connor, WE, Hoak, JC, Warner, ED: Massive thrombosis produced by fatty acid infusion. J Clin Invest, 42:860, 1963.

59. Thomas, DP, Wessler, S: Stasis thrombi induced by bacterial endotoxin Circ Res, 14:486, 1964.

60. Kingdon, HS, Lundblad, RL, Veltkamp, JJ, Aronson, DL: Potentially thrombogenic materials in Factor IX concentrates. Thromb Diath Haemorrh, 33:617, 1975.

61. Gitel, SN, Grieco, AJ, Wessler, S, Snyderman, SE: The thrombogenicity of 6-azauridine. Haemostasis, 8:54, 1979.

62. Wessler, S. Yin, ET: The experimental hypercoagulable state induced by Factor X: comparison of the nonactivated and activated forms. J Lab Clin Med, 72:256, 1968.

DISCUSSION

DR. GOLDZIEHER: Dr. Wessler, would you be kind enough to comment on factor X and the hypercoagulable state in pregnancy?

DR. WESSLER: Zymogens of the K-dependent proteins, are elevated in the pregnant state particularly in the second and third trimester. I do not know of any evidence that elevated zymogens, and we have studied infusions of zymogens in our model, can ever induce thrombosis. Therefore, I doubt that these elevations of the inactive molecules in the pregnant state can cause thrombosis. However, upon delivery, those levels do remain elevated and the proteins may become activated. That may be a partial explanation of the much higher incidence of postpartum deep vein thrombosis than during pregnancy.

DR: KNOPP: You have elegantly shown us the effects of estrogens on the clotting system in the rabbit model. I wonder if there is any evidence of similar or opposite effects of progestin, and if oral contraceptive preparations of varying estrogen-progestin potency will have different effects on the clotting system?

DR: WESSLER: I have really condensed here all that we ever did with contraceptives. We have not examined progestins, per se, but the model could very easily be used for these compounds.

Fifty percent of individuals with pulmonary emboli or heart attacks -- I am not including strokes -- have no known risk factors for thrombosis. They may either be taking drugs or there is something in the diet or in the environment not yet identified that is responsible for intravascular coagulation. It is this issue that we should like to address with the model.

DR. STADEL: There is a consistent finding in the epidemiologic literature that magnification of smoking effects is predominantly on the arterial side and the studies that have looked at smoking on the venous side have found at most a marginal relationship.

Perhaps something enters the arterial circulation when smoking a cigarette where the concentration is high. It then goes through the capillaries and so forth were is gets dissipated. Are you aware that this glycoprotein disappears largely by the time the blood reaches the venous side of the circulation?

DR. WESSLER: What Dr. Becker and our group have demonstrated in rabbits is the glycoprotein in tobacco smoke condensate enhances thrombosis in both the veins and arteries of animals pretreated with oral contraceptives. In so far as the veins are concerned, our findings conflict with the available clinical observations. I cannot explain the discrepancy.

DR. STADEL: There are a lot of recommendations based on epidemiologic studies that women who are to undergo surgery should discontinue oral contraceptives at least a month in advance. In your opinion, is it sufficient to give heparin?

DR. WESSLER: Yes, I think the physician and the surgeon have a choice. You may elect to wait two or three months for Xa inhibitory activity to return to normal values or, without delay, you may institute a low dose heparin regimen, 5000 USP units of heparin 2 hours prior to surgery subcutaneously and then every 12 hours (in a hemostatically competent patient not on aspirin), and eliminate the risk of postoperative thrombosis attributable to oral contraceptives.

Similarly, women on oral contraceptives who are subjected to major trauma with immobilization, as with leg fractures, should be considered for low dose heparin prophylaxis. You need only monitor the platelet count so that the one percent incidence of serious thrombosis cytopenia does not develop.

THE EFFECTS OF ORAL CONTRACEPTIVE USE ON LIPOPROTEINS: SIGNIFICANCE FOR ATHEROSCLEROSIS

Robert H. Knopp

Northwest Lipid Research Clinic
Seattle, Washington

INTRODUCTION

The purpose of this review is to summarize important aspects of lipoprotein physiology and how abnormalities in this process can lead to accelerated atherosclerosis. The effects of various oral contraceptive formulations on lipoprotein lipid concentrations will then be examined followed by consideration of the epidemiologic experience associating oral contraceptive use, progestin dose, and arteriosclerotic disease in premenopausal women. This experience will be contrasted with postmenopausal estrogen use and its association with arteriosclerotic heart disease. To determine if oral contraceptives produce changes in lipoprotein lipids that are different from a physiological elevation of estrogen and progestin, comparisons will be made between oral contraceptive use and pregnancy. The question of whether oral contraceptive preparations can be successfully evaluated for their potential risk for arteriosclerosis causation in animal models will be discussed and contrasted with the alternative option of carefully examining lipoprotein physiology in human subjects in the earliest stages of oral contraceptive evaluation. Regardless of the approach taken, the conclusion will be drawn that better and more definitive approaches are required to evaluate the potential significance of long-term oral contraceptive use on arteriosclerotic disease.

PHYSIOLOGY OF LIPOPROTEINS

Approximately 100g of triglyceride fatty acids and 150mg of cholesterol are absorbed from the human intestine daily. These lipids are incorporated into chylomicrons in the intestinal wall and enter the circulation via the lymphatic system. As shown in Figure 1, lipoprotein lipase (LPL) hydrolyzes triglyceride into fatty acids and glycerol at capillary endothelial surfaces abutting organs which can store triglyceride fatty acids such as adipose tissue and/or oxidize them such as muscle and liver. A smaller triglyceride poor particle or remnant results from this process (Figure 1). A surface component of this remnant, consisting of apoproteins C, A_I, A_{II}, and phospholipids, exchanges to HDL which serves as a reservoir for these components. The core remnants which are rich in cholesterol ester and apolipoproteins B and E are taken up by the liver mediated by hepatic triglyceride lipase (HTGL). Here, the

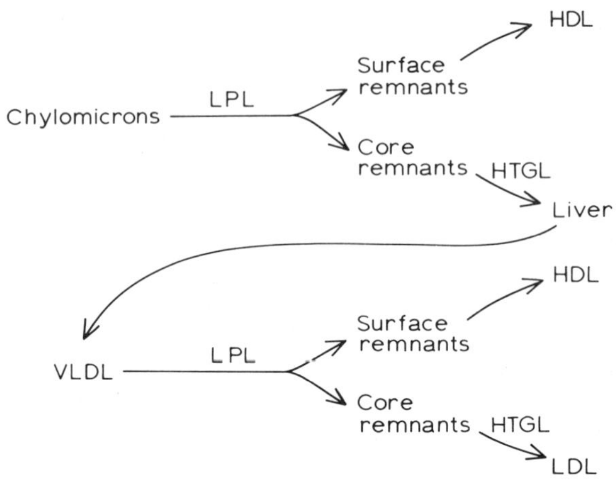

Figure 1. Metabolism of chylomicrons in very low-density lipoproteins.

cholesterol may have several fates such as secretion into bile, conversion to bile acids, or secretion into very low density lipoprotein (VLDL) triglyceride as shown in Figure 1. Here again this triglyceride rich particle is sequentially degraded to a less triglyceride rich particle under the action of LPL (Figure 1). Again, surface and core remnants result from this process with exchange of surface remnants to HDL. However, core remnants are now converted to low density lipoprotein (LDL) in the liver with recognition of apo E and hepatic triglyceride lipase playing a role. The primary carrier of cholesterol to tissues in the body is LDL where cholesterol is removed from the circulation via specific LDL receptors on cells using cholesterol for cell renewal and steroid hormone secretion.

The mechanism for removing cholesterol from cells in the body is illustrated in Figure 2. HDL_3, one of the subfractions of high density lipoprotein (HDL), is shown to receive apolipoprotein constituents from the liver, intestine, and the chylomicron and VLDL surface, as well as

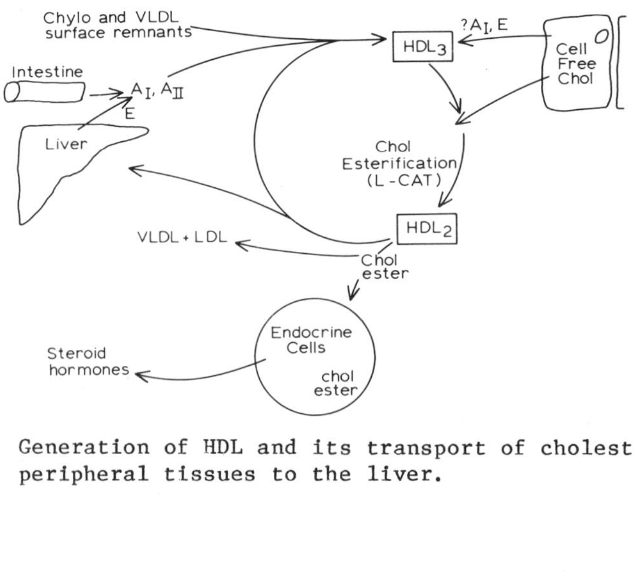

Figure 2. Generation of HDL and its transport of cholesterol from peripheral tissues to the liver.

possible peripheral tissues themselves. This HDL_3 acts as an acceptor for cellular free cholesterol and as a cofactor for cholesterol esterification by the lecithin cholesterol acyltransferase (LCAT) reaction converting HDL_3, a relatively cholesterol poor lipoprotein to HDL_2, a lipoprotein relatively rich in cholesterol ester. This cholesterol ester then can transfer to other cells such as the adrenal gland or the placenta[1] which may utilize cholesterol ester for steroid hormone synthesis or can be transfered to very low and low density lipoproteins. Another potential fate of HDL_2 is to deliver cholesterol to the liver itself where that cholesterol can be recycled or excreted in the bile.

Abnormalities in the pathways of lipoprotein metabolism described are associated with accelerated atherosclerosis. For instance, conditions where the clearance of remnants is impaired due to a lack of hepatic recognition as Type III hyperlipidemia, uremia and possibly, hypothyroidism and diabetes, are all associated with accelerated atherosclerosis. Equally well established is the association of elevations in low density lipoprotein concentrations with accelerated atherosclerosis from many epidemiologic studies. In these, such as the Framingham study[2], atherosclerosis increases exponentially with the rise in LDL cholesterol concentrations. Conversely, reductions in HDL concentrations are also associated with an exponential increase in cardiovascular disease susceptibility. More recently, studies have shown that individuals coming to coronary angiography for angina pectoris or those recently suffering a myocardial infarction both show selective reductions in HDL_2 as compared to HDL_3[3,4]. It would appear that any of these lipoprotein changes is sufficient to induce arteriosclerosis. Whether their combined effects are additive or synergistic is not known.

LIPOPROTEIN CHANGES ASSOCIATED WITH ORAL CONTRACEPTIVE USE

Since the first studies of Wynn and Doar, it has been known that oral contraceptive use is associated with an increase in plasma triglyceride concentrations. Since then the Collaborative Lipid Research Clinic Program studies have shown that triglyceride is increased on the average about 50% and cholesterol 5-7%[5]. In the aggregate, the use of oral contraceptives causes slight increases in LDL and in VLDL with no change in HDL[6].

In studies emanating from the Northwest Lipid Research Clinic, we have asked the question, how do these generally well described changes in oral contraceptives relate to estrogen, progestin composition and

Table 1. Oral contraceptive hormone composition and relative potencies.

	Type	Chemical Composition				Relative Potencies	
		Estrogen**	Dose (μg)	Progestin	Dose (mg)	Estrogen (M=1.0)	Progestin (Noreth=1.0)***
rtho-Novum	Combined	M	50,80,100	Norethindrone	1.0-2.0	50-100	1.0-2.0
novid	Combined	M	75-100	Norethynodrel	2.5-5.0	75-100	2.7-5.4
orlestrin	Combined	EE	50	Norethindrone acetate	1.0-2.5	60	2.0-5.0
vral	Combined	EE	50	Norgestrel	0.5	60	15
emulen	Combined	EE	50	Ethynodiol diacetate	1.0	60	15
vulen	Combined	M	100	Ethynodiol diacetate	1.0	100	15
racon	Sequential*	EE	100	Dimethisterone	25.0	120	1

*In the sequential formulation, EE is taken for 16 days and dimethisterone for 5 days.

*M = mestranol; EE = ethinyl estradiol.

**Noreth = norethindrone.

Table 2. Adjusted[a] lipids and lipoproteins arranged by ascending estrogen and progestin potency.

	mg/dl[b]									
	Cholesterol		Triglyceride		HDL-C		LDL-C		VLDL-C	
	Mean ± SD	Median	Mean ± SD	Median	Mean ± SD	Median	Mean ± SD	Median	Mean ± SD	Median
WOMEN 20-44 years										
Menstruating										
Nonusers	180 ± 30.9	176	79 ± 37.0	72	55 ± 15.4	54	113 ± 27.8	109	12 ± 9.0	11
Ortho-Novum	193 ± 25.9	193*	121 ± 47.7	113*	59 ± 14.5	58*	118 ± 26.7	118	16 ± 9.3	15*
Enovid	202 ± 29.4	198	130 ± 37.5	132*	75 ± 20.4	73*	112 ± 26.1	110	16 ± 7.0	14
Norlestrin	203 ± 45.4	195*	120 ± 57.3	111*	53 ± 14.3	54	134 ± 41.7	124*	17 ± 13.2	14
Ovral	194 ± 36.5	195*	109 ± 43.3	101*	45 ± 13.4	43*	133 ± 35.6	135*	17 ± 9.8	15*
Demulen	203 ± 45.6	209*	130 ± 47.3	128*	58 ± 14.4	57	124 ± 42.0	132	22 ± 10.6	20*
Ovulen	199 ± 29.7	194*	151 ± 68.2	141*	55 ± 14.7	54	124 ± 27.0	124*	20 ± 13.6	18*
Oracon	220 ± 41.8	219*	154 ± 58.8	128*	78 ± 28.4	73*	122 ± 34.8	122	21 ± 18.2	16
Nonmenstruating										
Nonusers	189 ± 58.1	192	93 ± 83.2	81	52 ± 11.9	55	123 ± 56.1	124	13 ± 10.9	12
Equine Estrogen	227 ± 52.7	222*	149 ± 59.9	130*	65 ± 18.9	67*	142 ± 51.6	139	20 ± 9.3	20*
WOMEN 45-65 years										
Nonmenstruating										
Nonusers	230 ± 44.3	226	114 ± 66.9	100	61 ± 15.6	61	154 ± 43.8	147	16 ± 13.8	13
Equine Estrogen	219 ± 33.9	218*	141 ± 71.5	126*	69 ± 17.7	67*	133 ± 33.9	131*	18 ± 12.5	16
Ethinyl Estradiol	229 ± 29.7	228	168 ± 56.7	157*	86 ± 19.3	83*	121 ± 23.7	119	22 ± 9.0	26
Diethylstilbestrol	236 ± 23.5	233	132 ± 64.0	120	93 ± 11.4	90*	127 ± 19.2	125	16 ± 15.2	18

[a] Adjusted for age, Quetelet's Index, smoking and drinking.

[b] To convert mg/dl cholesterol to mH/L, multiply by 0.02586; to convert mg/dl triglyceride to g/L, multiply by 0.01.

*Significantly different from nonusers at the 5% level.

potency. With respect to high density lipoprotein we have found that those hormone formulations that are progestin dominant (as shown in Table 1) have the lowest HDL cholesterol concentrations while those that are most estrogen dominant have the highest HDL cholesterol concentrations (Table 2). These results and the subjects comprising them have been recently published[7]. In general they confirm the studies of Bradley et al[8]. In addition, progestins in the 19-nortestosterone class lower HDL more than the C-21 progestins[9]. Recent studies from Finnish workers indicate that the total HDL reductions are specifically associated with HDL_2 fraction[10].

Less well appreciated is the fact that the same progestin dominant oral contraceptives that lower HDL can lead to increases in LDL cholesterol[7]. LDL cholesterol increases as much as 20% with the progestin rich oral contraceptive formulations (Table 2). In contrast, use of postmenopausal estrogens is associated with a reduction in LDL cholesterol concentrations.

With respect to VLDL, we have found that the most progestin dominant of the oral contraceptive formulations is associated with an increase in the VLDL cholesterol/triglyceride ratio. These results are shown in Table 3. In addition, LDL progestin dominant Ovral mediates a higher cholesterol triglyceride ratio than any of the other oral contraceptives evaluated. These results are taken from a previously published population survey of employees of the Pacific Northwest Bell Telephone Company[11].

In summary, oral contraceptives affect each of the lipoprotein classes in a manner that is associated with accelerated arteriosclerosis. These effects are not the same across all classes of oral contraceptives and are particularly associated with formulations that are dominant or potent in their progestin effect.

Table 3. Percentage of women in each hormone group with lipoprotein cholesterol/triglyceride ratios above the 50th percentile for nonhormone using controls.

Ratio/Hormone Group	n*	% Above Median	95% C.I. for p=.50
VLDL(C/TG)			
Ortho-Novum	58	44.8	(.37,.63)
Norlestrin	12	50.0	(.22,.78)
Ovral	26	80.8 †	(.35,.65)
Demulen	6	66.7	(.12,.88)
Ovulen	12	58.3	(.22,.78)
Oracon	5	40.0	(.07,.93)
Estrogen	27	63.0	(.32,.68)
LDL(C/TG)			
Ortho-Novum	53	34.0	(.37,.63)
Norlestrin	12	16.7 †	(.29,.71)
Ovral	24	64.3	(.31,.69)
Demulen	8	25.0	(.25,.75)
Ovulen	11	36.4	(.32,.68)
Oracon	5	40.0	(.11,.59)
Estrogen	31	54.8	(.44,.56)
HDL(C/TG)			
Ortho-Novum	64	31.2 †	(.39,.61)
Norlestrin	13	23.1 †	(.27,.73)
Ovral	19	17.2 †	(.33,.67)
Demulen	8	12.5 †	(.27,.73)
Ovulen	14	21.4. †	(.29,.71)
Oracon	4	50.0	(.01,.99)
Estrogen	39	38.5	(.35,.65)

*The number of women whose values are within the lipoprotein triglyceride concentration range for reference curve (see methods).

† Percentage of subjects above and below the median is outside the 95% confidence interval about the median.

EPIDEMIOLOGIC EVIDENCE OF CARDIOVASCULAR DISEASE IN ORAL CONTRACEPTIVE USERS

One of the first clues of enhanced arteriosclerosis risk in oral contraceptive users was the finding of increased prevalence of fatal myocardial infarction in older oral contraceptive using women, particularly those having other cardiovascular risk factors, such as smoking, hypertension, or hypercholesterolemia[12-14]. Meade and associates then found that death from myocardial infarction was associated with increasing progestin dosage in oral contraceptives used[15]. Subsequently, Slone and associates found that the risk of myocardial infarction was related to the length of time of oral contraceptive use and persisted even after discontinuation, a finding highly compatible with an arteriosclerotic basis for the coronary heart disease observed[16]. Evidence to further implicate the progestin component of the pill (rather than the estrogen) is the association of postmenopausal estrogen replacement therapy with diminished cardiovascular disease risk observed by Bain and collaborators[17]. This association is also compatible with the recently published study from the Lipid Research Clinics Program, indicating that all cause mortality is reduced in estrogen users postmenopausally[18]. Thus the case for enhanced risk for arteriosclerotic cardiovascular disease associated with progestin use appears to be quite strong. There are no studies yet available to indicate whether these effects are selectively associated with alterations in very low density lipoprotein composition, low density lipoprotein cholesterol increases, or HDL cholesterol decreases.

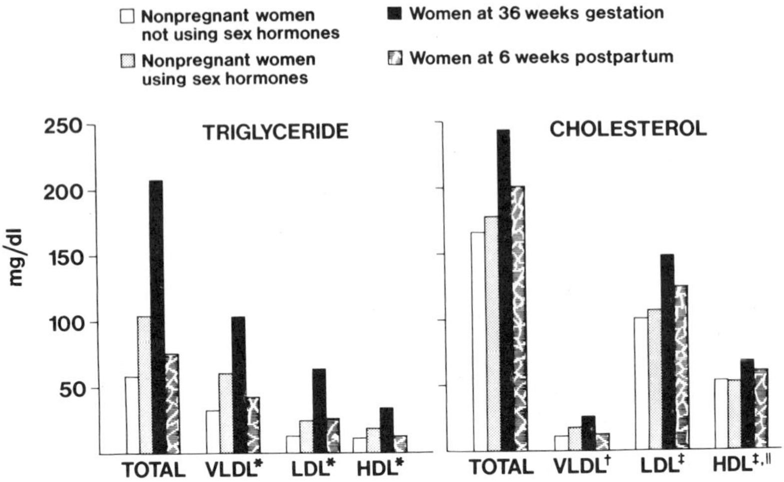

Figure 3. Effects of oral contraceptive use and pregnancy on median lipoprotein triglyceride and cholesterol concentrations. Differences among all groups are significant at $p < 0.01$ except as noted: *users vs. postpartum, † nonusers vs. postpartum, ‡ users vs. nonusers.

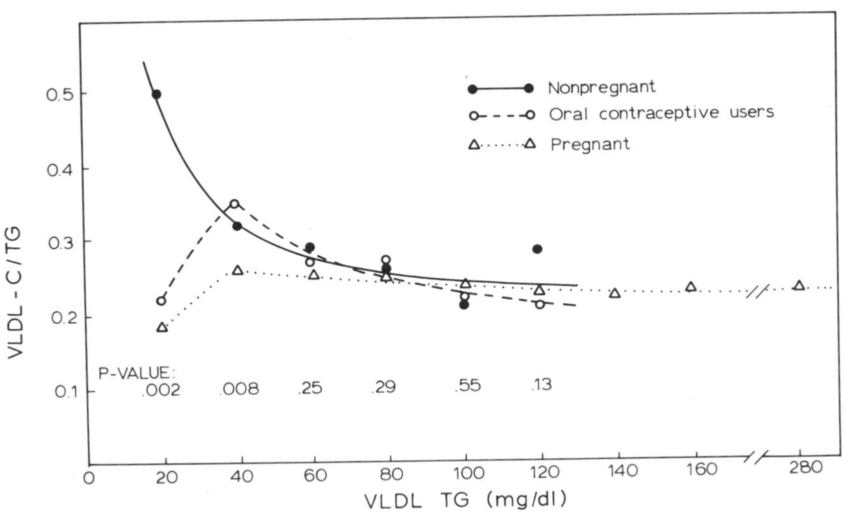

Figure 4. Effect of oral contraceptive use and pregnancy on the very low-density lipoprotein cholesterol to triglyceride ratio.

EFFECTS OF PHYSIOLOGICAL INCREASES IN NATURAL ESTROGEN AND PROGESTERONE

One possible approach to judge the significance of oral contraceptive induced changes in lipoprotein lipids is to compare oral contraceptive induced changes with those seen in a condition where natural estrogens and progesterone are physiologically elevated, namely pregnancy. We have performed such a comparison in human pregnancy comparing lipoprotein concentrations as well as cholesterol to triglyceride ratio[19]. As shown in Figure 3, oral contraceptive use in the aggregate differs from pregnancy with respect to the fact that HDL cholesterol concentrations are not elevated. However, increases in VLDL and LDL concentrations do occur in common and are in fact greater in pregnancy. In addition, there is an enrichment in LDL triglyceride relative to cholesterol in both pregnant women and oral contraceptive users. Shown in Figure 4 is a comparison of the cholesterol to triglyceride ratio in very low density lipoprotein expressed as a function of VLDL triglyceride (TG) concentration to determine if the ratio in oral contraceptives users differs from pregnancy. It can be seen that oral contraceptive users in the aggregate are between normal and pregnant subjects at lower VLDL-TG concentrations and are identical with normal and pregnant subjects at higher triglyceride concentrations. Such similarities also are seen in LDL and HDL (data not shown). Thus abnormalities in VLDL composition appear to be selectively associated with only certain classes of oral contraceptive concentrations, particularly the progestin rich[11]. There is little evidence to suggest that pregnancy, at least in the human, is associated with an acceleration of arteriosclerosis[19], although this is hard to prove. Perhaps the comforting point from this comparison is that apart from the adverse effect on HDL cholesterol, oral contraceptives comprised solely of the 19-nortestosterone series (an unnatural progestin to be sure) show as a class no differences from pregnancy.

In passing, it should be noted that some women show a greater degree of hyperlipidemia in response to pregnancy or oral contraceptive use than others. Thus another approach to the control of arteriosclerosis risk in oral contraceptive users is to identify women with abnormal responses to sex hormones by screening their lipids late in gestation or during the early stages of oral contraceptive use using established criteria[19,20] to preclude the use of sex hormone treatment. Studies of lipoprotein composition such as those described above as well as of lipoprotein metabolism in abnormal responders to sex hormones may reveal special abnormalities not seen in oral contraceptive users in general. Such abnormalities are in fact seen in VLDL composition in subjects with combined hyperlipidemia[21].

ANIMAL MODELS

While animal models have been used extensively to evaluate basic processes in lipoprotein physiology, numerous differences have also been established between the most commonly used animal models, such as the rat, rabbit and the subhuman primate, and man. As an example, the rabbit appears to be particularly susceptible to cholesterol feeding and has a limited capacity to clear remnants of chylomicron or VLDL catabolism. Thus the rabbit may be considered a model for remnant removal disease or conditions that might influence this process. For instance, it has been shown that estrogen treatment enhances the removal of cholesterol rich remnants in the rabbit model and diminishes the amount of arteriosclerosis that would otherwise occur[22]. The rat would appear to be a relatively poor model for evaluating oral contraceptive effects relevant to humans inasmuch as LDL cholesterol concentrations are generally very low, while HDL cholesterol concentrations are rather high and are particularly enriched with apolipoprotein E. None of these features are typical of the human species.

Cholesterol feeding studies have been successful in producing arteriosclerosis in numerous subhuman primates, but the one available study of oral contraceptive administration in the monkey has not so far been productive of accelerated arteriosclerosis[23]. The reasons for this finding may be related to the oral contraceptive preparation used, the duration of use, the monkey species observed, or the degree of hypercholesterolemia observed. Nonetheless, if particularly representative pathophysiologic processes could be selected using appropriate animal models, for instance remnant clearance in the cholesterol fed rabbit, the potential significance of different oral contraceptive formulations, for instance progestin rich versus progestin poor or low versus high dose progestin, might be profitably screened in an appropriate animal model. Clearly more work has to be done to characterize animal models that will provide useful information on effects relevant to human lipoprotein physiology. One important step would be to confirm in an animal model the hypothesis advanced above associating arteriosclerosis with use of progestin rich oral contraceptives.

PROPOSED HUMAN STUDIES

Perhaps a better approach to evaluating the effects on lipoprotein lipids of the newer oral contraceptive formulations and those under development is to obtain measurements on human lipoprotein fractions in the earliest phases of human testing. If in fact an oral contraceptive has an unfavorable effect on VLDL cholesterol to triglyceride ratio, or LDL or HDL concentrations, particularly in HDL_2, then further development of this formulation might be discouraged. Another important point is the need for ongoing surveillance of oral contraceptive use and postmenopausal progestin use in relationship to lipoprotein lipids and arteriosclerotic disease. Further studies are also needed to confirm and extend the relationship between ascending progestin dose and kind of progestin to coronary heart disease. The need for a better national reporting system of oral contraceptive use and heart disease occurrence might assume a higher priority in light of the need for more up-to-date information.

CONCLUSION

The accumulated evidence indicates that oral contraceptive use can be associated with acceleration of arteriosclerotic heart disease by several effects on lipoprotein metabolism which appear to be particularly sensitive to the relative dose and potency of the constituent progestins and estrogens in oral contraceptive formulation. The most ideal oral contraceptive preparation might in fact be that which maintains the minimum progestin and estrogen dose necessary for contraception and maintains a relative estrogen/progestin potency such that major changes in VLDL, LDL, and HDL concentration and composition are avoided. Early testing of lipoproteins in humans with focus testing of physiologically and pathophysiologically relevant questions in animal models will provide the most efficient development of safe sex steroid contraceptives in the future.

ACKNOWLEDGEMENTS:

This work is supported by the Lipid Research Clinics Contract HV-12157-L. The excellent secretarial assistance of Nanci Presley-Holley and Donna Fatland is gratefully acknowledged.

REFERENCES

1. Knopp, RH, Lawson, R: Effects of intracellular cholesterol depletion on human trophoblast progesterone secretion and the response to low and high density lipoproteins. Endocrinol (Program and abstracts of the 64th Annual Meeting, San Francisco, CA, Abstract #389), p 177, 1982.

2. Gordon, T, Castelli, WP, Hjortland, MC, Kannel, WB, Dawber, TR: High density lipoprotein as a protective factor against coronary heart disease. The Framingham Study. Amer J Med, 62:707, 1977.

3. Miller, NE, Hammett, F, Saltissi, S, Rao, S, Van Zeller, H, Coltart, J, Lewis, B: Relation of angiographically defined coronary artery disease to plasma lipoprotein subfractions and apolipoproteins. Brit Med J, 282:1741, 1981.

4. Ballantyne, FC, Clark, RS, Simpson, HS, Ballantyne, D: High density and low density lipoprotein subfractions in survivors of myocardial infarction and in control subjects. Metabolism, 31:433, 1982.

5. Wallace, RB, Hoover, J, Sandler, D, Rifkind, B, Tyroler, HA: Altered plasma-lipids associated with oral contraceptive or oestrogen consumption. Lancet, 2:11, 1977.

6. Wallace, RB, Hoover, J, Barrett-Connor, E, Rifkind, B, Hunninghake, D, Mackenthun, A, Heiss, G: Altered plasma lipid and lipoprotein levels associated with oral contraceptive or oestrogen use. Lancet, 2:111, 1979.

7. Wahl, P, Walden, C, Knopp, R, Hoover, J, Wallace, R, Heiss, G, Rifkind B: Effect of estrogen/progestin potency on lipid/lipoprotein cholesterol. New Eng J Med, 308:862, 1983.

8. Bradley, DD, Wingerd, J, Petitti, DB, Krauss, RM, Ramcharan, S: Serum high-density-lipoprotein cholesterol in women using oral contraceptives, estrogens and progestins. New Eng J Med, 299:17, 1978.

9. Hirvonen, E, Malkonen, M, Manninen, V: Effects of different progestogens on lipoproteins during postmenopausal replacement therapy. New Eng J Med, 304:560, 1981.

10. Tikkanen, JM, Nikkila, EA, Kuusi, T, Sipinen, S: High density lipoprotein-2 and hepatic lipase: Reciprocal changes produced by estrogen and norgestrel. J Clin Endocrinol Metab, 54:1113, 1982.

11. Knopp, RH, Walden, CE, Wahl, PW, Hoover, JJ, Warnick, GR, Albers, JJ, Ogilvie, JT, Hazzard, WR: Oral contraceptive and postmenopausal estrogen effects on lipoprotein triglyceride and cholesterol in an adult female population: Relationships to estrogen and progestin potency. J Clin Endocrinol Metab, 53:1123, 1982.

12. Radford, DJ, Oliver, MF: Oral contraceptives and myocardial infarction. Brit Med J, 3:428, 1973.

13. Mann, JI, Inman, WHW: Oral contraceptives and death from myocardial infarction. Brit Med J, 2:245, 1975.

14. Mann, JI, Inman, WHW, Thorogood, M: Oral contraceptive use in older women and fatal myocardial infarction. Brit Med J, 2:445, 1976.

15. Meade, TW, Greenberg, G, Thompson, SG: Progestogens and cardiovascular reactions associated with oral contraceptives and a comparison of the safety of 50-μg and 30-μg oestrogen preparations. Brit Med J, 280:1157, 1980.

16. Slone, D, Shapiro, S, Kaufman, DW, Rosenberg, L, Miettinen, OS, Stolley, PD: Risk of myocardial infarction in relation to current and discontinued use of oral contraceptives. New Eng J Med, 305:420, 1981.

17. Bain, C, Willett, W, Hennekens, CH, Rosner, B, Belanger, C, Speizer, F: Use of postmenopausal hormones and risk of myocardial infarction. Circulation, 64:42, 1981.

18. Bush, TL, Cowan, LD, Barrett-Connor, Ed, Criqui, MH, Karon, JM, Wallace, RB, Tyroler, HA, Rifkind, BM: Estrogen use and all-cause mortality. Preliminary results from the Lipid Research Clinics Program follow-up study. JAMA, 249:903, 1983.

19. Knopp, RH, Bergelin, RO, Wahl, PW, Walden, CE, Chapman, M, and Irvine S: Population-based lipoprotein lipid reference values for pregnancy compared to non pregnant women classified by sex hormone usage. Amer J Obstet Gynecol, 143:626, 1982.

20. Walden, CE, Wahl, PW, Knopp, RH, Warnick, GR, Ogilvie, JT, Hazzard, WR, Hoover, JJ, Albers, JJ: Hyperlipidemia in the Pacific Northwest Bell Telephone Company Health Survey: Part I Lipoprotein cholesterol and triglyceride concentrations. Arteriosclerosis, 3:117, 1983.

21. Walden, CE, Knopp, RH, Wahl, PW, Hoover, JJ, Albers, JJ, Hazzard, WR, Ogilvie, JT, Warnick, GR: Hyperlipidemia in the Pacific Northwest Bell Telephone Company Health Survey: Part 2 Lipoprotein lipid interrelationships. Arteriosclerosis, 2:125, 1983.

22. Kushwaha, RS, Hazzard, WR: Exogenous estrogens attenuate dietary hypercholesterolemia and atherosclerosis in the rabbit. Metabolism, 30:359, 1981.

23. St. Clair, RW, Henderson, GR, Heaster, V, Wagner, WD, Bond, G, McMahan, MR: Influence of dietary fats and an oral contraceptive on plasma lipids, high density lipoproteins, gallstones, and atherosclerosis in African green monkeys. Atherosclerosis, 37:103, 1980.

DISCUSSION

DR. BRENT: In the Bain study where you indicated that the rate of contraceptive use is related to risk of myocardial infarction, how do you correct for age? If contraceptive use for 10 years is compared with that for five years, the chances are good that the average age of the population is not the same. In other words, if you compared a group that is five years older than another, there will be a different incidence of disease.

DR. KNOPP: That was taken into account.

DR. BERENDES: It was a case-controlled study and it was included in the analysis.

DR. BRENT: Based on your knowledge, and not considering what you heard today, how would you design an oral contraceptive?

DR. KNOPP: Well, I think one rational approach would be to prepare an oral contraceptive with a minimum estrogen and progestin content, and then adjust the estrogen/progestin ratio to have the minimum or, hopefully, no effect on lipoproteins.

DR. BRENT: Well, what number? Is it the ratio that you discussed? Would you like it to be exactly the same as the ratio on metabolic effects that you observed in a nonuser, is that the end point that you would look for?

DR. KNOPP: You mean like the LDL to HDL cholesterol ratio?

DR. BRENT: Yes. Is it one number that you would seek to attain?

DR. KNOPP: No, I don't think so, because the ratio is very misleading. You could have a ratio of 2.5 to 1 with a LDL cholesterol of 200 and a HDL cholesterol of 80 but the significance for arteriosclerosis may not be the same for a LDL of 50 and a HDL of 20 where the ratio is still 2.5 to 1.

I would try to guide new oral contraceptives development to HDL concentrations in the physiologic range for women, which is 55, and for LDL about 100.

DR. EDGREN: I have two comments and a question. Some years ago Dr. Sturtevant and I reviewed the literature and pointed out that we didn't feel that the current potency concepts were really meaningful, and I am concerned this may effect the interpretation of your data.

My own personal feeling, derived from both original publications and what has been said today, is that androgenicity of the compound may be more relevant than its progestational activity.

Based on the earlier HDL data, the norethindrone containing oral contraceptives shift the HDL either slightly upward or are without effect, depending on which preparation was employed. Now, with the number of patients studied, did you ever classify them to determine whether, say, the 2 milligram/100 microgram preparation differed from the 1 + 80, and the 1 + 80 was the one that seemed to push them up slightly?

DR. KNOPP: We would have liked to have done that analysis. Unfortunately, when the data were originally obtained, they were gathered by category of oral contraceptive and not the specific dosage.

With respect to the relative progestin versus androgen potency, I would like to agree with you. I saw the data you presented yesterday showing the relative androgenicity of the progestins and they are quite compatible with the kinds of observations we presented today.

I would also indicate our potency criteria are not the best; potency probably needs to be couched in terms of the end points that are being studied.

DR. BARDIN: You just commented on what I really wanted to discuss. We did some studies a number of years ago where we ranked the potency of progestins in kidney, uterus and liver. The most potent, medroxyprogesterone acetate, is also a more potent androgen than levonorgestrel when assayed by effects on the external genitalia, mouse kidney and even on the prostate.

Yet, it has no effect. So, androgenicity as we measure it as defined in the dictionary isn't quite right, because the dose response effect of all progestins on the rodent liver, at least, does not correlate in any way with androgenicity on the male reproductive tract and progestational activity as measured by changes in the uterus.

In fact, they are in a totally different order. Now, this is not using lipoproteins as an end point; it is using microsomal enzymes and drug metabolites. So you could say, these observations might not hold for lipoprotein analysis, but I bet it would be somewhat similar.

The receptors are probably different. It may well be that the receptors for progestins in liver may be totally different than in the uterus. I think, in your analysis, you have not accounted for any bimodal distribution that could be created by ratios.

I would suggest that in your studies you add, even though it is an artificial situation, groups of patients treated with progestin only. You might be very surprised at what happens when you treat a patient with only levonorgestrel, because there is something about your data, the estrogen/progestin combination, that is not explained on the basis of high progestational potency.

I don't understand it myself, but I think you need that as a control. You do have an estrogen control. Finally, I would like to congratulate you on putting together this enormous body of data and making an attempt to organize it. While it could still be refined, it is some of the best data we have. I believe we will move forward to a better understanding of what this means.

DR. KNOPP: Wayne, I thank you for your comments and I agree about the imponderables raised by this analysis. We need surveillance studies using oral contraceptives currently being marketed.

DR. CLARK: I would just like to ask Dick if he has actually tested frank androgens and seen effects on LDL and so forth?

DR. EDGREN: We have not. But wasn't there an androgen in the Bradley study? Didn't they have a group of just androgenic materials?

DR. KNOPP: I don't think so.

DR. EDGREN: They had some medroxyprogesterone acetate in a series of oral contraceptives.

DR. KNOPP: There are studies of oxandrolone, which is an androgenic/

anabolic agent, that markedly reduces HDL cholesterol, raises hepatic lipase, and does all of the things that an androgenic progestin would do.

DR. EDGREN: It pushes the HDL's down?

DR. KNOPP: Yes.

DR. DICZFALUSY: I have two questions, Dr. Knopp. One is related to the other. Is there a difference in nonusers if you take blood samples at different parts of the cycle in estrogen dominant and progestin dominant periods. Is that significant and, if so, by how much?

My second question is, do you happen to have data in men treated with testosterone or a testosterone ester? How marked is that suppressive effect on HDL cholesterol?

DR. KNOPP: In response to the first question, there are very limited studies on the lipoprotein response to an oral contraceptive over time or even changes in lipoprotein lipids in the menstrual cycle. It appears that there are probably fewer changes over the four week oral contraceptive regulated cycle than during the natural menstrual cycle, when some small changes in LDL and HDL cholesterol have been observed.

We haven't the faintest notion at what point in the cycle the blood samples were drawn for our studies, but we do keep coming up with the same answer all the time. The results are compatible with cross sectional and longitudinal studies. So, I would like to know more about what you are asking, but I don't think it is a serious criticism of the data.

DR. DICZFALUSY: It was not criticism; it was information.

DR. KNOPP: Well, it is a potential criticism, indeed. I mean, I have asked the question critically in the same way. The answer to the second question, we have not used testosterone, but stanozolol, another anabolic steroid, has been studied by our group. Stanozolol reduces HDL cholesterol in men from an average of 45 to about 28 mg/dl, which is about the fifth percentile.

DR. SHELTON: I just want to say that I agree with your basic point which is that one does need to be concerned about the atherosclerotic process and the potential effect of progestins on that process.

But I think there are a couple of epidemiological points that must be brought out. First there are other studies of myocardial infarction besides the Slone study which indicate no increased risk in former contraceptive users, and there may be some methodological problems why that hasn't been demonstrated. But we must realize that, while it is a very good study, is the only one so far that I know of to report that.

DR. KNOPP: I am not sure that is the case, because I showed at least three studies that have.

DR. SHELTON: I guess I was referring to the issue of former users.

The other point with respect to the Meade study and Dr. Brent's question. I believe that study did not control for age and that is a very important confounding variable. There is a recent United States study that reports older women do use higher dose pills. Any study that does not control for that, and I believe the Slone study did, has a significant epidemiologic flaw.

DR. BERENDES: Are there any other questions?

DR. BLYE: Is the relationship between HDL cholesterol and sex steroids of sufficient concern to warrant including it as a parameter to be measured in the early assessment of new steroidal contraceptives in animal tests?

DR. KNOPP: Well, I believe the question of whether the evaluation of a new steroidal contraceptive in an animal would lead to changes in HDL or other lipoproteins that are interpretable is really open to question. I would think that one would have to be dealing with a very well characterized model where you knew what estrogen/progestin responses were before you would put that much credence in it.

I would prefer to agree with some of the other speakers who suggested that toxicologic screens be done for new agents to make sure they don't contain some inadvertent poison, and then go on to clinical studies where you know what to look for and what to deal with, e.g., in selected groups of 50 for six months. You could do a very careful examination of a number of lipoprotein fractions in such a study.

I think, at least with respect to lipoproteins, apart from specific questions that can be directed to the animal, the proper model for the study of man is man.

CYNOMOLGUS MACAQUES AS MODELS FOR EVALUATING EFFECTS OF CONTRACEPTIVE STEROIDS ON PLASMA LIPOPROTEINS AND CORONARY ARTERY ATHEROSCLEROSIS[1]

Donald Koritnik, Thomas Clarkson, and Michael Adams

Department of Comparative Medicine
Bowman Gray School of Medicine
Winston Salem, North Carolina

INTRODUCTION

One of the most interesting aspects of the natural history of human atherosclerosis is the relative sparing of white, premenopausal women from the development of coronary artery atherosclerosis. In Table 1 we have summarized the male female differences in deaths due to myocardial infarction in the United States in 1974.

There has been considerable investigative effort to determine if male female differences in coronary artery atherosclerosis can be explained by differences in exposure to the traditional risk factors. In Table 2 we have summarized the male female differences in major risk factors among the subjects in the Framingham study. In this, and most other population studies, premenopausal females have been found to have considerably higher plasma high density lipoprotein (HDL) cholesterol concentrations than do males. Since plasma HDL cholesterol concentrations are inversely related to risk for coronary heart disease, it is thought by many that this relatively large male female difference may account for much of the observed differences in risk of coronary heart disease.

Further evidence for this association can be seen in the clear inverse relationship between plasma concentrations of HDL cholesterol and rates of coronary heart disease among large groups of human females. We have summarized these observations in Table 3. As can be seen, rates of coronary heart disease increase with decreasing plasma HDL cholesterol concentrations, and increase dramatically at HDL cholesterol concentrations less than 35 mg/dl.

Several recent studies have demonstrated that some types of progestin containing oral contraceptives lower the plasma concentration of HDL cholesterol[1-3]. Plasma HDL cholesterol increases with increasing doses of estrogen and decreases with increasing doses and potency of progestin[4-8]. Derivatives of 19-nortestosterone (e.g., norethindrone and

---

[1]These studies were supported in part by grants from The Population Council and the National Heart, Lung and Blood Institute (SCOR HL-14164).

Table 1. Male-Female Differences in Myocardial Infarction Rate in the United States[1,2].

Age	Females	Males	Ratio
15-24	0.2	0.3	1.5
25-34	1.5	5.0	3.3
35-44	10.1	50.8	5.0
45-54	45.0	215.5	4.8
55-64	158.3	542.9	3.4
65-74	452.0	1091.4	2.4
75-84	1101.9	1888.4	1.7

[1] The data presented for males and females are deaths per 100,000 population.

[2] The data are obtained from National Center for Health Statistics, DHEW. Vital statistics of the United States, 1974. Volume II. Mortality. Part A. Hyattsville, MD, 1978.

norgestrel), common ingredients of combination oral contraceptives, exert the greatest HDL cholesterol lowering effect[2,6,9]; hydroxyprogesterone derivatives, e.g. medroxyprogesterone acetate, appear to have little or no effect on plasma HDL cholesterol[6,9,10]. Though population studies have found a relationship between decreased plasma HDL cholesterol and increased coronary risk, there is no experimental evidence to indicate whether this pharmacological lowering of plasma concentrations of HDL cholesterol influences the extent of coronary artery atherosclerosis. The difficulties in obtaining such evidence from human studies has suggested the need for testing contraceptive steroids in a suitable non human primate model[11]. Ideally, such a model would mimic man as regards gender differences in extent of coronary artery atherosclerosis and plasma lipoproteins.

Description of the Model

Male female differences in plasma lipids and lipoproteins of cynomolgus monkeys with diet induced hyperlipoproteinemia have been described by Rudel and Pitts[12]. Biochemical characterization followed the separation of plasma lipoproteins by agarose column chromatography. In both males and females low density lipoprotein (LDL) was the fraction that increased most significantly in response to a cholesterol containing diet. LDL mass concentrations were not different between males and females, but males were found to respond to increased dietary cholesterol with an

Table 2. Male-Female Differences Among Human Beings in Risk Factors for Coronary Artery Atherosclerosis*.

Risk Factor	Males	Females
Relative weight, %	122	121
Systolic blood pressure, mm Hg	139	139
Plasma Triglycerides, mg/dl	135	113
Plasma Low Density Lipoprotein Cholesterol, mg/dl	142	154
Plasma High Density Lipoprotein Cholesterol, mg/dl	46	58

* Data are from the Framingham Study, Examination 11.

increase in LDL molecular weight while females responded with an increase in the number of LDL particles. Cholesterol ester content was the factor which influenced the larger size of LDL in males. The females had higher HDL concentrations with a different composition than males; females had a higher percentage of protein and a lower percentage of free cholesterol and cholesterol ester.

Male female differences in the extent of diet induced coronary artery atherosclerosis in this species were described by Hamm et al[13]. Males were found to have significantly more extensive coronary artery atherosclerosis than females and this effect was independent of changes in plasma lipids and lipoproteins. The extensiveness of coronary artery atherosclerosis was found to be inversely correlated with plasma HDL cholesterol concentrations. An independent influence of a behavioral characteristic, competitive dominance, on the extensiveness of coronary artery atherosclerosis was described.

The effects of ovariectomy and social dominance on the extent of atherosclerosis were examined in a more recent study[14]. In that study, ovariectomy resulted in a more atherogenic plasma lipid pattern and increased the extent of coronary artery atherosclerosis. In intact females, decreased ovarian function (high frequency of anovulation; lower luteal phase plasma progesterone) was associated with low dominance status, a lipid pattern similar to ovariectomized females, and increased prevalence of advanced atherosclerosis of the coronary arteries. These findings suggest that the association between low social status and advanced coronary artery disease may be mediated by alterations in ovarian function.

Table 3. Relation of Plasma High Density Lipoprotein Cholesterol to Incidence of Coronary Heart Disease Among Human Females*.

Plasma High Density Lipoprotein Cholesterol Level (mg/dl)	Population at Risk	Coronary Heart Disease Rate/1,000
75+	199	20.1
65-74	216	13.9
55-64	353	39.7
45-54	386	49.2
35-44	220	54.5
25-34	67	164.2

* Adapted from Gordon, T., et al, Am. J. Med. 62:707-714, 1977.

Thus, female cynomolgus monkeys share with white, premenopausal females a relative protection against coronary artery atherosclerosis when compared to males of the same age. Also, as in human females, the premature loss of ovarian function seems to abolish this relative protection. HDL cholesterol is inversely correlated with the severity of diet induced coronary artery atherosclerosis in this species, an apparent parallel to the observed inverse correlation between HDL cholesterol and risk of ischemic heart disease in women. Thus, this animal model appears to be suited to answer some important questions concerning the occurrence of coronary heart disease in contraceptive steroid users. In this paper we describe our experience with this species in studies of the effects of contraceptive steroids on risk factors for coronary artery atherosclerosis.

Availability of Animals

Macaca fascicularis is one of a very few primate species which can be obtained in relatively large numbers from commercial importers. In addition, the National Institutes of Health support several domestic breeding colonies. There are some differences in the development of coronary artery atherosclerosis among animals from Indonesia and the Philippine Islands. Studies should use one or another of these sources but not mix groups.

Health Evaluation, Quarantine, and Acclimation

Upon arrival at our facility, monkeys are maintained in quarantine for a minimum of 90 days during which six intradermal tuberculin tests are administered at two week intervals. The animals must be free of contagious or zoonotic disease prior to release from quarantine.

Animal health evaluations include: initial physical examination, determination of blood pressure, characterization of an electrocardiogram recording, a determination of total and differential leukocyte count, a hematocrit measurement, a urinalysis, and quantitation of SGOT and SGPT. Additional clinical tests are prescribed as necessary to diagnose illness. Animals with diseases that might potentially interfere with experimental protocols are eliminated.

Since the acclimation of animals to new housing and environmental conditions is necessary, several months must be allowed prior to the start of experimentation. Some experiments necessitate housing animals in social groups and fight-inflicted wounds can cause substantial morbidity and mortality in the weeks following group formation. As will be described in detail, we utilize this acclimation period to evaluate cycling activity of the females and allow time for the serum lipid concentrations to stabilize after the introduction of the experimental diet. Since many of the animals have been undernourished prior to arrival, the weight gain during this initial period can be considerable. Our protocols allow for a seven month preexperimental period.

Training Monkeys for Non Stressful Sampling

Each monkey is trained to respond to a given signal by voluntarily presenting a leg for venipuncture or the perineum for vaginal swabbing. The training of subjects is accomplished by behavioral modification through negative reinforcement or avoidance training. Briefly, the movable back of a squeeze back cage is drawn tightly so that the subject is pressed against the cage front, one of its legs is grasped by the technician, pulled to the front of the cage, and extended completely. After the leg has been straightened, the ankle is then rotated so that the perineal area is forced against the cage front and directed toward the sampling area. As soon as the subject assumes this position, the restraining back of the sampling cage is released. Thus the animal quickly learns to associate the presentation of leg and perineum with the removal of a noxious stimulus. Based on our experience with this technique, approximately one month of daily training is necessary to have the animal voluntarily present itself for venipuncture and vaginal swabbing when given an appropriate cue.

In some experiments involving group housing, animals must be trained to enter a transport cage from the group cage. The animals are then transported to a sampling area where they enter squeeze back sampling cages. Training for these sampling procedures are more complex than those described above, but can be accomplished on a similar time scale.

Number of Animals and Variability of Response

The development of coronary artery atherosclerosis in this species is dependent on the hypercholesterolemic stimulus. There is much individual variability in the hypercholesterolemic response to a given diet as well as the degree of coronary artery atherosclerosis produced at a given plasma cholesterol concentration. Because of this variability and the fact that untreated intact females are relatively resistant to coronary artery atherosclerosis, the number of animals needed in experiments can be relatively large. In general, based on our studies comparing extent of coronary artery atherosclerosis in intact females to that of males or ovariectomized females, we have found that 20 to 25 animals are required in each treatment group to ensure a high likelihood (60-80 percent) of detecting a statistically significant treatment effect.

Type of Diet to be Utilized

The induction of atherosclerosis by dietary manipulation in cynomolgus monkeys depends to a large extent on cholesterol content and type and amount of fat in the diet. In the studies described below one can see the baseline differences in total serum cholesterol concentrations (TSC), HDL cholesterol, and triglyceride concentrations in females fed different diets. Although we have had experience with several different diet formulations[15], it seemed reasonable to formulate a diet which approximated the fatty acid composition and cholesterol content of the diet consumed by most North American women. These diets incorporate a natural products base (Purina Monkey Chow) with dry egg yolk (cholesterol) and lard (saturated fat) added.

Length of the Experiment

In several pilot projects in which contraceptive steroids were administered, significant changes in HDL cholesterol occurred in less than a month. Thus, the alterations in lipids and lipoproteins resulting from different treatments can be determined relatively quickly. Our experience with the endpoint of coronary artery atherosclerosis, on the other hand, has indicated that much longer time periods are needed. Both the extent of coronary artery atherosclerosis and characteristics of the lesions are dependent on the cholesterol and fat content of the diet. In most of our studies we have fed diets containing about 0.3 mg of cholesterol/Cal. which induces a moderate hyperlipoproteinemia with plasma cholesterol concentrations of about 300 mg/dl. With this relatively mild hypercholesterolemia 24-30 months is required to have sufficient coronary artery atherosclerosis to evaluate.

TYPE, DOSE, AND ROUTE OF ADMINISTRATION OF CONTRACEPTIVE STEROIDS

Once the nature of the contraceptive steroid to be tested is known, decisions can be made to deliver the preparation in a manner which mimics the situation in women. This can present some problems in nonhuman primate species.

Most contraceptive preparations are formulated for oral consumption. In women, the contraceptive preparation may be delivered for 21 days with seven days off the treatment; sequential contraceptives deliver doses of estrogen and progestin which change over 28 days to mimic the normal cycle. Such manipulations have been difficult in our experience with macaques, since these non human primates do not readily accept an oral contraceptive formulation in concentrated form, even when incorporated into a banana flavored tablet. Since the animals accept a banana flavored placebo, we have concluded that the ingestion in a single dose is accompanied by nausea. This interpretation is supported by the decreased intake of diet in those females that continue to consume the banana flavored contraceptive tablet. Other attempted methods of administration include the use of sugar cubes, apple slices, flavored gelatin, or applesauce, but these have also been unsuccessful. We have found that the incorporation of the contraceptive preparation into the diet dilutes the dose and solves many of the problems associated with taste preference. Thus, one pill is incorporated into each 1800 Cal of diet (the daily caloric intake of an average women). When the animals consume the amount of diet needed to maintain weight, they receive a proportional contraceptive dose. Changes in dosage or sequential administration is easily accomplished since the basic diet remains constant. We have chosen to feed the same contraceptive preparation (in the diet) continuously in our studies.

The administration of contraceptive preparations through other devices, such as intravaginal rings(CVR), can be accomplished without great difficulty. One must calibrate carefully the delivery from such a device, both in vivo and in vitro, so that the intended effect can be accomplished. Some female cynomolgus macaques (about 10 percent) repeatedly expel the rings. The loss of treatment rings is usually accompanied by breakthrough bleeding which can be detected by an alert technician; a new ring can be inserted with minimum difficulty. These rings can be left in place for periods greater than six months, however, periodic replacement is desirable to circumvent vaginal infection.

Plasma Lipids and Lipoprotein Changes

As we have mentioned, the plasma lipoprotein concentrations should be allowed to stabilize after the animals are fed the experimental diet before any steroid treatment is initiated. Three to four months is usually sufficient, but a longer period allows for four to five preexperimental evaluations of the lipids and lipoproteins. Prior to the experimental period, the females are distributed into groups based on their total serum cholesterol (TSC) and HDL cholesterol concentrations. This selection process also takes into account age, weight, and cycling history and results in experimental groups which have comparable means and variances for these parameters.

The concentrations of triglycerides, TSC, and HDL cholesterol are determined in blood samples collected from the animals bimonthly. We have conducted several different experiments which demonstrate the effect of different contraceptive treatments on the concentrations of TSC and HDL cholesterol.

In preliminary studies, ten sexually mature female cynomolgus monkeys from the colony were fed a diet that contained 40 percent of calories from fat and 0.1 mg/Cal of cholesterol[16]. Prior to the insertion of intravaginal rings containing levonorgestrel, blood samples were collected for plasma lipid and lipoprotein cholesterol determinations every week for one and a half months. After insertion the rings were left in place for 20 weeks. Rapid decreases were observed for both total plasma cholesterol (TPC) and HDL cholesterol concentrations after ring insertion. The ratio of TPC to HDLC was increased. Pretreatment concentrations of triglycerides (21 ± 7 mg/dl) decreased slightly after the initiation of treatment, but then increased at 12 weeks (31 ± 6 mg/dl). Concentrations of both TPC and HDL cholesterol returned to pretreatment values during the weeks following ring removal. When the percentage of HDL that was HDL_2 was evaluated before and after ring insertion, it was determined that among the majority of animals the change was from about 12 percent before ring insertion to 6 percent after insertion.

Changes in lipids and lipoproteins have been documented in a

Table 4. Lipid and Lipoprotein Cholesterol Changes after Administration of Levonorgestrel-Containing Treatments.

	TOTAL SERUM CHOLESTEROL (mg/dl)	HDL CHOLESTEROL (mg/dl)	TRIGLYCERIDES (mg/dl)
Pretreatment	369 ± 21	39.5 ± 2.3	16
2 Month Control	437 ± 65	43.9 ± 4.5	19
2 Month CVR	366 ± 25	25.4 ± 3.3†	9
2 Month OC	419 ± 56	32.9 ± 5.3†	41†
4 Month Control	397 ± 41	43.1 ± 4.4	12
4 Month CVR	394 ± 30	29.3 ± 3.1†	11
4 Month OC	466 ± 52†	25.1 ± 3.0†	33†

* TSC and HDL expressed as mean ± SEM, Triglycerides as median

† Concentrations are different than pretreatment value ($p<.05$)

collaborative study with the Population Council comparing vaginal ring versus oral treatment with levonorgestrel/estrogen. The experimental design included 4 groups of animals: 1) a control group of males; 2) a control group of females which received placebo vaginal rings; 3) a group of females that received vaginal rings calibrated to deliver 43 μg of norgestrel and 26 μg of estradiol per day; and 4) a group of females that received 75 μg of norgestrel and 7.5 μg ethinyl estradiol per day in their diet. The animals were fed a diet which contained 38 percent of calories as fat and 0.3 mg of cholesterol per Calorie. Initial results indicate that both treatments lower HDL cholesterol (Table 4). Total serum cholesterol is not changed by the treatments except in the fourth month when it is increased by the oral treatment ($p<0.05$). Triglyceride concentrations were increased by oral treatment ($p<0.05$; Wilcoxon Test), but the ring treatment was without effect.

Because of the interest in the chemical configuration of the progestin in relation to its ability to lower HDL cholesterol, a pilot project was designed to look at the effect of two 19-nortestosterone derived progestins (ethynodiol diacetate and norgestrel) compared to a 17-hydroxyprogesterone derivative (medroxyprogesterone acetate). These progestins were incorporated into the animals' diet as the commercial preparations Ovral (0.5 mg norgestrel + 0.05 mg ethinyl estradiol), Demulen (1.0 mg ethynodiol diacetate + 0.05 mg ethinyl estradiol), and Provera (50 mg medroxyprogesterone acetate). The study was conducted as a cross over design, with each of twelve monkeys receiving each of the preparations for one month with a one month period of recovery between treatments. A significant decrease ($p<0.05$) in HDL cholesterol was observed with all treatments

Table 5. Lipid and Lipoprotein Cholesterol Changes after Treatment with 19-nor-Testosterone vs. 17-Hydroxyprogesterone Derived Progestins.

	TOTAL SERUM CHOLESTEROL (mg/dl)	HDL CHOLESTEROL (mg/dl)	TRIGLYCERIDES (mg/dl)
Ovral:			
Pre-treatment	139 ± 7	68.0 ± 3.3	50 ± 7
Post-treatment	136 ± 7	48.3 ± 4.0†	52 ± 6
Demulen:			
Pre-treatment	143 ± 4	66.4 ± 4.7	54 ± 9
Post-treatment	160 ± 9	51.8 ± 3.4†	57 ± 7
Provera:			
Pre-treatment	144 ± 4	66.0 ± 3.3	55 ± 9
Post-treatment	130 ± 6†	57.7 ± 3.4†	41 ± 8

* Values given are mean ± SEM

† Denotes values which are different from pre-treatment ($p<.05$)

(Table 5), but the decrease was greatest with the Ovral and Demulen treatments. Total serum cholesterol was decreased in the animals treated with Provera ($p<0.05$), and the increase noted with Demulen approached significance ($p<0.1$). Triglyceride concentrations were not different in any of the groups after contraceptive treatment. The lowering of HDL cholesterol by Provera might be negated by combining an estrogen with the treatment.

Evaluation of Cycling Activity and its Interruption

It is desirable to know whether the contraceptive formulation under study is effective in disrupting the regular reproductive cyclic activity of the animals being studied. The reproductive characteristics of the individual study animals are determined during the preexperimental period and then periodically once contraceptive treatment is initiated. Both single caged and group caged females can be trained to present themselves for vaginal inspection. The detection of vaginal bleeding is aided by the insertion of a cotton tipped swab. Females are swabbed on a daily basis and the vaginal bleeding patterns for each animal are recorded. Less frequent monitoring of bleeding patterns is possible, since menstrual bleeding is usually of 3-4 days duration.

Additional information concerning ovulatory activity can be acquired by collecting periodic blood samples for the determination of progesterone

Table 6. Concentrations of Levonorgestrel (mg/dl) at Different Times Post-Feeding of Ovral Containing Diet.

Hour After Feeding	Animals Sampled #1320	#1324	#1338
1	0.5	2.1	1.2
2	1.0	3.1	1.4
3	1.3	3.2	1.8
4	1.5	3.2	1.5
5	1.6	2.7	1.4

* Animals had consumed diet by one hour post-feeding.

concentrations. Although the sampling in untreated females can be optimized by collecting the sample during the luteal phase (use of vaginal bleeding records), this is not practical in treated animals that have no regular bleeding patterns. We have found that the evaluation of samples collected twice a week is sufficient to detect a luteal elevation of plasma progesterone by radioimmunoassay.

We have documented the effective interruption in cycling activity with the above methods in our long term contraceptive studies. Some animals have experienced breakthrough bleeding upon initial treatment or after ring loss, but this is not usually accompanied by elevated progesterone concentrations.

Individual Differences in Contraceptive Steroid Effectiveness

Since there will be variability in the extent of atherosclerosis, it is important to determine whether these differences relate to the way in which individual animals metabolize the contraceptive steroids. The quantification of concentrations of the contraceptive steroids in the circulation at various times after ingestion has been used to characterize the dosage in women. These studies are more difficult in nonhuman primates because of the difficulty in delivering the dose in a concentrated form. Individual eating habits of the macaques have resulted in variable consumption of the diet related to the time of blood sampling, resulting in less confidence in circulating hormone concentrations as indicators of differences in drug metabolism. An example of the contraceptive concentrations after consumption of the diet in three females (Table 6) indicates the problems associated with sampling.

Another approach which has been used to estimate the individual sensitivity to treatment is the measurement of serum proteins which respond to steroid treatment in a dose response fashion. Sex steroid

Table 7. Binding Capacities of Sex Steroid Binding Globulin and Transcortin in Contraceptive Study.

	SHBG (μg/dl)	CBG (μg/dl)
Control Females	4.42 ± 0.37	2.55 ± 0.71
Contraceptive Vaginal Ring	1.14 ± 0.27*	3.06 ± 0.79
Oral Contraceptive	2.47 ± 0.27*	5.52 ± 0.99*

* Different from control levels (p<.05)

binding globulin (SHBG) increases with estrogen treatment and decreases after progestins or androgens[17,18], while transcortin (CBG) increases only in response to estrogen treatment[19]. Since the contraceptive progestins have some androgenic activity, changes in the binding capacity of these binding proteins can be used to reflect the relative androgen to estrogen nature of the contraceptive treatment. In our study, the binding capacity of SHBG was lowered ($p<0.05$) by both treatments, and the CVR treatment resulted in significantly lower values than OC treatment. The binding capacity of CBG was increased by the OC treatment ($p<0.05$), indicating the estrogenic nature of the treatment (Table 7).

Both serum thyroxine (T_4) and triiodothyronine (T_3) concentrations are elevated after some contraceptive treatments[20], a reflection of the influence of estrogen treatment on thyroxine binding globulin. Both T_3 and T_4 were elevated in the oral treatment group in our study (Table 8).

Metabolic Alterations Induced by Contraceptive Steroids

The insulin resistance which has been described in women using oral contraceptives (reviewed in 21) can also be studied in the cynomolgus macaque. We have determined that greater insulin concentrations are necessary to maintain similar glucose clearance in female macaques treated with some contraceptive preparations (Table 9). The relationship of insulin resistance after contraceptive treatment to the changes in lipid metabolism can be explored in this non human primate model.

Contraceptive treatment has been shown to result in changes in heparin releasable lipase activity in women (reviewed in 22). Since these hormone sensitive enzymes play an important role in the clearance and metabolism of lipids, it is important to study the changes induced by contraceptive treatment. Our initial data from such studies suggest that these measurements will be helpful in understanding the lipid changes during contraceptive treatment.

DESCRIPTION OF PATHOLOGICAL EVALUATIONS AT NECROPSY

Each animal is anesthetized with Ketamine and weighed, after which anesthesia is maintained with pentobarbital. The pericardium is

Table 8. Thyroxine and Tri-iodothyronine Concentrations in Contraceptive Treated Monkeys.

	Tri-iodothyronine (ng/ml)	Thyroxine (ng/ml)
Control Females	1.93 ± 0.17	103 ± 4
Contraceptive Vaginal Ring	1.76 ± 0.13	100 ± 5
Oral Contraceptive	2.77 ± 0.16*	155 ± 9*

* Different from control levels ($p<.05$)

Table 9. Glucose Clearance and Insulin Resistance in Contraceptive-Treated Cynomolgus Macaques.

	Glucose Clearance (K)	Maximum Insulin (μU/ml)
Control Females	2.84 ± 0.22	273 ± 44
Contraceptive Vaginal Ring	3.85 ± 0.30*	936 ± 141*
Oral Contraceptive	3.11 ± 0.24	583 ± 104*

* Denotes treatment means different than controls ($p<.01$)

incised and the circulatory system is perfused through the left ventricle with 0.1 M sodium phosphate buffer at 100 mm Hg for 5 minutes or until blood is cleared from the system.

The heart is perfused and fixed with 10% neutral buffered formalin in 0.1 M phosphate buffer for 60 minutes at 90 mm Hg. The aorta, femoral and carotid arteries are removed and opened longitudinally along the anterior surface; they are then fixed flat on cardboard in 10 percent neutral buffered formalin. The following organs are removed, weighed, and placed in formalin: kidneys, adrenals, spleen, pancreas, stomach, liver, gonads, reproductive system, lungs, brain, pituitary, thyroids, thymus, and eyes.

After approximately one week, the arteries are removed from the formalin and stained grossly with Sudan IV in isopropyl alcohol. The peripheral arteries are photographed (with all lesions demarcated) for gross evaluation and quantitation using the Zeiss MOP III Image Analyzer. The thoracic and abdominal aortas are both cut into six blocks and the common carotids and femorals are cut into three blocks each (plus one from the carotid bifurcation). The coronary arteries are sectioned as follows: one from the left main, five from each of the left anterior descending, the right coronary artery, and the left circumflex coronary arteries. The basilar and vertebral arteries of the brain are also sectioned. All the blocks are cut and sectioned for examination by light microscopy. Slides are stained with either hematoxylin and eosin stain using Harris's formula or Verhoeff van Gieson's technique for collagen and elastic fibers. Intimal areas are quantitated using the Zeiss MOP III Image Analyzer.

SUMMARY

Cynomolgus macaques appear to be suitable models for the study of effects of contraceptive steroids on coronary artery atherosclerosis and its risk factors. Frequently used contraceptive estrogens and progestins have effects on plasma lipids and lipoproteins of these animals that are similar to those observed in human females. Differences in extent of coronary artery atherosclerosis and risk factors among males, intact females, and ovariectomized females indicate that endogenous hormonal factors play a role in atherogenesis in this species. Thus, it is expected that exogenous contraceptive steroids may also influence atherogenesis in this species. The evaluation of circulating SHBG, CBG and T_3 or T_4 are useful in determining the androgenic/estrogenic nature of the contraceptive treatment. This nonhuman primate model is also suitable for study of the effects of contraceptive treatment on hepatic and lipase lipoprotein activities and insulin resistance and to understand better their interaction with lipid metabolism.

REFERENCES

1. Arntzenius, AC, van Gent, CM, van Der Voort, H, Stegerhoek, CI, Styblo, K: Reduced high-density lipoprotein in women aged 40-41 using oral contraceptives. Lancet, 1:1221, 1978.

2. Bradley, DD, Wingerd, J, Petitti, DB, Krauss, RM, Ramcharan, S: Serum high-density-lipoprotein cholesterol in women using oral contraceptives, estrogens and progestins. N Engl J Med, 299:17, 1978.

3. Larrson-Cohn, U, Wallentin, L, Zador, G: Plasma lipids and high-density lipoproteins during oral contraception with different combinations of ethinyl estradiol and levonorgestrel. Horm Metab Res, 11:437, 1979.

4. Wallace, RB, Hoover, J, Barrett-Connor, ED, Rifkind, BM, Hunninghake, DB, Mackenthun, A, Heiss, G: Altered plasma lipid and lipoprotein levels associated with oral contraceptive and oestrogen use. Lancet, 2:111, 1979.

5. Larsson-Cohn, U, Fahraeus, L, Wallentin, L, Zador, G: Lipoprotein changes may be minimized by proper composition of a combined oral

contraceptive. Fertil Steril, 35:172, 1981.

6. Hirvonen E., Malkonen, M, Manninen, V: Effects of different progestogens on lipoproteins during postmenopausal replacement therapy. N Engl J Med, 304:560, 1981.

7. Knopp, RH, Walden, CE, Wahl, PW, Hoover, JJ, Warnick, GR, Albers, JJ, Ogilvie, JT, Hazzard, WR: Oral contraceptive and postmenopausal estrogen effects on lipoprotein triglyceride and cholesterol in an adult female population: relationships to estrogen and progestin potency. J Clin Endocrinol Metab, 53:1123, 1981.

8. Wahl, P, Walden, C, Knopp, R, Hoover, J, Wallace, R, Heiss, G, Rifkind, B: Effect of estrogen/progestin potency on lipid/lipoprotein cholesterol. N Engl J Med, 308:862, 1983.

9. Tikkanen, MJ, Nikkila, EA, Kuusi, T: Different effects of two progestins on plasma high density lipoprotein (HDL_2) and postheparin lipase activity. Atherosclerosis, 40:365, 1981.

10. Silferstolpe, G, Gustafson, A, Samsioe, G, Svanborg, A: Lipid metabolic studies in oophorectomised women: Effects on serum lipids and lipoproteins of three synthetic progestogens. Maturitas, 4:103, 1982.

11. Baggett, B, Nash, HA: Effects of contraceptive steroids on serum lipoproteins and cardiovascular disease scrutinized at workshop in Bethesda. Contraception, 21:115, 1980.

12. Rudel, LL, Pitts, LL: Male-female variability in the dietary cholesterol-induced hyperlipoproteinemia of cynomolgus monkeys (Macaca fascicularis). J Lipid Res, 19:992, 1978.

13. Hamm, TE, Kaplan, JR, Clarkson, TB, Bullock, BC: Effects of gender and social behavior on the development of coronary artery atherosclerosis in cynomolgus macaques. Atherosclerosis, 48:221, 1983.

14. Adams, MR, Clarkson, TB, Kaplan, JR, Koritnik, DR: Ovariectomy, social stress and coronary artery atherosclerosis in cynomolgus monkeys. Atheriosclerosis, 3:476a, 1983.

15. Clarkson, TB, Hamm, TE, Bullock, BC, and Lehner, NDM: Atherosclerosis in Old World Monkeys. In: Strong, JP (ed): Primates in Medicine, Atherosclerosis in Primates. Karger, Basel, p 66, 1976.

16. Adams, MR, Rudel, LL, Clarkson, TB, Nelson, CA, Thau, RB, Moo-Young, AJ: Influence of a levonorgestrel-containing contraceptive vaginal ring on plasma lipids and lipoproteins in cynomolgus monkeys. Contraception, 28:253, 1983.

17. El Makhzangy, MN, Wynn, V, Lawrence, DM: Sex hormone binding globulin capacity as an index of oestrogenicity or androgenicity in women on oral contraceptive steroids. Clin Endocrinol, 10:39, 1979.

18. van Kammen, E, Thijssen, JHH, Rademaker, B, and Schwarz, F: The influence of hormonal contraceptives on sex hormone binding globulin

(SHBG) capacity. Contraception 11:53, 1975.

19. Moore, DE, Kawgoe, S, Davajan, V, Mishell, DR, and Nakamura, RM: An in vivo system in man for quantitation of estrogenicity. I. Physiologic changes in binding capacity of serum corticosteroid-binding globulin. Am J Obstet Gynecol, 130:475, 1978.

20. Weeke, J, Hansen, AP: Serum TSH and serum T_3 levels during normal menstrual cycles and during cycles on oral contraceptives. Acta Endocrinol, 79:431, 1975.

21. Wynn, V: Effect of progesterone and progestins on carbohydrate metabolism. In: Bardin, CW, Milgrom, E, Mauvais-Jarvis, P (eds): Progesterone and Progestins. New York, Raven Press, p 395, 1983.

22. Nikkala, EA, Tikkanen, MJ, Kuusi, T: Effects of progestins on plasma lipoproteins and heparin-releasable lipases. In: Bardin, CW, Milgrom, E, Mauvais-Jarvis, P (eds): Progesterone and Progestins. New York, Raven Press, p 411, 1983.

DISCUSSION

DR. BERENDES: Comments or questions?

DR. AKSEL: Of the initial group treated with Ovral, what was the length of treatment? This last group was treated only for four weeks. What was the length of treatment when you initially administered Ovral?

DR. CLARKSON: We are about 22 months into that study. We had originally planned to take them for two years, but I think we will try to take them for three. Of course, our aim is eventually to bring them to necropsy and quantitate atherosclerosis.

DR. GOEBELSMANN: Do you have data on the plasma levels of levonorgestrel for both the oral administration and vaginal rings in these monkeys? They could be considerably higher than those reported in women if you administer the same dose.

DR. CLARKSON: We do have data. I can't recall them, but perhaps Dr. Nash can.

DR. NASH: The animals with the vaginal ring receive a relatively constant dose of steroid. The levels in plasma are in the neighborhood of 2-1/2 to 3 nanograms per milliliter, not too different from what we see in human subjects and not too different from the data that Dr. Goebelsmann showed for Ovral users.

Insofar as the Ovral animals are concerned the values are not much different, possibly slightly lower. However, there is the problem of the time of sampling relative to the time the animals consume the Ovral, but the values are in the neighborhood of 2.5 nanograms per milliliter.

DR. KATZENELLENBOGEN: What do you think is the basis for the reduction in size of the LDL during oral contraceptive use?

DR. CLARKSON: I have no idea.

DR. KATZENELLENBOGEN: Do you think this is a good marker for hormonal effect?

DR. CLARKSON: I think it is much too premature to say. The only things that we know of that control LDL molecular weight are the gender differences that I referred to earlier and some effect of the relative saturation of fat. There is a strong correlation between LDL molecular weight and the cholesterol ester fatty acid composition.

This probably represents some differences in the cholesterol ester fatty acid composition of the LDL particles. I assume it is associated with the availability of the estrogen component of the Ovral pill, but it is much too early to speculate.

DR. CLARK: Ordinarily one would have to be insane to study rats as a model for LDL and HDL because they are generally considered not to reflect what occurs in humans. But we made some recent observations that suggest it more likely that the rat may become a valuable model. We have observed in male rats that, LDL does have a greater molecular weight and I believe it is shifted by the administration of estrogen.

In these animals we don't measure LDL or any other lipoprotein by the classical method, except we do flotation gradients instead of columns as you do. But we measure them by the binding of tritiated tamoxifen to LDL. While there is specific binding to LDL, the physiological significance is not known.

It readily detects LDL's. If we castrate an animal, LDL blood levels go up. If we replace with physiological amounts of estrogen, they decrease. There also is this shift in molecular weight which I believe you mentioned.

DR. CLARKSON: That is an interesting observation.

DR. KUZMA: I have two questions. The first one is on the type of diet you have chosen as the moderate atherogenic diet. Did you also, or are you thinking of using the normal Purina monkey chow, which is perhaps a preferred diet that some groups in the U.S. use?

Question number two. In Table 3, where you were pointing out Gordon's work on the increase in HDL and the reduced rate of coronary heart disease, did they take into account things like age, smoking and other things that are related to heart disease mortality?

DR. CLARKSON: Let me answer your questions in reverse order. I showed Tavia Gordon's Framingham data as just one of many examples of that inverse relationship. It has been carefully controlled for age, sex, smoking and other epidemiologic criteria.

It has been so carefully reviewed by the epidemiologists that no one questions the inverse relationship between HDL and coronary heart disease risk.

I have some definite notions about diet. Atherosclerosis investigators and nutritionists either use diets containing no added fat and cholesterol like monkey chow, unlike the diet of any population in the world, or add a tremendous amount of cholesterol to their experimental group, again, unlike any population in the world.

You have two groups unlike any that exist in primate biology, and in the middle group, where we really need information about how primates react to diet, we have no studies. So, we tried to avoid this by using diets that mimic the human experience as closely as possible.

We do allow monkey chow to be fed in our facility, but hesitatingly. The pilot study data I showed you are obtained from animals fed monkey chow, so the effect is there when they are fed monkey chow. But if one wishes to evaluate coronary artery atherosclerosis, which is really more important than guessing about what lipoprotein changes mean, you must measure plasma lipid concentrations in the range of human values.

Most monkeys fed monkey chow have cholesterols around 120 mg/dl and will not develop coronary disease. You must achieve levels of about 220 mg/dl to develop experimental lesions.

DR. BERENDES: Thank you very much.

CONTRACEPTIVE STEROID EFFECTS ON SERUM LIPOPROTEINS AND LIPOPROTEIN SUBCLASSES

Ronald M. Krauss

Donner Laboratories
University of California
Berkeley, California

INTRODUCTION

This report describes the application of methods recently developed in our laboratory to study changes in human serum lipoproteins and lipoprotein subclasses associated with use of contraceptive steroids.

Several years ago it was observed that variation in levels of high density lipoprotein (HDL) cholesterol in users of these steroid preparations resulted from the tendency of the estrogen component to increase HDL cholesterol and certain of the progestins to decrease HDL cholesterol[1]. In Figure 1 is shown a summary of results taken from data analyzed as part of the Walnut Creek Contraceptive Drug Study[1]. The various contraceptive and noncontraceptive steroid preparations used by groups of women in this study were ranked according to mean HDL cholesterol levels adjusted for age, relative body weight, alcohol intake, and cigarette use. Higher levels of HDL cholesterol tended to occur in individuals taking either pure estrogens or the sequential ethinyl estradiol dinorethisterone preparations, while lower HDL cholesterol levels were associated with use of combinations containing higher doses of progestins, particularly norethindrone acetate and levonorgestrel, with the lowest HDL cholesterol levels observed in a group of users of norethindrone acetate alone. The effects of progestins appear to relate in a general way to their relative androgenic or antiestrogenic effects[2], but one could also argue that effects on HDL cholesterol provide a bioassay for metabolic effects in humans, the mechanisms of which remain to be determined.

The cross-sectional observations have been confirmed by more recent studies in which treatment with progestins either alone or in combination with estrogens have been shown to lower HDL cholesterol, most strikingly in the case of levonorgestrel[3-8].

Studies in our laboratory and by others were subsequently carried out to assess in more detail the effects of estrogenic and progestational agents on serum lipoproteins with a view towards how these effects might help us to understand physiological and pathological mechanisms of lipoprotein metabolism in humans. In the case of HDL we initially focused

HORMONE PREPARATION				
Estrogen	Dose (mg)	Progestin	Dose (mg)	N
Ethinyl Estradiol	.10	Dimethisterone	25 (seq)	18
Ethinyl Estradiol	.02	None		32
Ethinyl Estradiol	.05	None		25
Mestranol	.08	Norethindrone	2.0 (seq)	16
Mestranol	.10	Norethynodrel	2.5	13
Conjugated Est.	≥ 1.25	None		455
Conjugated Est.	≤ .625	None		258
Ethinyl Estradiol	.05	Ethynodiol Diac.	1.0	15
Mestranol	.10	Ethynodiol Diac.	1.0	68
Mestranol	.08	Norethindrone	1.0	138
Mestranol	.10	Norethindrone	2.0	35
Ethinyl Estradiol	.05	Noreth. Acetate	1.0	21
Mestranol	.05	Norethindrone	1.0	135
None		None		3422
Ethinyl Estradiol	.02	Norgestrel	0.3	14
Ethinyl Estradiol	.05	Norgestrel	0.5	14
Ethinyl Estradiol	.05	Noreth. Acetate	2.5	21
None		Noreth. Acetate	5.0	12

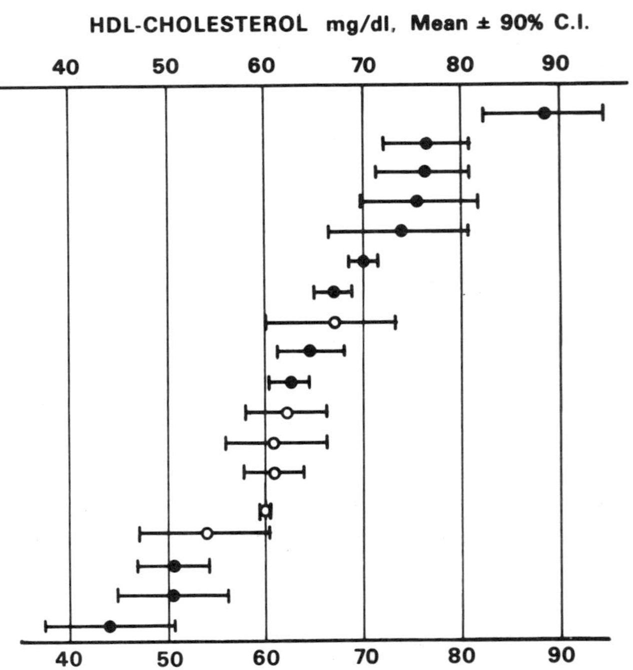

Figure 1. HDL-cholesterol measurements in groups of women using contraceptive and non-contraceptive steroid preparations and in non-user controls. Results have been adjusted for influence of age, relative body weight, alcohol intake and cigarette use. Data adapted from reference 1.

on studies of hormonal effects on three major subclasses of HDL which are structurally and metabolically related (Figure 2, reference 9). These species form a spectrum, with HDL_3, the most dense and protein enriched, HDL_{2a}, the more lipid and cholesterol enriched, and finally HDL_{2b} which is the most lipid enriched and most buoyant of the three species described here. In the ultracentrifuge the flotation or F rates of these particles increase as one goes from HDL_3 to $_{2a}$ to $_{2b}$ as a result of their progressive decrease in buoyant density and increase in particle size.

The metabolic interrelationships among these subclasses are complex and include cholesterol ester enrichment by the action of the enzyme lecithin:cholesterol acyltransferase, and also by transfer from other lipoproteins[10-12]. More recently it has been shown that HDL_2 phospholipids can be catabolized by an enzyme present in the hepatic endothelium (hepatic lipase), such that if one incubates hepatic lipase with HDL one can measure a loss of phospholipid from the HDL_2 fraction[13,14], and it has been hypothesized that levels of HDL_2 may be related, at least in some circumstances, to activity of hepatic lipase[15]. In other studies, levels of HDL_2 have been positively correlated with levels of another enzyme, lipoprotein lipase, which is involved in the catabolism of triglyceride rich lipoproteins[16-18]. The mechanism for this relationship is as yet unclear, but may involve, in part, a transfer of lipid and protein components from triglyceride rich lipoproteins to HDL during the course of lipolysis, with accretion of lipid by HDL_2 precursors.

Because levels of HDL_2 are generally increased in individuals with high levels of HDL cholesterol, particularly women vs men[19] and endurance athletes vs sedentary controls[20], and because HDL-cholesterol levels are inversely related to risk of coronary artery disease[21,22], it has been supposed that HDL_2 may be the major HDL species that act to "protect" against development or progression of coronary artery disease. More recently, Miller and colleagues have reported that levels of HDL_2 cholesterol were significantly depressed in a group of patients with severe coronary artery disease compared with individuals with less severe disease, in contrast with levels of total HDL cholesterol or HDL_3 cholesterol which were only minimally depressed[23]. While this is as yet a preliminary observation, it is consistent with the consensus that is developing around the role of HDL_2 as an "antiatherogenic" lipoprotein class.

Measurements of HDL subspecies in our laboratory were initially carried out by analytic ultracentrifugation[24] and more recently this

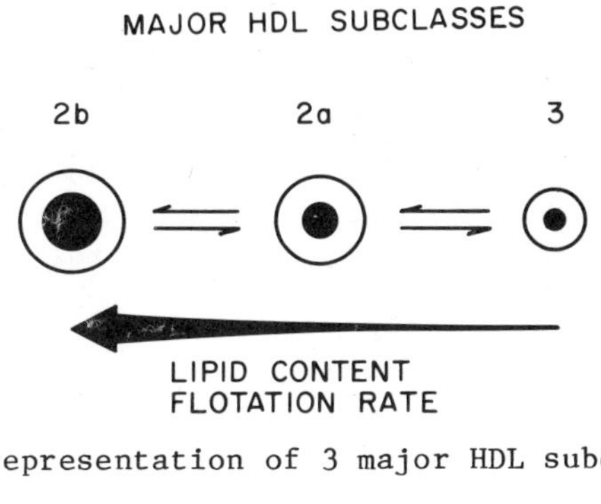

Figure 2. Schematic representation of 3 major HDL subclasses in humans[9].

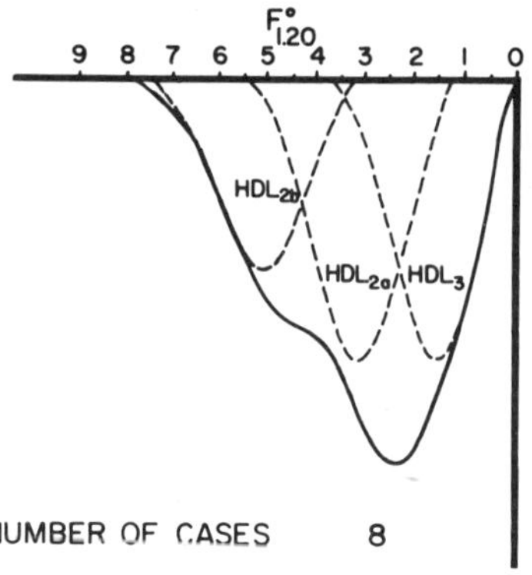

Figure 3. Computer-derived and corrected analytic ultracentrifuge schlieren profiles of total HDL mass (solid line) and 3 major HDL subclasses (taken from reference 9). $F°_{20}$ = corrected analytic ultracentrifuge flotation rate at d = 1.20 g/ml, 20°C.

analysis has been refined using computer techniques[25] to yield a corrected schlieren curve representing the distribution of HDL particles according to their flotation rates (Figure 3). Shown within the curve are component curves fitted by computer techniques used to estimate the concentrations of HDL_3, HDL_{2a} and HDL_{2b}[9].

Using analytic ultracentrifuge measurements we have compared HDL subclass distribution in postmenopausal women using conjugated estrogens with the results in a group of control women not using estrogens (Figure 4, reference 26). The difference in HDL distributions is more clearly

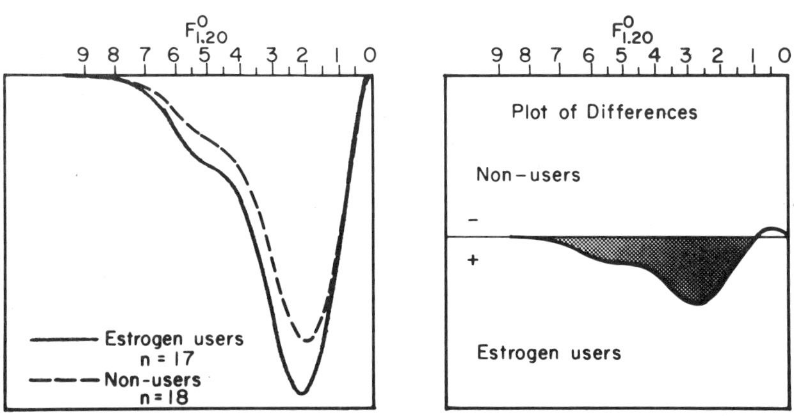

Figure 4. Analytic Ultracentrifugation of HDL. Left: Averages of analytic ultracentrifuge measurements of HDL in 17 post-menopausal estrogen users and 18 non-user controls (Data from studies in reference 26). Right: Computer-derived plot of differences in analytic ultracentrifuge measurements of HDL shown in left panel, performed as described previously[9,33]. Shaded are below baseline represents net increase in HDL mass in estrogen users vs non-users.

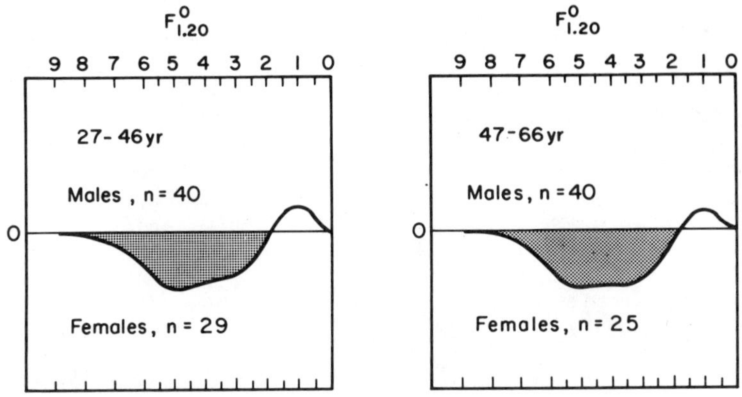

Figure 5. Differences in high density lipoproteins. Differences in mean of HDL analytic ultracentrifuge measurements of HDL in healthy men vs women. Difference plot computed as in Figure 4. (Data from reference 30).

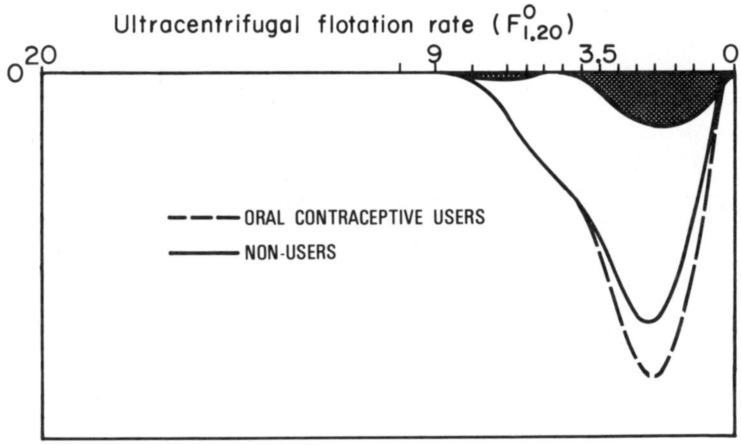

Figure 6. Averages of analytic ultracentrifuge measurements of HDL in a group of oral contraceptive users (n = 17) and in a group of non-user controls (n = 18). The shaded area represents the difference between the two curves and indicates the net increase in HDL mass in oral contraceptive users (Data taken from reference 31).

illustrated in the right panel where a plot of the difference has been computed as described in reference 9 to show that the higher levels of HDL in estrogen users fit a bimodal distribution which corresponds closely to the ultracentrifugal characteristics of the HDL_{2a} and 2_b subspecies, whereas the HDL_3 lipoproteins are not significantly different in the two groups. While these observations were conducted in groups of women that were matched as closely as possible for age, body weight and other factors, they do have the limitation of being cross section observations.

However, recent longitudinal studies have confirmed an estrogen induced increase in HDL_2[27,28], and we have also found the differences in another study population[29].

Interestingly, the difference in levels of HDL subspecies in estrogen users vs controls parallels closely, although not exactly, the differences in HDL subspecies between normal men and women in a random subset of a normal population studied earlier in our laboratory (Figure 5, reference 30). Again this illustrates higher levels of HDL_{2a} and $_{2b}$ in women compared with men both younger and older age groups. The estrogen effect is additive upon the sex difference, so that estrogen use results in additional increases in HDL_2 subspecies beyond those seen in the comparisons of women vs men[26,29].

These observations of estrogen effects of HDL subspecies take on particular interest when compared with previous studies involving analytic ultracentrifugation measurements of HDL in a group of 18 women oral contraceptive users, most treated with norethindrone-estradiol combinations, compared with 19 nonuser controls (Figure 6, reference 31). Rather than the predominant increase in HDL_2 subspecies found with estrogen use, the difference between users and nonusers is confined to HDL_3, with a slight overlap into HDL_{2a} region. We have concluded from this and from subsequent longitudinal studies[29,32] that progestin use can shift the estrogen mediated increase in HDL from more buoyant to more dense HDL subspecies.

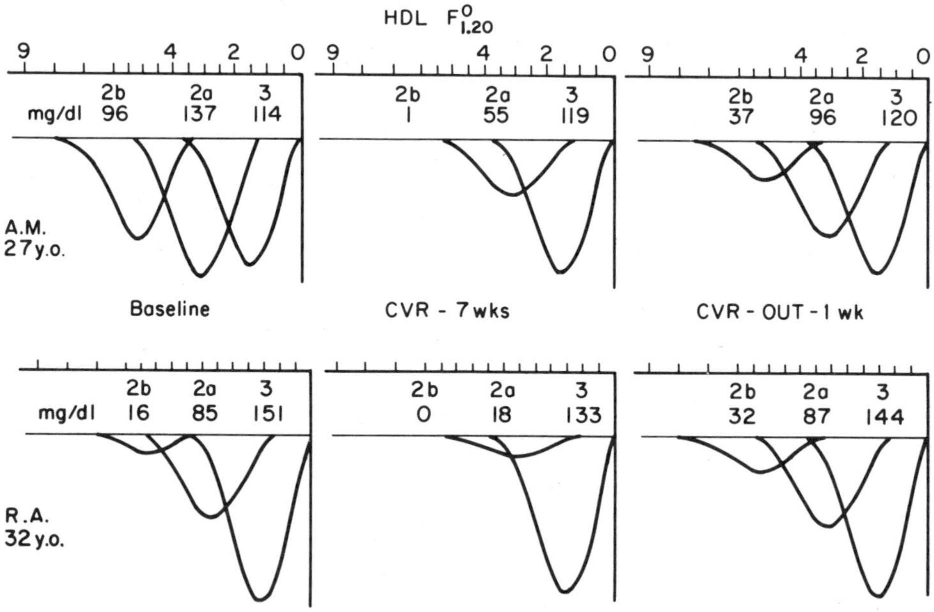

Figure 7. Measurements of three major HDL subclasses (HDL_{2b}, HDL_{2a}, HDL_3) derived from analytic ultracentrifugation results in two women at baseline (left panels), 7 weeks after insertion at estradiol-levonorgestrel contraceptive vaginal rings (middle panels) and 1 week after removal of the rings (right panels). (Data from reference 33).

Recently in collaboration with Drs. Roy, Pike, Mishell and Casagrande at the University of Southern California, we had the opportunity of examining changes in serum lipoproteins associated with administration of a potent progestin preparation, a contraceptive vaginal ring containing levonorgestrel and estradiol[33]. In Figure 7 are shown changes in HDL measured by analytic ultracentrifugation in 2 of the 9 women that we studied who are representative of the results seen in the group as a whole. After seven weeks of use there was a sharp reduction in total HDL, restricted to the HDL_2 components, with a rapid return toward baseline after one week following removal of the vaginal ring. The effects on HDL_{2b} were particularly dramatic, involving essentially complete obliteration of this species in these two subjects and a highly significant reduction in the group as a whole, whereas there were no significant effects on levels of HDL_3. The effects on HDL and HDL_2 are consistent with other data that indicate that the levonorgestrel-estradiol vaginal rings are strongly progestin dominant in their biological effects[33].

Recently in our laboratory we have focussed attention on hormonal effects on the low density lipoproteins, which transport the bulk of cholesterol in humans, and are felt to be directly involved in the atherosclerotic process. Again we initially employed analytic ultracentrifugation to provide detailed information regarding lipoproteins in the lower density classes. In Figure 8 are shown typical analytic ultracentrifuge schlieren profiles of very low density lipoproteins (VLDL) and low density lipoproteins (LDL) in women compared with men[30]. Although the centrifugation conditions differ somewhat from those used for study of high density lipoproteins, the flotation rate (S°) remains a function of density as well as size of the particles. VLDL are lipoproteins of S° 20-400, LDL have S° 0-12, and intermediate density lipoproteins (IDL) are in the S° 12-20 interval. Adopting an approach analogous to that used for examining differences in HDL between the sexes, we plotted the

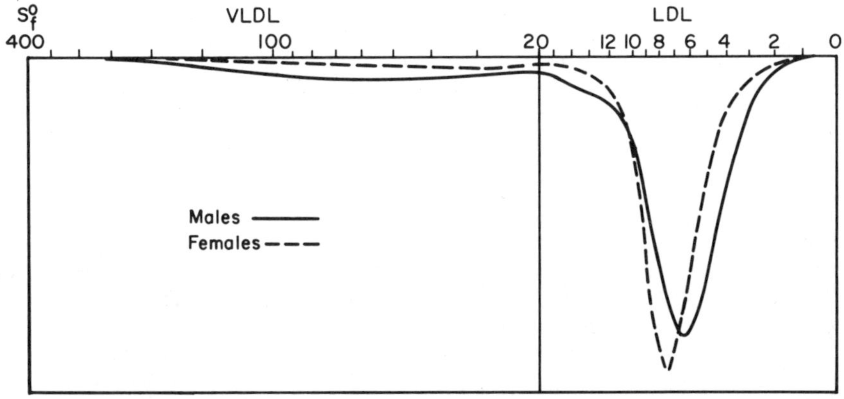

Figure 8. Low and very low density lipoproteins in normal males and females, 27-46 yr. Averages of analytic ultracentrifuge measurements of serum very low density lipoproteins (VLDL) and low density lipoproteins (LDL) in groups of healthy men and women. (Date from reference 30). S° = corrected analytic ultracentrifuge flotation rate at d = 1.063 g/ml, 20° C.

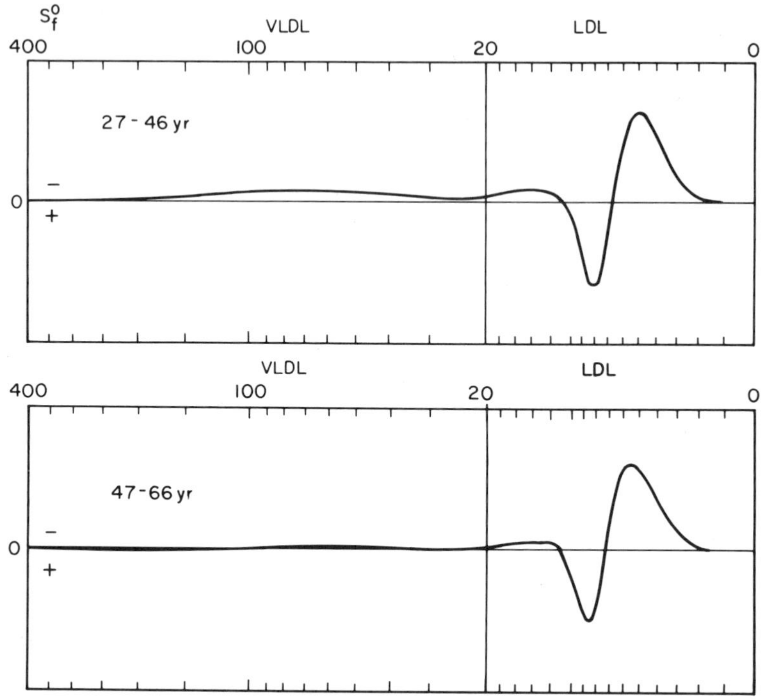

Figure 9. Plot of differences in the average analytic ultracentrifuge profiles of VLDL and LDL in women vs men shown in Figure 8. Areas below the baseline represent mass of lipoproteins higher in women than men, and areas above baseline represent mass of lipoproteins lower in women than men.

differences across the LDL flotation spectrum, and found that the curve defined differences in four intervals (Figure 9, reference 30). Levels of VLDL and of IDL were slightly lower in women, while the difference in LDL of S° 0-12 was biphasic, with mean levels of LDL in the S° 0-7 flotation intervals significantly lower in women than in men, and levels of LDL in the S° 7-12 region significantly higher.

In more recent studies we have shown that these sex differences in LDL defined by analytic ultracentrifugation can be ascribed to differences in concentration of specific LDL subspecies that have been separated and characterized by equilibrium density gradient ultracentrifugation[34,35]. A photograph of the centrifuge tube containing LDL separated by this procedure from plasma of a healthy menstruating female (Figure 10) shows the presence of four major isopycnic bands in the LDL density region, which have been designated as LDL I-IV in order of increasing density and decreasing size, flotation rate, and molecular weight[35]. LDL-I is included in the LDL of S° 7-12 as measured by analytic ultracentrifugation, and LDL-III is included in LDL of S° 0-7[35]. In a series of normal subjects we have shown that LDL mass in density fractions from band I tends to be higher in women vs men, while mass in fractions from band III tends to be lower, although the small number of subjects in these studies precluded

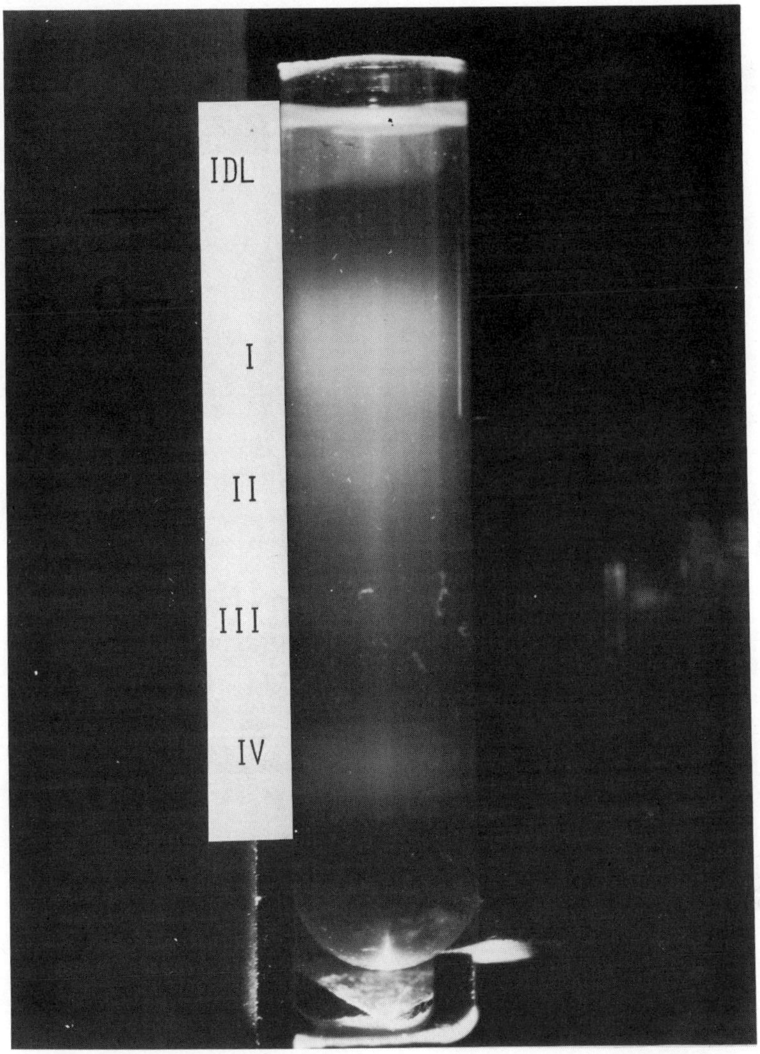

Figure 10. Tube showing separation of IDL (top) and multiple bands of LDL after equilibrium density gradient ultracentrifugation using the procedures described in references 34 and 35.

statistical significance of these differences[36].

We have also shown using measurements of LDL subfraction mass by both analytic ultracentrifugation[30] and preparative equilibrium density gradient ultracentrifugation[34], that levels of LDL-I are strongly correlated with levels of HDL_2 in both sexes, and there is more highly significant negative correlation between levels of LDL-III and HDL_2. Of the remaining LDL species, those in band II tend to overlap in physical and biological properties with LDLI, and to a lesser extent with LDL-III, while the LDL in band IV is distinguished not only by its higher density

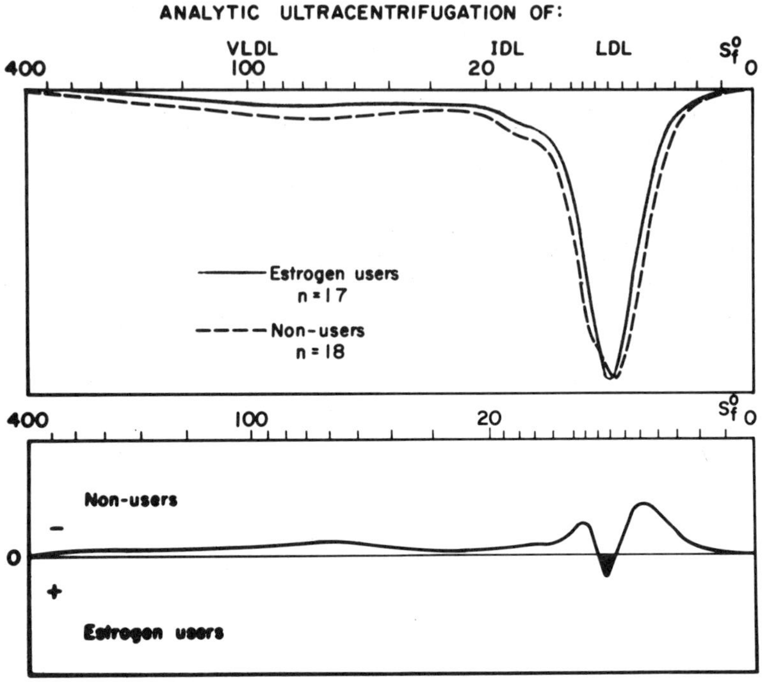

Figure 11. Top panel: Average analytic ultracentrifuge measurements of VLDL, IDL, and LDL in groups of estrogen users and non-users described in Figure 4 and reference 26. Bottom panel: Plot of differences in analytic ultracentrifuge results shown in top panel.

but also by smaller size and relative increase in protein and triglyceride content compared with LDL in bands II and III [34,35]. LDL-IV tends to be a minor component in most normolipemic individuals, but represents the major form of LDL in patients with moderate to severe hypertriglyceridemia[36].

The sex differences in concentrations of LDL subclasses, coupled with the reciprocal relationships of LDL-I and LDL-III with levels of HDL_2, led us to examine the possibility that gonadal hormones may affect levels and distributions of these LDL subspecies. In Figure 11 are shown the analytic ultracentrifuge schlieren patterns of the S° 0-400 lipoproteins in the groups of postmenopausal estrogen users and nonuser controls whose HDL schlieren profiles were shown in Figure 4. Differences across the LDL spectrum are seen more clearly in the difference plots shown in the lower panel of this figure. Within the LDL, there is a reduction in mass in the region of S° 2-5, as well as a reduction in the more buoyant LDL-I. While these changes were not of sufficient magnitude to reach statistical significance in this study, a similar pattern of differences was found in another comparison of postmenopausal estrogen users and non-user controls who showed differences in levels of HDL subspecies that were reported previously[29]. Thus, the differences in LDL associated with

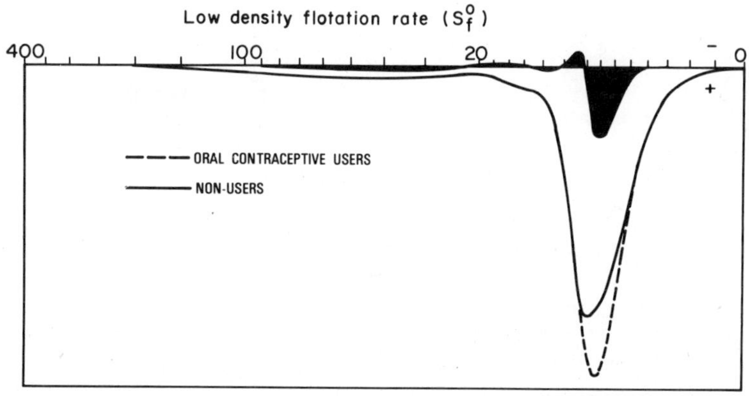

Figure 12. Average analytic ultracentrifuge measurements of VLDL, IDL, and LDL in groups of oral contraceptive users and non-users described in Figure 6 and reference 31. Shaded curve represents differences between the users and non-users.

estrogen use do not strictly parallel the differences between the sexes (Figure 9), although a relative reduction in the S° 2-5 lipoproteins, corresponding to LDL-III[35], is a common feature.

In order to examine alterations in LDL subclasses associated with oral contraceptive use, we turned to the groups of contraceptive users and nonuser controls whose HDL results were described above (Figure 6, reference 31). The S° 0-400 schlieren profiles for these groups are shown in Figure 12, along with the difference plot, depicted by the shaded curve. The users, the majority of whom were taking norethindrone-estrogen combinations, are here shown to have on the average increased levels of LDL confined principally to the region of S° $<$ 7. Thus in contrast to estrogen use, combination oral contraceptive use is associated with apparent increases rather than decreases in levels of LDL-III. The observations also suggest that the recently reported increases in levels of LDL cholesterol in groups of oral contraceptive users[37], may reflect higher levels of the smaller, denser LDL subspecies.

Based on the differences between the effects of estrogens and combination oral contraceptives on LDL, it seemed reasonable to suppose that the progestin component of oral contraceptives could act to oppose or otherwise modify estrogenic effects on LDL subspecies. An opportunity to examine the progestin effect was created by the studies described above (Figure 7) in which lipoproteins were measured serially by analytic ultracentrifugation in women using the progestin-dominant contraceptive vaginal rings that result in marked reductions in HDL_2. Comparison of the difference in the S° 0-400 lipoprotein distribution before and after seven weeks of contraceptive ring use in a representative subject are shown using the difference plot technique in the upper panel of Figure 13. Most striking is the increase in levels of LDL in the S° 0-7 region with an almost reciprocal reduction in the higher molecular weight, less dense LDL species, as well as parallel reductions in IDL and VLDL levels. Furthermore, within one week following removal of the ring (Figure 13, lower panel) these changes in lipoprotein classes reverted in a near

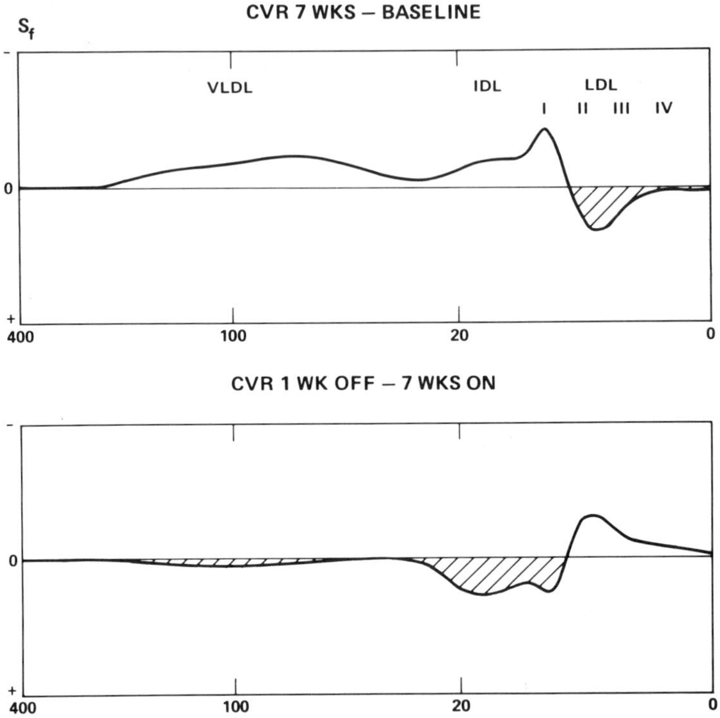

Figure 13. Top panel: Plot of differences in analytic ultracentrifuge measurements of VLDL, IDL, and LDL in a representative subject before vs 7 weeks after using a contraceptive vaginal ring (CVR) containing estradiol and levonorgestrel. Shaded area below baseline represents net increase in lipoprotein mass associated with CVR use. Subject is from study group described in reference 33. Bottom panel: Plot of difference in analytic ultracentrifuge measurements of VLDL, IDL, and LDL in subject from upper panel after 7 weeks of CVR use vs one week after removal of CVR.

mirror image manner to levels present at baseline. Thus with use of this potent progestational preparation there can be major and rapidly reversible changes in LDL subclasses that appear to occur in conjunction with reductions in HDL_2. This linkage of changes in LDL and HDL subclasses is consistent with the correlations in levels of these subclasses described previously[30,34]. Furthermore, the changes within the LDL were not reflected in significant net changes in total LDL concentration[31]. Thus a full appreciation of the potential metabolic and pathologic consequences of contraceptive steroid administration may not be revealed without consideration of changes in specific forms of lipoproteins, particularly LDL and HDL subspecies, within the lipoprotein spectrum. In this instance, a potent progestin with associated androgenic and antiestrogenic properties[1,2], produces changes in lipoproteins and lipoprotein subclasses that appear to be predictive of increased coronary risk, particularly reduction of HDL_2[23] and an increase in the LDL/HDL ratio[21,22]. The reciprocal relationship between HDL_2 and LDL-III raises the additional possibility

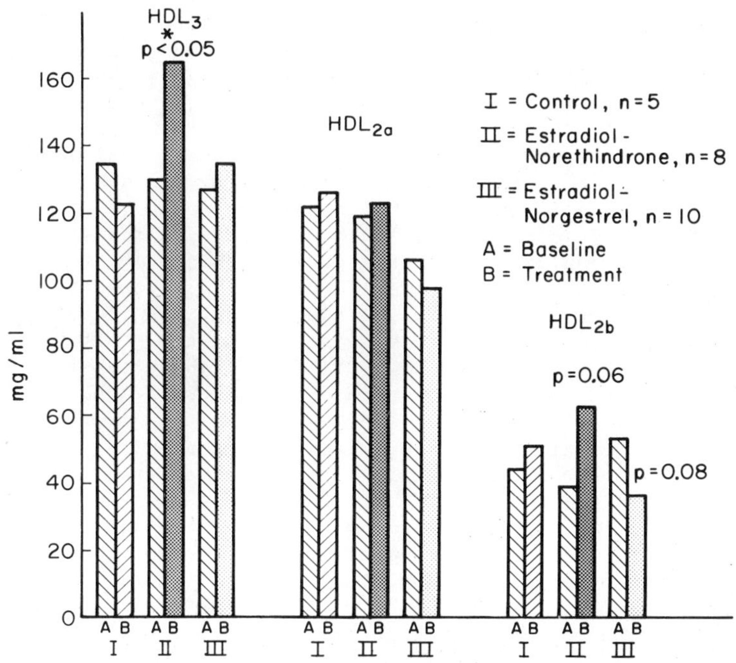

Figure 14. Analytic ultracentrifuge measurements of HDL subclasses in groups of women using no hormones (A), and using contraception with norethindrone 0.4 mg, ethinyl estradiol 0.035 mg (B), or norgestrel 0.3 mg, ethinyl estradiol 0.03 mg (C). Left bar in each bar represents value in follicular phase of pretreatment cycle, and right bar represents value after 7 weeks of hormone use. Data for HDL_3 are means, and for HDL_{2a} and HDL_{2b}, data are median values due to non-normal distribution of these two parameters. Results from reference 32.

that this subclass of LDL may contribute to any increase in risk associated with reduction of HDL_2. It should be recalled, however, that no studies have as yet demonstrated that induced changes in any lipoprotein parameters are associated with increased coronary risk. Furthermore, as described below, it appears to be possible to design lower dose estrogen-progestin preparations which minimize these pharmacological effects on serum lipoproteins.

A study aimed at examining this possibility was carried out in collaboration with Drs. Roy, Mishell, and Pike at the University of Southern California[32]. Changes in serum lipoproteins were examined in normal menstruating women randomly assigned to use of ethinyl estradiol, 0.035 mg, plus norethindrone, 0.4 mg (n = 10); use of ethinyl estradiol, 0.03 mg, plus norgestrel, 0.3 mg (n = 11); and no hormone use (n = 5). Serum lipids and lipoproteins were measured in the follicular phase of the menstrual cycle preceeding oral contraceptive treatment, and again seven weeks later. In the group of norethindrone users, levels of total cholesterol and cholesterol in HDL increased significantly with treatment, while in the norgestrel users there was a slight and insignificant reduction in HDL cholesterol[32]. The difference in change of HDL cholesterol with use of the two different estrogen-progestin combinations was statistically significant. Figure 14 shows the changes in HDL subclasses associated with oral contraceptive use. There was a significant increase in HDL_3 in users of the norethindrone preparation, and a slight and insignificant increase in users of the norgestrel preparation. These findings confirm the cross-sectional data presented above (Figure 6) showing that in a group of women using oral contraceptives, predominantly preparations including norethindrone, levels of HDL_3 were significantly higher than in nonuser controls[31]. In the present longitudinal study, levels of HDL_{2a} showed no changes using either of the contraceptive formulations. Changes in HDL_{2b}, however, showed an interesting divergence, with an increase in users of the norethindrone preparation, and a decrease in users of the norgestrel preparation. While neither of these changes in themselves reached statistical significance, the difference in the response in these two user groups was significant at the $p < 0.05$ level.

In the case of LDL analyses, total LDL concentration increased significantly in the norethindrone users, but ratios of LDL/HDL were not altered[32]. In the norgestrel group, there was a significant increase in this ratio, largely due to the reduction in the HDL_2 subspecies, since the ratio was also significantly higher if one used HDL_2 as the denominator[32].

SUMMARY AND CONCLUSIONS

In summary, these recent longitudinal studies confirm previous cross sectional data showing that individual progestins may differ in their effects on lipoprotein metabolism, even in the lower dose formulations. However, as in the case of the norethindrone containing preparations studies here, as well as in other low dose preparations studied recently[15,38], it may be possible to ameliorate potentially deleterious changes in HDL_2 and LDL/HDL ratios.

In conclusion, while we still have a great deal to learn about the clinical significance of lipoprotein subclasses, particularly those recently described within the low density lipoproteins, the findings reviewed here indicate that measurements of changes in subclasses associated with contraceptive steroid administration place us one step closer to a better understanding of biochemical mechanisms and possible pathologic consequences of these steroid effects. The development of recent microelectrophoretic techniques for analyses of both HDL and LDL subspecies[35,39] has made it more feasible to recommend that these measurements be included in studies designed to evaluate the metabolic effects of oral contraceptives. Consideration should also be given to measurements of other biochemical parameters that may be involved in the oral contraceptive effects on lipoprotein metabolism, such as changes in lipase activities which have been linked to changes in levels of HDL_2[13,18]. Finally, comparison of the results of these more detailed lipoprotein measurements in various experimental animal systems should improve our ability to examine possible differences and similarities with the lipoprotein distributions in humans, and to assess the possible relevance to humans of potentially pathologic lipoprotein changes demonstrated in these species.

REFERENCES

1. Bradley, DD, Wingerd, J, Petitti, DB, Krauss, RM, Ramcharan, S: Serum high-density-lipoprotein cholesterol in women using oral contraceptives, estrogens and progestins. New Engl J Med, 299:17, 1978.

2. Edgren, RA, Jones, RC, Peterson, DL: A biological classification of progestational agents. Fertil Steril, 18:238, 1967,

3. Goldzieher, JW, Chenault, CB, de la Pena, A, Dozier, TS, Kraemer, DC: Comparative studies of the ethynyl estrogens used in oral contraceptives. VII. Effects with and without progestational agents on ultracentrifugally fractionated plasma lipoproteins in humans, baboons, and beagles. Fertil Steril, 30:522, 1978.

4. Larsson-Cohn, U, Wallentin, L, Zador, C: Plasma lipids and high density lipoproteins during oral contraception with different combinations of ethinyl estradiol and levonorgestrel. Horm Metab Res, 11:437, 1979.

5. Rossner, S, Frankman, O, Marsk, L: Effects of ethinylestradiol/D-norgestrel combinations on serum lipoproteins. Acta Obstet Gynecol Scand, 59:255, 1980.

6. Hirvonen, E, Malkonen, M, Manninen, V: Effects of different progestogens on lipoproteins during post-menopausal replacement therapy. New Engl J Med, 304:560, 1981.

7. Tikkanen, MJ, Nikkila, EA, Kuusi, T, Sipinen, S: Different effects of two progestins on plasma high density lipoprotein (HDL_2) and postheparin plasma lipase activity. Atherosclerosis, 40:365, 1981.

8. Krauss, RM: Effects of progestational agents on serum lipids and lipoproteins. J Reprod Med, 27:503, 1982.

9. Anderson, DW, Nichols, AV, Pan, SS, Lindgren, FT: High density lipoprotein distribution. Resolution and determination of three major components in a normal population sample. Atherosclerosis, 29:161, 1978.

10. Nicoll, A, Miller, NE, Lewis, B: High-density lipoprotein metabolism. Adv Lipid Res, 17:53, 1980.

11. Glomset, JA: High-density lipoproteins in human health and disease. Adv Intern Med, 25:91, 1980.

12. Krauss, RM: Regulation of high density lipoprotein levels. Med Clin N Am, 66:403, 1982.

13. Shira, K, Barnhart, RL, Jackson, RL: Hydrolysis of human plasma high density lipoprotein-2-phospholipids and triglycerides by hepatic lipase. Biochem Biophys Res Comm, 100:591, 1981.

14. Groot, PHE, Jansen, H, van Tol, A: Selective degradation of the high density lipoprotein-2 subfraction by heparin releasable liver lipase. FEBS Lett, 129:269, 1981.

15. Kuusi, T, Saarinen, P, Nikkila, EA: Evidence for the role of hepatic endothelial lipase in the metabolism of plasma high density lipoprotein-2 in man. Atherosclerosis, 36:589, 1980.

16. Nikkila, EA, Taskinen, M-R, Kekki, M: Relation of plasma high-density lipoprotein cholesterol to lipoprotein lipase activity in adipose tissue and skeletal muscle of man. Atherosclerosis, 29:497, 1978.

17. Kekki, M: Lipoprotein-lipase action determining plasma high density lipoprotein cholesterol level in adult normolipaemics. Atherosclerosis, 37:143, 1980.

18. Taskinen, MR, Nikkila, EA: High density lipoprotein subfractions in relation to lipoprotein lipase activity of tissues in man - evidence for reciprocal regulation of HDL_2 and HDL_3 levels by lipoprotein lipase. Clin Chim Acta, 112:325, 1981.

19. Nichols, AV: Human serum lipoproteins and their interrelationships. In: Lawrence, JH, Gofman, JW (Eds): Advances in Biological and Medical Physics, New York, Academic Press, 1967, Vol. II, p 109.

20. Krauss, RM, Lindgren, FT, Wood PD, Haskell, WL, Albers, JJ, Cheung, MC: Differential increases in plasma high density lipoprotein subfractions and apolipoproteins (APO-LP) in runners. Circulation 55/56, Supp. III:III4, 1977.

21. Castelli, WP, Doyle, JT, Gordon, T, Hames, CG, Hjortland, MC, Hulley, SB, Kagan, A, Zukel, WJ: HDL cholesterol and other lipids in coronary heart disease: the cooperative lipoprotein phenotyping study. Circulation, 55:767, 1977.

22. Gordon, T, Castelli, WP, Hjortland, MC, Kannel, WB, Dawber, TR: High density lipoprotein as a protective factor against coronary heart disease: the Framingham study. Am J Med, 62:707, 1977.

23. Miller, NE, Hammett, F, Saltissi, S, Rao, S, van Zeller, H, Cottart J, Lewis, B: Relation of angiographically defined coronary artery disease to plasma lipoprotein subfractions and apolipoproteins. Br Med J, 282:1741, 1981.

24. Lindgren, FT, Nichols, VA, Freeman, NK: Physical and chemical composition studies on the lipoproteins of fasting and heparinized human sera. J Phys Chem, 59:930, 1955.

25. Ewing, AM, Freeman, NK, Lindgren, FT: The analysis of human serum lipoprotein distributions. In: Paoletti, R, Kritchevsky, D (Eds): Advances Lipid Research, New York, Academic Press, 1965, vol. 2, p 25.

26. Krauss, RM, Takaki, N, Lewis, SB: Relation of serum high density lipoproteins (HDL) to gonadotropin and estrogen levels in postmenopausal estrogen users and non-users. Fifth International Symposium on Arteriosclerosis, Houston, Texas, November, 1979.

27. Fahraeus, L, Wallentin, L: High density lipoprotein subfractions during oral and cutaneous administration of 17 β - estradiol to menopausal women. J Clin End Metab, 56:797, 1983.

28. Schaefer, EJ, Foster, DM, Zech, LA, Lindgren, FT, Brewer, HB, Levy, RI: The effects of estrogen administration on plasma lipoprotein metabolism on premenopausal females. J Clin End Metab, 57:262, 1983.

29. Krauss, RM, Lindgren, FT, Wingerd, J, Bradley, D, Ramcharan, S: Effects of estrogens and progestins on high density lipoproteins. Lipids, 14:113, 1979.

30. Krauss, RM, Lindgren, FT, Ray, RM: Interrelationships among subgroups of serum lipoproteins in normal human subjects. Clin Chim Acta, 104:275, 1980.

31. Krauss, RM, Lindgren, FT, Silvers, A, Jutagir, R, Bradley, DD: Changes in serum high density lipoproteins in women on oral contraceptive drugs. Clin Chim Acta, 80:465, 1977.

32. Krauss, RM, Roy, S, Mishell, DR, Jr, Casagrande, J, Pike, MC: Effects of two low-dose oral contraceptives on serum lipids and lipoproteins: differential changes in high-density lipoprotein subclasses. Am J Obstet Gynecol, 145,446, 1983.

33. Roy, S, Krauss, RM, Mishell, DR, Jr, Casagrande, J, Pike, MC: The effect on lipids and lipoproteins of a contraceptive vaginal ring containing levonorgestrel and estradiol. Contraception, 24:429, 1981.

34. Shen, M, Krauss, RM, Lindgren, FT, Forte, T: Heterogeneity of serum low density lipoproteins in normal human subjects. J Lipid Res, 22:236, 1981.

35. Krauss, RM, Burke, DJ: Identification of multiple subclasses of plasma low density lipoproteins in normal humans. J Lipid Res, 23:97, 1982.

36. Krauss, RM, Musliner, TA, Unpublished data.

37. Wahl, P, Walden, C, Knopp, R, Hoover, J, Wallace, R, Heiss, G, Rifkind, B: Effect of estrogen/progestin potency on lipid/lipoprotein cholesterol. New Engl J Med, 308:862, 1983.

38. Briggs, M, Briggs, M: A randomized study of metabolic effects of four low estrogen oral contraceptives: I. Results after 6 cycles. Contraception, 23:463, 1981.

39. Blanche, PJ, Gong, EL, Forte, TM, Nichols, AV: Characterization of human high-density lipoproteins by gradient gel electrophoresis. Biochim Biophys Acta, 665:408, 1981.

DISCUSSION

DR. BERENDES: Are there any questions?

DR. KNOPP: I am pleased to see that our studies are in such agreement. I think the similarities that exist provide a basis for making a statement about the relative estrogen and progestin potency on the basis of lipoproteins alone. I am fascinated by the observation that HDL_3 increases in your estradiol and norethindrone treated group. From what I gather this seems unlike anything else you have observed, either with estrogen alone or with progestin alone. Do you have any insights into that? I mean, how do you square that observation with progession from HDL_3 to HDL_2 as we understand it now?

DR. KRAUSS: I can only speculate, but since we have seen this difference cross-sectionally and longitudinally, I have had to pay more serious attention to it. I think the neatest way to explain it is to say estrogen induces an HDL increase, probably by increasing HDL synthesis, at least in part, directly. There is some evidence for that.

If the estrogen effect is dominant, then HDL becomes lipid enriched and more buoyant and becomes an HDL_2 species. Somehow the progestin, perhaps by stimulating hepatic lipase activity, changes the properties of that HDL. There could be other effects as well, but basically the progestin shifts the estrogen-induced HDL from more buoyant HDL_2 to more dense lipid depleted HDL_3 type particles.

If the balance is just right, there can be an increase in HDL_3 mass. If the progestin is more potent, there can be a net decrease of total HDL mass, and that is what happens with the norgestrel preparations.

SECTION 4

PANEL OF INTERNATIONAL DRUG REGULATORY AGENCIES

Moderator: Solomon Sobel

PANEL OF INTERNATIONAL DRUG REGULATORY AGENCIES

John A. Donohoe[1], Klaus-Wolf von Eickstedt[2], Partha Das Gupta[3], Solomon Sobel[4,5], Donald Sutherland[6]

[1] Drug Evaluation Center
Canberra, Australia

[2] Institut fur Arzneimittol des
Bundesgesundheitsamtes
Berlin, Federal Republic of Germany

[3] Central Drug Standard Control Organization
Ministry of Health and Family Welfare
New Delhi, India

[4] Director, Division of Metabolism and
Endocrine Drug Products
Food and Drug Administration
Rockville, Maryland, USA

[5] Moderator

[6] Bureau of Drugs
Vanier, Ontario, Canada

DR. SOBEL: In order to get some perspectives on the positions of agencies other than the FDA, we have invited representatives from other countries to discuss their requirements for preclinical testing and their general attitude concerning oral contraceptives.

This panel consists of Professor von Eickstedt from the Federal Republic of Germany, Dr. John A. Donohoe from Australia, Dr. D. J. Sutherland from Canada and from India Dr. P. Das Gupta. I think the most profitable way to proceed is for each panel member to make an introductory statement concerning the regulatory requirements in his country. We can start with Professor von Eickstedt.

PROFESSOR VON EICKSTEDT: There are some general differences between American and the Federal Republic of Germany's drug laws. In the United States, the requirements for the different phases of clinical trials are prescribed by the FDA. In the Federal Republic of Germany the laws prescribe that the principal investigator must be informed before the clinical trial about all pharmacological and toxicological data by the specialist responsible for these data. In addition, all pharmacological and toxicological data must be provided to the government office and a copy of the experimental design sent to the regional administrative office of the state in Germany where the study will be performed.

The clinical study must be based on the current state of knowledge and science concerning the new drug. If any serious adverse reactions occur attributable to the new drug, information in the regulatory offices will be provided to the prosecutor.

One has to understand the regulation; the clinician's responsibility for the patient is the main consideration throughout the clinical trial. The drug company must be cognizant of any potential adverse reactions before clinical trials are initiated.

In the case of an hormonal contraceptive, a whole spectrum of pharmacological characteristics of the new drug must be documented and provided to the clinician. Our preclinical testing requirements established by the Government Drug Institute are only recommendations and not binding. Their existence does not relieve drug company responsibility for developing new experimental designs for novel drugs.

Endocrinologic and pharmacologic effects are known before a Phase I study is initiated from the many tests available by which a hormone may be characterized. The minimal requirements which Dr. Zbinden mentioned yesterday include a broad spectrum of investigations which must be completed before a Phase I study can be started.

Preclinical investigations include short term liver function tests in beagles. While long-term beagle studies are not required for approval of new progestagens in our country, investigations of blood clotting factors in relation to pharmacokinetics and long-term metabolic studies must be undertaken.

These studies of a new hormone must go beyond the establishment of blood level curves and must include excretion patterns as well as identification and hormonal activity of the main metabolites. Once the Phase I clinical trial pharmacokinetics have been determined, they should be compared to those of the animal species used for long-term toxicological studies. The most relevant species will often be a primate.

Rhesus monkeys captured in the wild are usually unsuitable for safety studies. Their ages and diseases are unknown and cannot be accurately determined. Millions have been spent for the breeding of beagle dogs for long-term hormone studies. If some of this money could have been allotted for the investigation of monkey species available world wide, perhaps we would have a better basis for discussion of animal models. I believe that some day in Germany monkeys from modern breeding colonies will represent the best animal model. Companies which cannot provide data derived from such animals probably will not obtain new drug approval.

I have some comments concerning the questions which the participants of this workshop have been asked to address. The general pharmacokinetics of a new hormone should be established in more than one species before a Phase I trial is initiated. The pharmacokinetic data derived from the clinical trial may then serve to establish the best animal model in which to obtain additional pharmacokinetic and metabolic data. In this manner, the most suitable animal representation of the human may be acquired.

Each new hormone requires special guidelines. Scientists with knowledge of these drugs must provide guidelines for research workers and clinicians involved in the investigations.

Modifications of study design depend upon the most available animal models. In my opinion, short term studies in relevant monkey models are more useful than long-term studies in hundreds of rats. This does not mean, however, that studies in rodents or carcinogenicity studies are not needed.

Adverse reactions should be identified by means of "safety-pharmacology" which includes dose response curves and a whole spectrum of possible effects of the new hormone. Many different animal models are available for these tests and new ones are still in development.

Breeding studies and research in more than a half dozen monkey species should be initiated in an effort to identify additional relevant animal models.

The alternative to long-term studies in non-rodents are well designed, controlled, clinical studies which include all laboratory investigations which can establish the safety of the new drug under consideration.

DR. DONOHOE: In Australia, the evaluation of the safety and efficacy of drug products is required prior to a clinical trial or general marketing approval. The existing Australian requirements for preclinical testing of systemic contraceptives, progestogens and estrogens for long-term use are virtually identical to those in the United States.

The selection of the most suitable species to provide significant predictive data was a potential problem when the guidelines were first being considered and now has become a serious one. At the time of writing the existing guidelines, little data were available concerning differences in the metabolism, pharmacokinetics and physiological characteristics of the various steroids in animal species and man.

More importantly, with regard to the beagle bitch, few objections to the use of this animal in carcinogenicity bioassay were reported. We realize that the use of the beagle as model is receiving continuous criticism and, indeed, it may not be the most appropriate model for the testing of systemic oral contraceptives. Nevertheless, it may not be prudent to disregard the positive results obtained from this species or the wealth of data that are now available.

The existing requirements for the testing of systemic contraceptives may be criticized for their empirical nature in that there are rigid requirements for studies in specific species at specified doses and for specified periods of time. To this extent they are cumbersome and may inhibit innovation.

Further potential problems may arise because the only long-term toxicity and carcinogenicity assay completed prior to large scale use is a two-year study in rats. The long-term dog and monkey studies each have a number of years to run after marketing approval has been granted and definite evidence of toxicity or carcinogencity may not surface until the end of the study. Consequently, human exposure may be extensive by the time the substance has been shown to have a carcinogenic or significant toxicological effect in an animal species. For these reasons, it has been decided that the Australian guidelines should be revised.

When formulating the new guidelines, various general criteria were considered. It was thought that the guidelines should have an acceptable scientific basis with regard to current knowledge. They should indicate the minimum studies that would be expected and should not exclude the possibility of requiring additional species if data indicated that such studies were necessary.

They should allow each study or each substance to be considered individually on its own merits and be based on the expectation that compounds with widely varying structures will be investigated. Therefore, it cannot be assumed that any one species will be more appropriate than any other to demonstrate toxicity and carcinogenicity.

It was thought that the guidelines should provide flexibility in decision making, both for the pharmaceutical manufacturer in designing the tests and for the regulatory body, but that they should not reduce the level of safety which the present requirements were intended to provide.

Lastly, at the present time it is thought that they should not reject previous studies or previous results of long-term dog and monkey studies.

To achieve these aims, it was decided that a greater emphasis should be placed on the choice of the species for toxicity and carcinogenicity assessment with a valid choice being dependent on the pharmacologic, pharmacokinetic and metabolic properties of each compound in various species, including man.

Animal studies should be conducted to provide data that allow species suitability to be considered for long-term toxicology and carcinogenicity studies prior to the commencement of clinical trials.

It has been proposed to amend the current Australian guidelines by abolishing the obligatory seven-year study in dogs and 10-year studies in monkeys, but to require that the results of metabolic, pharmacokinetic and pharmacologic studies in the dog and in a species in which it is intended to conduct carcinogenicity studies be available before clinical trials commence, and that the results of two-year toxicity studies in the dog and carcinogenicity studies in two species be available prior to the commencement of Phase III clinical trials.

These proposed guidelines would, however, not preclude requiring seven-year carcinogenicity dog studies if chemical or pharmacological similarity to drugs known to be carcinogenic in the dog were found or to require tests in monkeys or other species if they were considered to be suitable and appropriate.

DR. SOBEL: Thank you. Dr. Sutherland?

DR. SUTHERLAND: Before proceeding with an overview of the history, safety and efficacy of steriodal contraceptives in Canada, I should mention that this paper was prepared by Dr. Lucis, Chief of the Division of Endocrinology and Metabolism, and be presented as he wrote it, although I am sure he would probably have revised it, in light of new information that has been provided.

All drugs intended for marketing in Canada are subject to the requirements of the Food and Drug Act and Regulations. These require the product to be safe and efficacious for the purposes indicated, when used under the conditions recommended.

The onus to secure the data for the purpose of meeting these requirements rests with the drug manufacturer or sponsor. The Health Protection Branch of the Department of Health and Welfare is responsible for facilitation of availability of safe and effective drugs but, at the same time, is obliged to secure the Canadian public from all perceived hazards and forms of fraud in relation to drugs. Ensuring a capable benefit-to-risk ratio for all drug products is a task which requires thorough evaluation of safety and efficacy profiles obtained from both animal and clinical studies.

In 1981, the Bureau of Human Prescription Drugs developed updated Preclinical Toxicological Guidelines which in general terms outline tests that are deemed acceptable to determine the toxicity of drugs and/or their metabolites in various biological systems. These guidelines indicate the type of information which is generally required by the Health Protection Branch for most drugs before clinical trials or general marketing can be undertaken.

It is considered that steroidal contraceptives represent a special class of prescription drugs in that they are intended for use by a healthy population strictly for the maintenance of temporary and reversible infertility. From the public point of view, this segment of the population generally has a long life expectancy and thus lengthy exposure to agents which have even a questionable safety profile is considered both risky and undesirable.

Ever since the early 1960s when the first steroidal contraceptives were approved for marketing, intensive safety surveillance has been maintained in Canada. In 1970, when the tumorigenic and carcinogenic potential of certain progestogens became known in canine species, a requirement for seven-year dog and 10-year monkey studies for all steroidal contraceptive products was adopted.

Since the 1970s there have been five progestogens on the Canadian market; norethindrone, norethindrone acetate, norethynodrel, ethynodiol diacetate, and dl-norgestrel. These are marketed as combination products either with ethinyl estradiol or mestranol.

Over the past 10 years, no new steroidal derivatives have been introduced as contraceptives. Injectable progestogens or their hormonal derivatives are available in Canada with labeled indications for several therapeutic uses, but not for contraception. Apart from a progestin containing intrauterine device, Progestasert, there are no other implantable hormonal products on the Canadian market.

In retrospect, the oral contraceptives which have passed the long-term animal safety requirements have performed well. Since 1969, both clinical and epidemiological experiences with marketed contraceptives have been periodically reviewed by a nongovernmental Special Advisory Committee on Reproductive Physiology. In consultation with this committee, a number of revisions and directions for use have been completed and at the same time the availability of lower dose estrogen-progestin combination products has been facilitated.

After several cases of endometrial carcinoma were reported to be associated with the use of sequential oral contraceptives in the United States in 1976, these products were summarily phased out of the Canadian market.

In 1978, all combination oral contraceptives containing 100 micrograms of estrogen were restricted. The label indication now reads as follows: "For contraception control only when lower dosage estrogen formulations prove to be unacceptable."

Several reviews of oral contraceptive market trends in Canada reveal that since the mid-1970s oral contraceptive prescriptions have swung almost exclusively towards products that contain 50 or less than 50 micrograms of estrogen per unit, with abundance of the latter. Estrogen-free products, i.e., low-dose progestin only pills, one containing dl-norgestrel, 75 micrograms, and the other norethindrone, 350 micrograms, which were introduced on the market during the early 1970s have not gained any significant acceptance.

The oral contraceptives currently available in Canada offer various choices of products, with a high degree of efficacy and a minimum of side effects.

The public not only expects but is beginning to demand that new products approved for marketing should not only be equivalent to existing products but in some ways be better and/or safer than those presently available. This has not yet been incorporated into Canadian drug law. Nevertheless, it would not be acceptable to offer the public a product with demonstrably less efficacy or less safety than those already marketed. During the early 1980s we approved only two additional oral contraceptives, one biphasic, Ortho 10/11 and the other a triphasic, Triphasil.

Since these products contain known progestogen and estrogen components, no additional short-term or long-term animal testing was required. Instead, data on clinical pharmacology along with evidence of clinical safety and effectiveness and an investigation concerning endometrial histology were evaluated and accepted.

Against this background and because of our experience in this field, we must weigh the scientific wisdom, the medical advantages and disadvantages of any revision and any relaxation of any of our policies that concern new contraceptive safety requirements.

We are constantly aware that users of these products are young, normal healthy individuals with long life expectancy and their exposure to any questionable agent carries an undue degree of health risk.

As in the past, we shall maintain a flexible and open attitude towards guidelines on pharmacology and toxicology. It is our belief that the ultimate objective of animal testing is to assess the probability that drugs will not produce adverse reactions when restricted to specific indications for clinical use.

This can be accomplished from a data base that includes adequate preclinical and clinical pharmacokinetic and metabolic profiles facilitating the selection of species for long-term safety studies. In the design of future animal studies such factors as the route of administration, dosage, dosage interval, cycling, and several other factors which we have all heard today, will have to correlate with the intended mode of proposed use in man.

DR. DAS GUPTA: The Indian preclinical norms do not differ substantially from those of the FDA or the Committee on Safety of Medicines of the United Kingdom. We generally do not ask for additional preclinical data because we are a developing country and since preclinical studies are very expensive we rely heavily on data generated in other countries. However, when required, we try to communicate with other regulatory agencies to confirm the authenticity of these data.

I want to make it clear that we do insist on clinical trials in India including both clinical pharmacology studies and the longer Phase II and III studies. In many cases we have observed, not only with steroids, large differences in the optimum effective dose of new drugs in the Indian population.

Our current requirements for steroidal contraceptives do not differ much from those of the American FDA. We request acute toxicity studies, both in rodents and nonrodents, to compare the LD_{50} values by different routes of administration. This also provides information of their absorption kinetics and differences between the LD_{50} and ED_{50}.

Subacute toxicity studies are requested in more than two species and if satisfactory, we may allow clinical pharmacology studies with emphasis on pharmacokinetics which provides enough information to modify or redesign the long-term toxicity studies.

These data are vital because of species differences in the biological half life, both by single and repeated dose, protein binding and the steady state of the drug.

Before we allow further prolonged clinical studies, we require two-year studies both in rodents and dogs. The more demanding studies of five and seven years duration are not being conducted in India and we depend on the results from abroad.

Because family planning is a top priority national program in India, there is a heavy pressure for clinical trials of new devices including the silastics and the vaginal ring. Implants are undergoing a late Phase II study under the supervision of the Indian Council of Medical Research and the early Phase II studies of the vaginal ring containing steroids are being evaluated in two or three Indian centers.

The preclinical requirements prescribed by the Indian Government have been determined in consultation with an expert group called the Drug Technical Advisory Board, a statutory body under the Act. We are trying to establish specific requirements for each new contraceptive such as silastics and vaccines to prevent pregnancy and leprosy.

DISCUSSION

DR. SOBEL: I was interested in asking Dr. Donohoe under what circumstances he would recommend the seven-year beagle and 10-year monkey studies? You said you would favor such studies with certain agents related to drugs that have proven carcinogenic in these models. Did I understand that correctly?

DR. DONOHOE: With regard to when we would apply them to any compound that was closely related to known estrogens and progestogens, the effect of the changes will put an emphasis on prior agreement between the regulatory authorities and the pharmaceutical companies with regard to the choice of species so as to avoid some of the problems that have occurred with the beagle bitch in regard to its appropriateness as a model.

We want to be able to discuss with the sponsor what would be a suitable assay for long-term toxicity and carcinogenicity on the basis of adequate pharmacology, pharmacokinetics, and metabolism. As to specific requests for dog and monkey studies, it would, to some extent, be up to the companies themselves to decide which models are most appropriate. Perhaps they would decide the proper species.

PROFESSOR VON EICKSTEDT: I would like to ask our Australian colleague which species are normally used for carcinogenicity studies in your country? You mentioned two species.

DR. DONOHOE: For most pharmaceutical products it would be the rat and the mouse.

DR. BRENT: Could the panelists give us a feeling for the number of contraceptive preparations which have been rejected under application to your agencies and what were the reasons for the rejection?

Secondly, how many Phase I preparations were voluntarily withdrawn by the pharmaceutical house itself and the reasons for rejection.

DR. DAS GUPTA: Related to steroids alone?

DR. BRENT: Related to the topic today. In other words, what I am asking is, how many contraceptive preparations have been formulated, submitted, and rejected, and what were the reasons for the rejection?

DR. DAS GUPTA: Well, in my country there has been no recent introduction of new contraceptives for eight or nine years.

DR. SOBEL: Well, I speak for our experience in the United States. We have, on the basis of the beagle studies, rejected chlormadinone, megestrol and a drug under a code name of MK655, a derivative of norethindrone. We withdrew a combination oral contraceptive containing Provera, Provest. We withdrew the sequentials, but not strictly on animal studies. The first sequential removed was on the basis of the chlormadinone content and subsequently Oracon was removed primarily on the basis of epidemiologic studies.

I think that is a sampling. I don't know if my list is complete, but these animal studies have provided a screening device. Certainly the best example and the drug in the public eye is Depo-Provera which does not have a contraceptive indication in the United States, based primarily on animal model studies.

DR. BRENT: So, pharmacokinetics, changes in the serum lipoprotein cholesterol, all of that area has never been used for either the rejection or the acceptance of a contraceptive; it has been primarily carcinogenic studies in the beagle?

DR. SOBEL: That is how it has worked out. We have moved as an Agency only in those circumstances. Certainly, we have some good drugs out there that are serving the public well and their efficacy is undoubted.

If research takes any tack, I would say it would be directed to better models in regard to things we discussed today, the lipid-altering and coagulation altering effects. This would inspire a new generation of drugs that are aiming for greater safety in this regard and that would be profitable.

But to answer your question precisely, no we haven't removed drugs or blocked drugs on this basis in the past, primarily because I don't think we have had a good enough model.

The state of the art has come to the point where I think we can search for meaningful models and perhaps inspire a new thrust in research. Right now most of the research, if one can call it that, consists of the manipulation of regimens in OCs in varying dosages in different parts of the cycle to improve control of bleeding patterns.

This is a laudatory aim as far as acceptability, but it is certainly not a major advance in the area. A side effect of this workshop might be that with better models there may be stimulation of research to create drugs freer from cardiovascular and thrombotic problems.

DR. DAS GUPTA: Although we are thinking of better models or additional models, we know that many of the clinical trials were prematurely terminated because of reduced acceptability of the drug for one reason or another. Therefore, in spite of the absence of alterations in lipid metabolism or hypercoagulability and liver and tumorigenic parameters, a new drug may cause as yet unknown and unexpected side effects in field trials.

DR. KUZMA: I have a question for Professor Von Eickstedt. You suggested two things. One is to start with animal studies, proceed to human studies and then return to preclinical investigations. Has that been tried in Germany and if so what has been its success?

You also suggested that several monkey species be used for testing. Has that been tried with success?

PROFESSOR VON EICKSTEDT: Our drug law does not specify the animal studies which must be done before Phase I, Phase II or Phase III clinical studies. These are my proposals made after a decade of developing steroids in the Federal Republic of Germany.

For instance, cyproterone acetate was a new steroid which introduced many problems for both company scientists and regulatory officals. It is not a typical progestogen and has marked antiandrogenic effects.

Initial clinical pharmacology must serve as the basis for Phase II studies, and human pharmacokinetics should be taken into account when designing long-term animal studies. We get irrelevant data from animal studies if the species selected metabolizes the steroid in a different way than man.

In addition to pharmacokinetics, the endocrinology of the animal model must be considered.

I rejected two estrogens because they really hadn't been tested adequately. Preclinical broad spectrum testing is now essential in the Federal Republic of Germany. The New Drug Act of 1978 places legal responsibility on the research workers of the company as well as the clinicians.

DR. AKSEL: I have a question for Dr. Sutherland. When you listed the number of contraceptives available in Canada, you stated that another contraceptive would have to be proven more efficacious and safer than the ones that are already in existence. What type of testing would your regulatory agency require to prove that the new contraceptive proposed for marketing is better than the existing ones?

DR. SUTHERLAND: I believe the way it was phrased was that the public expects or demands it. As far as the Canadian regulation is concerned, it isn't law. Nevertheless, in any review process, if a product doesn't provide, either by life tables or Pearl Index, efficacy equivalent to products that are currently available, or if cycle control isn't as good, then we will judge this product, in a sense, to be not as acceptable as those that are currently available.

The manufacturer might well be asked to clarify this point. I have seen this occur with one drug submission and there are submissions that did not proceed further.

DR. AKSEL: In other words, you use the same route of testing on any type of new drug being offered and have not changed your route of testing?

DR. SOBEL: One more quick question and one quick answer.

DR. EASTERLING: I was just curious, Dr. Donohoe, what the nature of the movement was in Australia that created the new proposals and a move away from the old guidelines.

DR. DONOHOE: There was no particular movement. It was just a general revision of our requirements.

DR. EASTERLING: It originated within your agency?

DR. DONOHOE: Yes

DR. SOBEL: One more question?

DR. HEYWOOD: I don't think it will be a simple question for you to answer. I am always perturbed about developing better models.

As a toxicologist, I am awfully sorry to have to tell you that there are no better models coming along. We have rats, mice, dogs, and monkeys.

Elephants, kangaroos, and nine-banded armadillos are not suitable for toxicology.

There is an intelligent use of animals in toxicology, which brings me to the second point. I wasn't quite sure what Drs. Donohoe and Sutherland were saying about the beagle model. Once you have given progestogens to beagle dogs at 25 times the human dosage level on a milligram per kilogram basis and developed an endocrinologic cripple, I am not sure what you can extrapolate, and I think it is very foolish for intelligent people to try and extrapolate from such a model to man.

And I am not quite sure what you were saying, therefore, about the new regulations in Australia and Canada, unless you are paying attention to receptor affinity. But then you are making the wrong comparisons. You can't compare apples with oranges. You have to compare the compounds in a proper manner, and this means taking into consideration pharmacokinetics and also receptor binding.

Then maybe you will find, like we all think, that all progestogens, including progesterone, are carcinogenic to the mammary gland of the beagle dog.

SECTION 5

DISCUSSION AND RECOMMENDATIONS

Moderator: William Andrews

DISCUSSION AND RECOMMENDATIONS

William Andrews

Department of Obstetrics and Gynecology
Eastern Virginia Medical School
Norfolk, Virginia

INTRODUCTION AND QUESTIONS

The function of an FDA, Bureau of Drugs Advisory Committee is to provide recommendations that will assist the Agency in making regulatory decisions. Agenda items presented to a Committee are accompanied by questions designed to elicit well-defined responses regarding specific Agency concerns.

Accordingly, the Division of Metabolism and Endocrine Drug Products, FDA, and the Center for Population Research, NIH, submitted the following six questions to the Fertility and Maternal Health Drugs Advisory Committee for consideration during this workshop.

1. How can the knowledge of pharmacokinetics, metabolism, and steroid hormone action be utilized in the design of meaningful animal safety studies?

2. Should guidelines for preclinical animal safety studies be amended to allow earlier Phase I clinical pharmacology studies?

3. How can the current long-term animal safety requirements be modified to consider the drug's chemical structure, pharmacology, and mode of administration for extrapolation to humans?

4. Should dose levels in animal safety studies consider an end organ's responsiveness? How can the results of these studies be extrapolated and predictive of potential human adverse reactions, e.g., thromboembolic and other vascular disorders.

5. What research should be undertaken to make data interpretation and evaluation predictive of potential clinical problems?

6. What are the alternatives to long-term animal studies that the FDA can rely on for the assessment of safety of steroid contraceptives?

Specific responses to the questions were provided by C. Wayne Bardin, M.D., Director, Center for Biomedical Research, The Population Council, and Professor Egon Diczfalusy, Special Programme of Research in Human

Reproduction, WHO. Both of these organizations were co-sponsors of the workshop.

Advisory Committee discussion, responses and recommendations concluded the workshop.

RESPONSE BY PROFESSOR EGON DICZFALUSY (WHO)

You have also asked me to provide my personal views on the six questions posed to the Advisory Committee and I shall outline them here.

1. The participants indicated how pharmacokinetics should and must play a central role in the design of meaningful studies; I can't see how you could avoid them.

2. There was indeed a consensus that earlier Phase I clinical pharmacology is essential.

3. I would propose that it may not be too hazardous to shorten considerably some of the long-term toxicological assessments. The question is what kind of information can be obtained after one year's toxicology which was not obtained after six month studies.

4. End organ responsiveness is a must. Predictive tests for vascular complications need to be refined.

5. Indeed, I feel strongly that research must be funded on the development of specific animal models as soon as possible. Don't wait too long. It is an obligation of the public sector to provide funding for this type of mission oriented research. I am not proposing a cross sectional study or a comparative pharmacological study in the hope of finding a perfect model but to find specific experimental conditions in well known animal models.

6. In the final analysis, the proper study of man is man. There is no substitute for careful clinical and epidemiological investigations. Animal studies will never provide the same answer.

AND THREE SUGGESTIONS

It is not a good excuse that large animals are expensive and therefore only a few of them can be used, with the consequence that findings cannot be interpreted statistically. By designing the studies in a proper way, this can be remedied. Research methods developed during the past 20 years involve a statistician in the planning of studies.

Furthermore, I feel it is no longer sufficient to base the assessment of endocrine profiles exclusively on reproductive organ weights. It was a very useful technique during the past 20 years, but today a variety of sensitive and specific analytical methods exist to measure the hormones produced by these organs or acting upon them. The incorporation of such methods in the assessment of endocrine profiles may add valuable information to the understanding of the effects obtained.

The second suggestion is that NIH and WHO make available necessary reagents for pharmacodynamic studies in several animal species. It would assist the development of improved animal models if specific and reliable reagents were available for growth hormone, FSH, LH, prolactin, etc. in a variety of species. NIH and WHO have started collaboration on the development of reagents for the assay of monkey gonadotrophins, but a much greater effort is needed. Such reagents would also enable investigators to assess species differences in endocrine response to new drugs better than they can do it today.

The third suggestion: Dr. E. Umberger of the FDA had a poster in his office stating that "the expert is seldom in doubt, but frequently in error." It is difficult for scientists to give good advice if they don't have access to basic information and I refer here to the animal toxicological data submitted to FDA by the pharmaceutical industry.

Everything has a useful life, be it a patent, classified information, a state secret or a trade secret. It ought to be possible to find a mechanism by which vital toxicological information could be made available - after the lapse of a certain number of years - to the scientific community. After a number of years, a state secret will become a curiosity of historical interest, but animal toxicological data will always remain of more than historical interest. By blocking indefinitely free access of scientists to such information we are damaging the very essence of the scientific process. As Professor George Sarton of Harvard once said: "the acquisition and systematisation of positive knowledge is the only human activity which is really progressive." Hence I would like to urge you, Mr. Chairman, to explore the various procedural, legal, or even legislative possibilities to remedy this situation.

Mr. Chairman, I started by quoting from the Sestri Levante document. With your permission I would like to close this summary with another quotation from the same publication. "Absolute safety is unattainable, and its pursuit regardless of other considerations is achieving more harm than good."

RESPONSE OF WAYNE BARDIN, M.D., THE POPULATION COUNCIL

In responding to question 1, I believe such studies are useful in determining how to test drugs at comparable bioavailability. Phase I studies in humans can yield pharmacokinetic data as well as information on biological activity. From these observations one can know roughly the dose range that will eventually be needed in the human and can design meaningful animal toxicological studies based upon biological activity and pharmacokinetic data.

The answer to the second question, it is absolutely essential if we intend to complete meaningful toxicological studies that early human studies be required. This will permit proper design of the toxicology study.

The third question is, "How can the current long-term animal safety requirements be modified with respect to the drug's chemical structure?" I think this will vary enormously among different drugs. If one is interested in a steroid that has been tested extensively in animals and has been in clinical use for many years, extensive toxicology may not be essential if the drug is administered by a different route. For example, if a drug is to be given which has been tested in the oral mode, then studies need to be designed for that situation rather than starting all over as if it were a totally new compound. This is particularly true when there is already a substantial background of experience in animals and humans.

The specific issues will relate to the new dosage form. For example, if it is a vaginal dosage form, vaginal toxicology, should be addressed. There may be less concern about hepatic toxicity since it has already been thoroughly investigated during, say, oral administration when the liver receives a large dose due to the first pass effect.

I have addressed the fourth question in my presentation: many unusual effects will be observed that are not related to the biological activity of the agent being tested if very high doses are used.

With regard to the fifth question, I think research should attempt to identify why some individuals exhibit adverse reactions to steroids. For example, androgens produce multiple metabolic effects, but only a few subjects will have actual side effects such as thrombosis. Some understanding of the individuals with the problems would provide great insight into the side effects of contraceptives. Knowledge of adverse reactions will not accrue in animal studies. Side effects such as thrombosis are not general biological phenomenon; they represent individual responses, and should be studied as such.

I think the answer to the last question is really one that can be discussed extensively. In my view, it has to do with distinguishing between epigenetic and genotoxic agents. Steroids are thought to be epigenetic. They are promoters and the fact that all promoters are not the same should be addressed.

DR. DICZFALUSY: Thank you very much. May I ask you the last question? What is your position, vis-a-vis the proposition of Dr. Humpel, that instead of chronic toxicity, subchronic toxicity studies should be done using the parenteral route of administration?

DR. BARDIN: I think if a drug is going to be given parenterally, one has to test it that way. I don't know that I would ignore the route of administration especially with regard to local effects. For example, if one is going to give a drug orally, the greatest local effect, or the organ that is exposed to the highest concentration is the gastrointestinal tract and the liver. In addition, I don't think if you were going to test a steroid bearing IUD that you would want to forego some kind of local toxicity study examining the histopathology of the uterus in at least one species that has comparable steroid binding. Ultimately, the best test is the human.

DR. DICZFALUSY: Thank you very much.

COMMITTEE DISCUSSION AND RECOMMENDATIONS

DR. ANDREWS: Summarizing of the data presented, certain concepts have been clearly identified. One is the need to ascertain the proper dosages and animals for a given test. Additional concepts include the use of existing applicable data, consideration of different routes of administration, drug serum levels and clearance rates.

In most situations the high doses used are irrelevant and probably misleading. The toxicological studies should be based on known chemistry and untoward effects.

Flexibility is to be strongly emphasized. Now, all this raises some broad questions. Should the basic animal testing requirements be modified? Should time requirements before initiating the Phase III studies be altered or shortened?

QUESTIONS 1 and 3

To begin discussion, I suggest a statement which is basically the answer to the first FDA question, and an answer partially to question three. The proposed answer is "basically the knowledge of steroid pharmacokinetics and metabolism should be used in the design of animal safety studies including appropriate doses and considering bioavailability, serum levels, clearance rates, and idiosyncratic responses of the test animal. Different species may be appropriate in evaluating different risks. Multiples of the effective threshold dose and not multiples of the equivalent human dose should be employed. Avoid megadose trials which may be misleading, with paradoxical results. Use available data from different serum levels and clearance rates following different routes of administration, but rely on human data when available."

With that as a start, I would like to encourage the Committee to comment on the first question:

"How can the knowledge of pharmacokinetics, metabolism, and steroid hormone action be utilized in the design of meaningful animal safety studies?"

Question 3: "How can the current long-term animal safety requirements be modified to consider the drug's chemical structure, pharmacology, and mode of administration for extrapolation to humans?"

DR. BRENT: I think these are very difficult questions to answer. Under pharmacokinetics, I just wonder about when, if ever, we are going to take into consideration and utilize the information that has been developed with regard to receptors. With the synthetic progestational agents, each has a different spectrum of effects as we elevate the dose, and when we use a multiple of many times the human dose, they no longer have the effects that we actually see clinically.

For instance, when medroxyprogesterone acetate and some of the masculinizing hormones are administered at very high dosages their major effect may be at the glucocorticoid or the androgen level. Is it time now that, using pharmacokinetics, we begin to determine when a drug dose in animals is no longer having the desired clinical effect?

Certainly, at least in the area of congenital malformations, when we observe an increased incidence of cleft palate at very high dosages of these compounds, it is primarily a glucocorticoid effect. When a drug reaches a certain blood level and saturates other receptors and no longer functions as a progestational agent but as an androgen or glucocorticoid, it is no longer being tested for its intended use.

DR. ANDREWS: And it is no longer an appropriate dose. I think this is probably one of the major concerns that must be addressed.

DR. LIPSETT: Dr. Diczfalusy spoke very lucidly about pharmacokinetics, but I haven't heard anything about comparing the peripheral effects of one steroid hormone with another.

For example, using species where you observe similar increases in one of the hepatic alpha-globulins, or the same decrease in a gonadotropin, or the same increase in the estrogen-sensitive neurophysin, you may be getting closer to equivalent doses.

I think these are very important indices that add to any study of steroid effects on the organism.

DR. AKSEL: Considering end organ responsiveness, which is really the basis of establishing the animal models, if the hormone to be used is for contraception and the purpose is blocking ovulation, then at least the testing should be performed on that animal at a dosage that actually blocks ovulation without going into ten-fold and fifty-fold studies that are highly pharmacologic.

DR. BERENDES: I wish we could add something else to question number one. It seems to me, when trying to relate the current animal safety requirements to what we currently know about adverse effects of contraceptive steroids, I can't relate our knowledge of animal toxicology to our knowledge of adverse clinical effects of contraceptive steroids.

In the discussion by representatives from other regulatory agencies, someone had suggested that maybe new steroid contraceptives should be safer and better. At least that was one of the desires expressed. I wonder how we could ever get to that point. I don't know to what extent animal safety studies, as we currently conduct them, would ever lead us to that point.

As far as I am concerned, my advice is very different. I don't think you would ever know, unless you had that particular compound in clinical use, and the extensive experience we currently have with marketed contraceptives.

I submit that new animal safety studies should attempt to incorporate the perceived or known adverse effects from organ receptors of contraceptives already in use. These adverse effects are basically in the cardiovascular system.

Dr. Wessler introduced a potentially very useful animal model in his presentation and Dr. Clarkson may have a model in macaques which could address the meaning of these lipid marker changes in terms of atherosclerosis.

I don't think, from what we know about adverse effects on organ receptors, that we can expect to identify the sort of clinical adverse events in studies involving only 10 or 20 monkeys.

DR. CORFMAN: I have a question for Dr. Sobel. What we are considering are the possibilities of making the procedure of dealing with the FDA more flexible, with some adjustments in the testing process of new drugs and the interchange between applicants (developers of these drugs) and the FDA.

Do you believe that is feasible and the FDA would be able to respond to a more flexible system?

DR. SOBEL: I am not quite sure about some parts of the question, but certainly we are prepared to change our procedure in testing oral contraceptives, if that is the question. It is really the purpose of this meeting. If we can develop ways to test these drugs more expeditiously without sacrificing any of the safety considerations, we are certainly open to that.

PROFESSOR VON EICKSTEDT: We know that nearly all the progestogens exhibit dose dependent effects on the liver of different test animals but we can't directly correlate morphological changes to metabolic or even protein synthetic effects. We should invest in more research on this complicated system and try to relate it to the different functions of the liver. This should be strictly related to the pharmacokinetics and metabolism of the substances we have to compare in animal models and humans.

DR. KUZMA: Were the initial guidelines accepted after as much thought, discussion and effort by as large a representative group of scientists as we appear to have today?

DR. SOBEL: The original guidelines were not subjected to as much extra-Agency discussion. There was a great deal of inter-Agency discussion and input from industry. Introduction of the beagle was based on a pharmaceutical manufacturer's approach to the problem and we felt at that time (I was not in the Agency at the time) that since the model which this company developed had apparently been able to detect with great sensitivity the development of mammary carcinomas with a derivative of norethindrone, that this probably was a reasonable model.

The 10-year primate and the 7-year beagle studies were not chosen arbitrarily. These time spans were an attempt to be analogous to the half-life span of the possible maximum exposure of women to OCs.

At that time there was no reason to believe this was an unreasonable approach; even the multiples of dosages that seem large in view of our current knowledge of receptor effects followed classic carcinogenic modeling.

It was believed to be a reasonable approach even though we did not have the vast knowledge of bioavailability, serum levels, etc. that we have now.

That essentially is the background. We did the best we could. In 1967 Congressional legislation required us to issue guidelines and assist industry in the performance of the preclinical studies. The recommendations made at that time were reasonable in view of the state of the art.

Now, some 16 years later, I think we can modify some of the positions taken at that time, however, the passage of time has fortified the strength of some of the models, just by our knowledge of the findings in different species.

When I said I don't think we should discard the beagle model, I meant that we have acquired a great deal of information about it and that we really don't know what to replace it with that would be that much better. I think Dr. Heywood was right when he said "what shall we look for, armadillos, or what-have-you?"

DR. SCHAFFENBURG: We have discussed dose and multiples of doses. I don't think we should lose sight of the manner of administration. These drugs have been given continuously and it has been emphasized here that some of the carcinogenic effects seen are due to constant exposure, particularly in the case of estrogen.

I think we should contemplate studies administering the drug in the same manner in which it is intended for clinical use, i.e., orally if it is to be given orally, and given cyclically in cycling animals, not continously.

For example, if you administer peptide hormones like LHRH continuously, the effect is totally different from that when given in a pulsing fashion. So, if you are going to use oral contraceptives cyclically, then they must be tested cyclically.

DR. EASTERLING: I think at some point in the consideration of these six questions we should address the waiving of safety requirements for known drugs, and I suspect this first question may be the best place to do it.

DR. ANDREWS: I suggested using available data on different serum levels and clearance rates with different routes of administration on different species and, also, to rely on human data when available.

Is the Committee in agreement that one doesn't have to go back to square A for new administration routes of compounds with known pharmacokinetics?

(Nods of assent)

DR. TAGATZ: I think when this was discussed before, the issue considered whether or not we were dealing with truly a new compound as opposed to a derivative or a new delivery system of a previously tested compound. I think the derivatives should be treated more like a new compound than a new delivery system for an old compound.

We must be careful that the derivative compounds administered by a new route do not have different pharmacokinetics, that they be evaluated early and clinical studies initiated as soon as possible.

DR. PERLMUTTER: I would like to suggest that perhaps, with a new mode of delivery for an existing drug, that as long as it can be established that bioavailability and pharmacokinetics are similar that completed studies should be accepted.

DR. BRENT: Dr. Sobel, on what basis have oral contraceptives been rejected? I think you indicated the majority of unapproved drugs were based on the beagle results. In other words, the beagle results have been the most useful or most utilized in rejecting the application of a new oral contraceptive.

Dr. Stadel told us that the human epidemiological literature indicates exactly the opposite, i.e., oral contraceptives are almost protective against breast disease. Therefore, in a sense, results in the one experimental model that has been used to reject use of particular preparations are almost diametrically opposite that of the clinical findings with marketed oral contraceptives.

DR. ANDREWS: Let Dr. Stadel clarify his statement.

DR. STADEL: I do not agree with the interpretation that has just been presented. My position is as follows. The oral contraceptives that were used extensively in the United States in the sixties and seventies were mainly the 19-nortestosterone progestogens in combined formulation with 50 micrograms of estrogen. For the most part there is very scant representation of 17-acetoxy progestogens in these data.

There is not really a suggestion of protection for the breast, there is simply no impact. The protection data pertain only to the endometrium and ovary. Now, what I further said with regard to the issue of 17-acetoxyprogestogens is that it will be possible to do some reasonable evaluation of the beagle model in a year or two when the data from the World Health Organization study in Thailand, which does have a good deal of information on DMPA exposure, become available. Those data will provide a framework for placing the beagle findings on proper perspective.

DR. SOBEL: I agree with what Dr. Stadel says. The protective effect shown by all our epidemiologic data, essentially, is based on the 19-nor derivatives. Our exclusion of many of these 17-acetoxy derivatives as components of oral contraceptives may have saved the country a great deal in regard to mammary carcinoma. We don't know.

We may get some answers from the World Health Organization analysis of populations exposed to medroxyprogesterone acetate. If it shows that there is no increased incidence in women who have taken it for an appreciable time, then we say that the model has been excessively stringent and perhaps not allowed us to introduce otherwise valuable drugs.

But we don't know. There is a possibility of an increase in mammary carcinoma. Certainly some mention was made of greater mitotic activity associated with this type of agent. I don't know. I would just say that we have good epidemiological data in regard to carcinogenesis. Is this a result of our screening procedures?

DR. BRENT: Do you agree with Dr. Heywood, who described the high dose beagle as an endocrine cripple?

DR. SOBEL: Well, at this high doses it is not only an endocrine cripple, but subject to renal amyloidosis, a diabetic effect and infectious processes in the uterus (pyometra). It certainly has a lot of ill effects at 25-times the human dose. Those effects are of interest, of course, but whether they are pertinent is the subject of this meeting.

MR. HALL: Can I just add a point of clarification to the statements made about the WHO neoplasia and steroidal contraception study. There will be preliminary data published in the summer and I did point out to you that on initial analysis of breast cancer data with DMPA in Thailand there certainly is not an increased relative risk and there may well be a protective effect.

I also stated that we will continue surveillance in the future as we accumulate epidemiological data over a long period. We will not be able to answer the question with certainty, but I think even in the preliminary analysis you will see a decrease rather than an increase in relative risk of mammary cancer.

DR. BLYE: I would like to direct a few comments to you about the dog. For over 40 years the dog has been known to respond uniquely, not uniquely sensitive, but uniquely to sex steroids.

Long before the first oral contraceptive was ever perceived, endocrinologists knew that the dog responded to both estrogens and progestins in an unusual manner and thus the results found in the long-term dog studies were not really unexpected. As far as induction of beagle mammary tumors, Depo-Provera was one of the most potent progestins tested and it is the drug on which we have more clinical experience than any other C-21 progestin.

With regard to the dog, one must take into consideration its unique responsiveness to sex hormones including the fact that progesterone itself causes the same effects. Depo-Provera has had extensive usage and, as Mr. Hall has pointed out with the preliminary WHO studies, there does not seem to be any evidence whatsoever that these conditions we see in the dog extend to man.

DR. BRENT: So, what is the bottom line? I am not clear, because I happen to agree with what you are saying. You would recommend a lowering of the dose in the beagle, the use of the beagle, or not use of the beagle?

DR. BLYE: I would like to ask Dr. Sobel what he considers to be useful features of employing the dog in safety studies of steroidal contraceptives.

(Laughter)

DR. SOBEL: Well, I think it is important to realize that the beagle dog does not respond to some of the derivatives of 19-nortestosterone by production of mammary carcinomas. The dog does discriminate amongst the steroids. A discriminating ability is the hallmark of a good model, of course. It does respond in differential ways.

Controlled studies of DMPA with progesterone show differentials. Progesterone causes a very low order of tumor formation, whereas DMPA in equivalent dosages causes a very high dose related response in the beagle. This model has screened and differentiated between steroids.

Whether the differentiation is a valuable one, we do not know. The massive data that we have reviewed in regard to DMPA is characterized primarily by the large numbers. We have explored this with epidemiologists internally as well as outside the Agency and the quality of the data no where approaches what we have for contraceptives containing the 19-nortestosterone derivatives. We have nothing that approaches the British cohort studies, nothing at all.

We have not been able to analyze the WHO data, in fact, we have been enjoined not to discuss it by the Depo-Provera Public Board of Inquiry. I am sort of at a disadvantage. The data will be analyzed and we hope to make some decision based on the quality of the WHO data and what they show. I don't have the dim view that Dr. Blye has of the beagle model. I have seen it has an ability to differentiate amongst the progestational agents. We have a very good experience in this country in regard to carcinogenesis, although, I don't know if it can be attributed to the the screening ability of the beagle. Perhaps it is the most maligned animal in history at this point.

DR. BLYE: Just one quick point. We have heard in the last three days that one approach to the discrimination in the dog might be clarified if these drugs were given in equivalent progestational doses. We all know that the 19-nor steroids are far less potent progestational agents than the C-21 steroids. Thus the discrimination provided by the dog may actually be a discrimination of progestational potency rather than a discrimination based upon molecular structure.

DR. GABELNICK: I just wanted to add an important point, I think, that relates not only to the beagle model but to all models, and that is your suggestion, Dr. Andrews, that the data be normalized to the minimal effective dose. If we keep that in mind when we are looking at the multiples, I think we can avoid a lot of problems in comparisons.

DR. ANDREWS: Our answer to question one is basically that the knowledge of steroid pharmacokinetics, metabolism, and steroid hormone action should be utilized and the test(s) should employ appropriate doses, considering bioavailability, serum levels, clearance rates, and idiosyncratic responses of the animals. Different species may be appropriate for evaluating different risks.

Use multiples of the effective threshold dose, not equivalent human dose. Avoid megadose trials which may be misleading with paradoxical results. Use available data on different serum levels, clearance rates, with different routes of administration. Rely on human data where available.

DR. BRENT: Since the most dramatic effect is in the area of clotting rather than carcinogenesis I think that the pharmacokinetics and the alterations in the serum at least be slanted in that direction at the present time.

DR. ANDREWS: Yes, the appropriate dose, and so on.

DR. BRENT: Then I would support the motion.

DR. ANDREWS: Is there any other question on this?

(No response)

If not, all in favor of accepting this, raise your hands.

(Show of hands)

Opposed?

(No response)

QUESTION 2

"Should guidelines for preclinical animal safety studies be amended to allow earlier Phase I clinical pharmacology studies?"

DR. ANDREWS: I would also propose an answer to question two, and then I am going to call on each of you for comments. The answer is yes, including toxicity studies of a limited duration permitting early Phase I clinical investigation to establish the appropriate human therapeutic dose and pharmacokinetics and then additional animal studies based upon these findings.

Comments and suggestions on that?

DR. PERLMUTTER: Do you want to add a time to that or do you want to leave it flexible?

DR. ANDREWS: I am open to suggestions.

DR. PERLMUTTER: There were several speakers here who suggested that we would gain no further information after six months of studies, and I can see no reason why we need two years if the general consensus is six months.

DR. ANDREWS: Current regulations require 90 day studies in rats, dogs, and monkeys prior to initiation of Phase I studies limited to 10 subjects up to 10 days. Phase II studies utilizing approximately 50 subjects for three menstrual cycles require the completion of one-year studies in rats, dogs, and monkeys.

I think the question is when do you move to Phase III and how much do you do prior to that? Phase I requires just 90 days now. The question is how to get to Phase II and III. Should requirements be shortened to 90 days or six months, what is the recommendation?

Dr. Perlmutter, do you want to make a specific recommendation?

DR. PERLMUTTER: Well, I would say that evidence presented here in the last few days has been that six months should be adequate for initiation of Phase III trials.

DR. AKSEL: I think the answer to question two is just a simple yes. I wouldn't add anything else.

DR. ANDREWS: Okay, then we need to address Phase III requirements as another question and it looks like this is where that should be addressed.

DR EASTERLING: I would like to suggest that we include Dr. Perlmutter's comment in answer to number two.

DR. ANDREWS: May we modify that, Dr. Sobel, to include moving to Phase III. Phase I is really fairly short-term right now.

DR. SOBEL: Yes, I just want to clarify what the implications of moving to Phase III studies - these are large field clinical trials. The Committee would be willing to move to those on the basis of six months toxicology? Is that what the Committee is voting?

SPEAKER: Six months toxicology in animals.

DR. SOBEL: Of course. The Committee agrees to that? I just want to be sure you know what the implications are.

DR. McKENZIE: Question two relates to Phase I. I am not sure what the Committee's decision is as to the duration of studies that would be necessary to support Phase I clinical studies.

DR. ANDREWS: I think there was discussion on one of the presentations that possibly that could be shortened. Dr. Diczfalusy, did you mention six weeks?

DR. DICZFALUSY: Yes. The recommendations made by Professor Zbinden that, in fact, if the Phase I study involves only the administration of very small amounts to a limited number of subjects for a short period of time, then he said a month's toxicology in two species, such as rat and monkey, in his opinion, would be sufficient.

I was more wary in my recommendations and said say four to six weeks or so.

DR. ANDREWS: Would the Committee be agreeable to a recommendation of six weeks for Phase I studies before moving to Phase II, and then six months for both animal and human studies in Phase II before moving Phase III? All in favor of that recommendation, please signify by raising their hands.

(Affirmative answer)

I basically intended to answer question III in the previously submitted statement. Is there anything else that we need to address in question three, or should we move to question four?

QUESTION 4

"Should dose levels in animal safety studies consider an end organ's responsiveness?"

(Affirmative response)

"How can the results of these studies be extrapolated and predictive for potential human adverse reactions, e.g., thromboembolic and other vascular disorders?"

Appropriate testing is needed in appropriate animals. I am sure a lot of this must be determined in the human.

DR. AKSEL: Also, utilizing the previous information on some of the adverse side effects, and directing the establishment of the experiment towards those adverse reactions.

DR. BRENT: Well, does this mean it involves the development of different animals models? I think Dr. Lipsett said he had to specifically evaluate the particular pharmacological effect under consideration in an animal model. From what I recall, we didn't have very good animal models for the two major adverse effects that have been reported in the human.

MS. WEST: Well, in response to that, perhaps the data will just have limited usefulness if, in fact, the best study of man is man, and you already have data in humans that is probably more useful.

DR. BERENDES: The discussion of question three brings up the problem of sample size. I submit that unless you have an unusually responsive animal model the known adverse effects of oral contraceptives probably aren't as clear as let's say, clinical events.

Can you use biochemical responses? Can you use effects on the thrombogenic system of the kind that Dr. Wessler discussed yesterday, substituting for an end organ response, which you may not be able to identify under the constraints of sample size?

DR. DICZFALUSY: Mr. Chairman, if I may quote again Professor Zbinden, in his opinion, after the Phase II studies, he said, I would make the drug widely available at that stage as soon as possible and start very careful monitoring. He felt that from that point on it is the clinical, the human, the epidemiological study, which matters.

As soon as something disturbing occurs during a study, you then attempt to go back with the specific question and determine if it can be answered in an animal model. I agree that it may not. That is why I suggested that we should see to it that the next generation which will follow us will not be bound by these problems and more models should be available.

DR. PERLMUTTER: I would like to echo that, because if you go back in the history of oral contraception, of all the reported side effects, not one of them was really predicted by the animal models.

Although I want to make sure that the drug is safe for human use, indeed we won't identify these side effects until there are large scale clinical studies.

DR. BARDIN: I want to encourage the interpretation of metabolic studies. They are very important and furnish clues as to what to look for epidemiologically. Most metabolic changes observed in patients receiving steroids occur in all of them. All subjects that receive a certain progestin show a change in insulin tolerance; all patients who get estrogens show a change in clotting factor(s).

But the clinical consequence of those changes are rare and, in a way, they give us a hint that something might occur epidemiologically. But they are not predictive. I think this is the problem of trying to transfer a few metabolic studies, whether in an animal model or in a small group of patients, into a clinical interpretation.

Ultimately it will have to be ascertained in a large population, provided there are no acute or subacute toxicological effects. Nonetheless, metabolic studies can give you a hint, based on all our past experience, of what to look for.

DR. ANDREWS: Thank you. Can we bring this question to the floor.

DR. BRENT: It was stated that in any animal model there are certain maximum levels with regard to ratio to therapeutic dose. Are we accepting those to be continued?

Dr. Heywood believes that doses beyond 10 times the therapeutic dose are of limited value. But yet there are some animal models where we go to 100 times the therapeutic dose. Should, therefore, the consideration of the maximum exposure in any animal model be a consideration in the modification of the regulation?

DR. ANDREWS: Possibly this should be addressed. The original statement used "appropriate dose," and "avoiding megadose." Now, do you want to make further specific recommendations?

What we basically have proposed to say in answer to question four is to answer the first part yes, and the second part "by appropriate animal and epidemiologic studies, directing the studies on the basis of previous findings."

All in favor of that, please raise your hands.

(Show of hands)

Opposed?

(No response)

DR. ANDREWS: Before moving on the last two questions, there are clarifications that have been suggested on two of the points we have already covered. Dr. Easterling, do you want to discuss the first one?

DR. EASTERLING: Thank you, Mr. Chairman. This deals with the issue of waiving new drug requirements for old drugs that are simply being administered by a different route.

I believe the Committee's feeling about this is that as long as there is comparable bioavailability that these new drug requirements should be waived. Secondly, where the major metabolite of a new derivative has been studied extensively, we would recommend that the new drug requirement be waived.

DR. ANDREWS: I believe that was the intent and it is well to spell that out.

All in favor, raise your hands.

(Show of hands)

Opposed?

(No response)

Thank you, Dr. Easterling. During discussion of multiples of dose with a specific recommendation as to the upper levels, a proposal was made that this be 10 times the effective threshold dose.

DR. HUMPEL: I would like to comment on this. You should be aware that 10 times threshold dose in each animal species may result in a lower level than human.

DR. ANDREWS: We are trying to do this on an equivalent, not just on milligram-per-kilogram, therapeutic basis.

DR. HUMPEL: If you give the rat ethinyl estradiol, the effective threshold level is lower than in humans. I think one should be aware of that.

DR. ANDREWS: The proposal is that this be tailored to individual species and still have multiples doses. The intent was that the multiples not be so high that it would give distorted responses.

DR. BLYE: I believe what Dr. Humpel is saying is that 10 times the threshold dose in one species may give you 100 times the human dose in terms of milligram-per-kilogram. It might be meaningful to discuss whether or not this threshold is important. It is essential if you are evaluating efficacy, but is it equally important for safety?

With safety, it may be more significant to consider how much of the drug is in the body irrespective of its pharmacological or physiological activity. Currently, the regulations stipulate the use of fixed multiples of the human dose so you are concerned more with the body burden of the drug, irrespective of its physiological activity or potency in that species.

DR. ANDREWS: Thank you. Is the Committee ready to consider this question?

DR. BLYE: With the understanding that in some cases this is going to go beyond the 50 times human dose.

DR. ANDREWS: I think we have discussed the need for flexibility, and obviously the Agency is going to use judgment. Flexibility contemplates guidelines that do not include high doses which overwhelm the liver.

All in favor of recommending that the maximum dose be limited to 10 times the animal threshold dose -

DR. AKSEL: In that species.

DR. ANDREWS: In that species. All in favor?

(Affirmative response)

Thank you.

QUESTION 5

"What research should be undertaken to make data interpretation and evaluation predictive of potential clinical problems?"

DR. EASTERLING: I would suggest that our recommendations include that we develop animal models as soon as possible to meet these needs.

DR. BRENT: You mean for the known effects that we already have observed in the human?

DR. PERLMUTTER: I don't know that question five can be answered as is, because I don't know of anything that is predictive of potential clinical problems in the future. Actually, we are dealing with retrospective analysis and a better definition of the problems encountered. I don't know how to anticipate potential clinical problems on the basis of available animal data.

But as to predictive of potential clinical problems, that is really quite impossible, as we have seen from past experience.

DR. EASTERLING: It seems that we have leads for new animal models for cardiovascular effects of the oral contraceptives, an area that we are most concerned about. If we pursue developing models specific to that organ system, then we would certainly be in a better position to predict potential problems in the future.

DR. ANDREWS: Dr. Diczfalusy suggested funding development of specific animal models which could be expanded for study of specific problems. Would that be a reasonable answer to that question?

All in favor of that answer please raise their hands.

(Affirmative response)

QUESTION 6

Our last question: "What are the alternatives to long-term animal studies that the FDA can rely on in the assessment of steroid contraceptives?"

Dr. Diczfalusy's response was "careful epidemiological studies." I think that is a reasonable response. Are there additions to that?

DR. BERENDES: We can talk about Phase IV, which some of us know as postmarketing surveillance. An effective postmarketing surveillance system would include appropriate case-controlled studies done at certain intervals repeatedly, and certain follow-up studies.

It may answer the question. Certainly you get around the problem of having a drug out in the field for a number of years before someone begins to look for possible adverse effects.

DR. CORFMAN: I wanted to ask whoever formulated the question whether "alternative" means "instead of," or "in addition to?" That is a rather important distinction.

DR. SOBEL: Well, I don't think "instead of" would be a very easy question to answer. Most of us feel that we can't really abandon animal studies. I would interpret this question to mean supplement or provide ancillary information.

DR. AKSEL: Dr. Sobel stated yesterday that some of the long term animal studies were based on the life expectancy of the animal, i.e., half of their life. I assume that the dog lives 14 years and the study is for seven years. Now, I think this needs to be looked at more realistically from the point of a woman's reproductive life and the number of years oral contraceptives or similar steroids are actually taken. Hardly any women use oral contraceptives for half their reproductive life.

So, I think those studies can be shortened very reasonably.

DR. ANDREWS: This actually implies that they use steroid contraceptives their whole reproductive life which, as you correctly state, is rarely ever the case.

DR. EASTERLING: I suppose now is the time to go back to my earlier comment that deals with Dr. Zbinden's rather adamant statement that long-term studies should now be no more than two years in duration.

I raise that for discussion.

DR. SOBEL: I asked Dr. Andrews for a few minutes to present the Committee with information concerning FDA's experience with the long-term studies and perhaps help you arrive at a more appropriate time for the length of the studies.

As far as the appearance of neoplastic effects in the beagle, we start to observe them about the fourth and fifth year with acceleration thereafter. As far as the endometrial carcinoma is concerned, we have observed this in our rhesus model at about 100 months.

In general, correspondence between clinical observation following use of the 19-nortestosterone derivative containing oral contraceptives and findings in our dog and monkey models has been good. We haven't seen any dose related effects. There have been sporadic tumors that we have discounted, or felt could be in line with a spontaneous occurrence.

But the real dose-response carcinogenic effects have been seen primarily with the 17-acetoxyprogesterones. As far as saying our beagle model is overly sensitive, one of the acetoxyprogesterones has shown hyperplastic changes in the mammary gland of the monkey, a species which is resistant to development of mammary gland cancer.

The monkey endometrial carcinomas occurred a bit later. I don't know if it is well-known but a beagle study was repeated, and showed, with a progesterone control, a very clear dose-related response to Depo-Provera.

DR. CORFMAN: Well, if the definition of alternative is in addition to, the answer to six is simply careful epidemiological studies.

DR. ANDREWS: Possibly adding postmarketing surveillance.

DR. CORFMAN: That would be part of it. I wonder if Dr. Donohoe would be willing to tell us why the Australian regulatory agency has decided to drop the seven and ten year studies. You did say that yesterday, didn't you?

DR. DONOHOE: The proposed guidelines we are currently discussing with industry have suggested that they may be dropped. There is still the problem that we would like long-term studies in two animal species. While one species may be the rat, the other species would undoubtedly be the monkey, so we still would probably have long term studies.

DR. PERLMUTTER: How many years?

DR. DONOHOE: I am not sure at the moment just what we would require. That hasn't been settled. Our present guidelines are most concerned with what should be available before Phase III clinical trials rather than prior to actual marketing.

DR. HUMPEL: I would like to comment on the experience we have with C-19 and C-21 steroids in seven year dog studies. There are drastic differences in kinetics between the two types of steroids in the beagle but not in humans.

MR. HALL: Mr. Chairman, if I may make one or two points. This is an issue that WHO's Special Programme of Research in Human Reproduction has addressed at length over many years, and as many of you may be aware, the program does have a Toxicology Review Panel which assesses all animal data and gives considered opinions regarding toxicological requirements for drugs or delivery systems that are being developed under the auspices of the organization.

This question of the beagle model has been considered at length and in depth for many years. Drs. Zbinden and Heywood are at this meeting and are ex-members of the Toxicology Review Panel. Dr. von Eickstedt is currently a member.

They unanimously came to the decision that the beagle is an inappropriate model for testing of all steroids with regard to its special mammary situation, with regard to the acromegaly that develops and with regard to a special situation with progestogen receptors.

One of the problems we are faced with is something that has been drawn to everyone's attention during this meeting and that is the lack of access to information. We understand, although we don't know where the information is or how we can get at it, that it isn't just the 17-hydroxyprogesterone derivatives that can give rise to mammary tumors in the beagle. The 19-nortestosterone derivatives can do it as well.

Finally, I might just add that we have no idea of the age of the monkeys used in safety studies. Wild caught monkeys have been used in these studies to date. To test an old monkey for the remainder of its lifetime compared with one that is just mature gives a totally different picture, and if there was any way of getting around this, I think that you might find that it is possible to test for shorter periods in well-defined and well-controlled animal models.

PROFESSOR VON EICKSTEDT: We think the beagle is inadequate for long-term studies. This does not mean that we think the monkey is inadequate, and I think the monkey is the species to be considered if well bred animals are available.

DR. ANDREWS: Thank you very much. The beagle keeps running back into the discussion. I was trying to get our questions answered first before going back to the animals, but I gather we have some consensus on question six. The answer to question six is "careful epidemiological studies with postmarketing surveillance."

DR. BRENT: I am just wondering whether we couldn't make a stronger statement. We so infrequently have an opportunity to make major advances in certain aspects of medical care or medical surveillance in our country.

Part of our recommendation should be that this is an important area and we need much better clinical surveillance, not only in this area but in monitoring all drugs.

DR. ANDREWS: It is certainly highly desirable. I believe CDC is trying to do this. It comes down to available dollars.

DR. BRENT: But they (CDC) get their budget cut. Actually this fiscal year they have had a reduction in their resources to monitor adverse effects.

DR. BERENDES: I have just a very brief comment on what Dr. Brent just said. Would it be appropriate to recommend that Dr. Sobel convene a few experts in this area to advise him or how to set up a more appropriate postmarketing surveillance system combined with certain epidemiological studies?

DR. SOBEL: We have a group at the FDA that meets with several groups that are funded by us, including the Boston Collaborative Surveillance Program and Boston University. I don't think we have to form a new group but we certainly could expand the membership of the group to get more input from, say, NIH.

DR. STADEL: I have very strong feelings about what kind of mechanism would be most efficient and that is registration of exposure. I was informed by FDA lawyers that they didn't think the Agency had the legal power to require that at the present time.

DR. SOBEL: The registration route specifically for DMPA was brought up years ago, actually, in a Federal Register notice in 1974. The mandatory registration of use was suggested. At that time it was felt, at least from the Agency side, that it was within the statute.

The real problem is interference with the practice of medicine. That Federal Register notice, as you know, was stayed during October of 1974, and the registration part of it was never tested in the courts. So at least nine years ago the Agency felt that it was not contrary to the Food and Drug Law to have such a procedure. But since it has never been subjected to a court test I really don't know.

DR. BARDIN: Registration would be difficult. Can you imagine the kind of follow-up that would be required to obtain meaningful data, and what the consequences of only 50 percent follow-up would impose on interpretation of such data?

If you want to do it, it must be a formal setting to perhaps limit the problem of follow-up.

I think registration couldn't be a recommendation just because you have a drug marketed. It must be a systematic study in which you have a strong follow-up.

DR. ANDREWS: I think the details are something that would have to be discussed later.

DR. CORFMAN: What was recommended for DMPA over 10 years ago was not a registration of patients, but a registration of pharmacists, clinics and physicians who would prescribe it. Part of the strategy was simply to impress on the medical professional the seriousness of using DMPA as a way to compromise making it available to them.

DR. ANDREWS: Could I call for the recommended answer to number six?

(The question was called)

All in favor or this, please raise your hands.

(Affirmative response)

DR. ANDREWS: A couple of other questions have been suggested. One is the duration of Phase III studies. We had presentations here in the last two days encouraging going to larger scale clinical studies as soon as feasible. The current requirements are two years for Phase III. This is usually at the manufacturer's expense and limits the number of cases.

I wonder if there are any thoughts as to whether it would be feasible to shorten the requirements for Phase III trials? I think we recognize that a certain number of things are only going to be detected with careful clinical surveillance.

DR. SOBEL: Just to give you a frame of reference at what we look at with OC's, we feel that the requirements that demonstrate efficacy can be done well in six months if one is just looking at efficacy and safety is not a consideration.

For safety considerations at present, we are looking at something like 200 women for two years. For efficacy considerations one could condense 600 women for a period of six months. So, we have some flexibility in an OC study where safety is not a great concern.

These are not formal guidelines, but this is what the medical review staff looks at, usually, as a minimum for establishing the basis for a new drug application.

I don't want you to think that these are written and formally defined, but that is roughly the frame of reference for an oral contraceptive evaluation for a new drug application.

DR. KUZMA: Has anyone looked at the data to see if you have learned anything in the second year that you had not learned in the first year?

DR. SOBEL: That is a very good question. We have a project in the Agency with a staff fellow working on that. Do you know more after 1000 patients than you know after 500 patients? I haven't seen the results of the analysis.

If the Committee feels that these guidelines should be more elaborate or don't agree with them, that is perfectly all right. When a manufacturer comes to us, they want to know, "What would you like to look at to know about the safety and the efficacy of this drug." These are really informal guidelines, but they have worked quite well and I don't think they have represented a major impediment to drug development.

DR. BERENDES: This is a substantial problem, at least with some of the Phase III studies. It is not a question of time, it is a question really of knowing whether you have adverse effects. I am aware that some of them, at least, have no comparison group. I would submit that it might be much more useful to shorten the period of exposure and to have a comparison group.

DR. SOBEL: I think you have a lot of sympathetic thinkers in our Agency. As you know, our biometricians believe, a good number of them within the FDA, that although the concept of a control group for the testing of an OC in regard to efficacy is really not necessary, that perhaps controlled studies should be done on safety.

It would be perfectly all right, as far as I am concerned, to strengthen that stand, because it is a stand that does have a great deal of support within the Agency. Many of these informal guidelines have developed over the years in response to a compromise between over regulation and safety considerations.

But, certainly, in regard to safety, controlled trials with OC's is quite a reasonable approach. If the Committee would like to move in that direction, it is certainly not blazing new ground as far as our thinking within the Agency.

DR. ANDREWS: My personal thought is that you might be limiting the clinical exposure by doing that and what you may need is numbers.

PROFESSOR VON EICKSTEDT: I would like to support Dr. Sobel's presentation concerning the need for two year studies. The question was raised, what do you see after one year? We are in contact with a company with whom we are discussing problems concerning an oral contraceptive for which they are trying to get data from more than one year's treatment. Are there, for instance, delayed effects on the endometrium? How can one find out about the return of fertility with a new contraceptive?

I think that after treatment for one year has been finished, the second year can be of great interest.

DR. KUZMA: At one time it may have been necessary to make an arbitrary decision of two years, but now that there is experience and data, either with the FDA or with the pharmaceutical firms, there is no need to make an arbitrary decison. Maybe you should go to three years, or five years. Let's look at the data and see if indeed it is useful to remain at two years. If it is, fine. If not, let's change it to a time that is adequate, but based on some evidence that hopefully exists some place.

DR. SOBEL: I think everybody realizes that for the types of events we are looking at, i.e., serious events, 200 subjects is not an adequate sample. We are certainly not going to pick up rare or serious cardiovascular events with that population.

Looking at the data would tell us that you need 100,000 women to define attributable risks of cardiovascular events.

DR. KUZMA: If it is a token time period, why not change it?

DR. SOBEL: I am not quarreling with that. I confess that it is arbitrary. It seemed to be a number that might pick up rather high incidence events. It has not proven to do so, because fortunately there are no serious high incidence events. The events that we are looking for can't even be picked up with fairly large cohorts as you know from the Walnut Creek analysis and even with the very good British cohort studies.

When we really want to look at these events, we fall back on case-control methodology. So, it is a very difficult situation. What you are saying is that in the case of a new molecular entity we are not going to pick up serious cardiovascular mortality, but 200 subjects will be perhaps enough to pick up unexpected side effects of higher incidence.

DR. KUZMA: My suggestion would be that since we don't have the data, perhaps you ought to go to your staff or call on appropriate people who have access to these data and look at what would be a more reasonable duration and number of patients.

DR. SOBEL: I can tell what the data are; they are fairly well known in the literature. We are not going to reach a meaningful base until we go up several orders of magnitude, and that is not feasible economically.

DR. STADEL: You are not going to identify any epidemiologic end points in these early studies. That is impossible. I think there are some things you can do, though.

For steroid contraceptives that are similar to the ones that we are now using, you can get a lot of information from a one-year study in which you look at certain biochemical parameters which may be predictors of a cardiovascular effect.

Determine the effects of a new steroid on antithrombin function, lipoproteins for any unusual reactions, compared to the results with one or another of the currently marketed formulations as a standard.

That could be either done as a randomized trial or, as a nonrandomized cohort study.

I think a one-year study of reasonable size, say 200 women, would give you quite a bit of information about how a new formulation compared with one of the widely use formulations in terms of its effects on antithrombin function, lipoproteins, and perhaps a few other carefully selected variables which give us some measure of confidence about its potential for the major problem with the currently available pills.

DR. EDGREN: Phase III trials require more than 200 subjects. We initially enrolled between 2000 and 3000 women to have at the end of two years approximately 200 patients. I think it may even be a little higher now. These are estimates that I made a decade ago.

Such a study, would require a minimum of two years to initiate, enroll patients and gather the investigators together. It would require another two to four years to complete the study another couple of years to complete analysis of the data. This would require a minimum of about five years. On the basis of current prices in the clinic, and this is just a guess--I think we are talking about $4-5 million for the study.

MR. HALL: Drs. Stadel and Edgren have brought up some of the points that I had intended raising. You can't convert an ongoing Phase III study into an epidemiologically sound investigation of safety. Dr. Sobel has clearly stated that the FDA accepts quite a lot of flexibility in this area.

I think you mentioned earlier that is necessary to have well designed, case-controlled studies following epidemiological events at a later date. WHO's experience with later multicenter worldwide Phase III clinical trials and involving tens or hundreds of thousand women months of use of both oral contraceptives and injectable contraceptives indicate that by the end of one year there is a 50 percent dropout, however good your follow-up facilities are in those particular clinics.

In a highly developed country you should be able to obtain follow-up procedures that yield better follow-up rates than that, but it is not possible. We have seen this consistently throughout the developed and the developing world with both injectibles and OC's. Fifty percent follow-up is about all you expect at the end of the first year.

Phase III studies evaluate use effectiveness, efficacy and the reasons for drop out, i.e. is it a bleeding problem, etc. These studies do have a useful role.

But they must be compared with another drug. You have to be very careful how you do a controlled study; you can't randomize an IUD with an oral contraceptive. We have tried to randomized maybe four different OCs and two injectibles in some of our studies and even then there is a problem, because the two injectibles are given at two different time periods.

If you are going to retain a Phase III study, there are some useful outcomes. You have data on how the recipient is perceiving that particular drug for the first time and why there are dropouts. We have attempted to build studies around these Phase III trials for example, one goes back and starts specific metabolic studies and follows up subjects for, say, a period of one year.

This must be done in addition to the standard Phase III studies. For example, our program has studies of effects on lipids, lipoprotein metabolism, and coagulation factors. However, if you set up specific studies to look for too many end points, you may ruin your original study design.

DR. ANDREWS: Thank you, Mr. Hall. I think all of these comments are pertinent and will be part of the record. My opinion is that the most we can do at the moment is recommend flexibility in consideration of how long these studies should be, recognizing that getting to clinical usage will really give us the most information. But safety certainly does have to be assured.

DR. KUZMA: Well, I feel strongly enough to propose a motion that we cut it down to at least one year, until better scientific evidence is available to indicate that it should be 18 months or 24 months, or whatever.

I would like to move that the current two year Phase III studies be limited to one year study.

(The motion was seconded)

DR. ANDREWS: Any other discussion of the motion? We have not spelled out the subjects. I presume that would stay at the present --

DR. KUZMA: Two hundred, or it could be increased to whatever.

DR. ANDREWS: It would be easier to get 200 at the end of the pipeline if you had a shorter time.

All in favor of that, please signify by raising your hand.

(Affirmative response)

DR. SOBEL: Do you want to make a recommendation regarding the use of controls for these studies?

DR. ANDREWS: The problem of controls in contraceptive studies is expense, which eventually gets passed to the consumer.

DR. BLYE: What is the matter with using pre-treatment and post-treatment clinical chemistries, the subjects serving as their own controls?

DR. ANDREWS: That is an option.

I would like to open up the last subject now and that is the appropriate test animal.

DR. NELSON: I have one question. There seems to be a conflict in whether 19-nortestosterone steroids caused breast tumors in beagles. Dr. Humpel said they did and I thought Dr. Sobel said they did not.

DR. SOBEL: There is one 19-nor derivative, chlorethinyl norethindrone. Every one on the market does not cause tumors in beagles.

DR. HEYWOOD: Lynestrenol actually causes mammary gland nodules and tumors in the beagle dog, and that is a 19-nortestosterone derivative.

DR. SOBEL: I am talking about drugs marketed in the United States.

DR. HEYWOOD: Oh, sorry.

DR. HUMPEL: Lynestrenol is actually a prodrug of norethisterone.

DR. DICZFALUSY: Mr. Chairman, this is very interesting information because we have good evidence that, at least in the human, lynestrenol is almost quantitatively converted into norethisterone. I have evidence from Organon, the company which makes the drug, that in every species they have tested so far, lynestrenol was converted into norethisterone.

I don't know whether or not they have tested the conversion in the beagle dog but that would certainly be worthwhile doing.

DR. ANDREWS: One possibility is that if the appropriate doses were used, whether these tumors might turn up in the beagle at multiples of threshold dose considering the beagle's sensitivity and peculiar reaction to progestins.

DR. SOBEL: I will not get into specifics, but we have some evidence that a nonmarketed norethindrone given parenterally produced an increase in mammary tumors and at least one carcinoma, but not the same order of magnitude and dose-related response that we have seen with the 17-acetoxyprogesterones.

It is our belief that in regard to carcinogenesis, as far as we know, the beagle model perhaps has served us well. On the other hand maybe it has kept off the market some drugs which also would be carcinogenic in man. But that information is still lacking.

Those products in the U.S. market that have undergone the current animal screening have not caused carcinoma.

DR. PERLMUTTER: One of the other terms we have heard over the last couple of days is "bioavailability," and whether or not we are giving equivalent drugs to beagle dogs, and that the 19-norprogestins are much weaker drugs. I wonder if you gave equivalent doses, you wouldn't get tumors and cancers in beagle dogs with all progestins.

DR. AKSEL: I would really like to poll the Committee. What we have heard in the last two days about results in the beagle dog with contraceptive steroids has demonstrated to me that the data cannot be extrapolated to the human or even to other animals. The beagle is a species that has a unique response to progestational agents.

I am interested in polling the Committee, how many of you think that maybe we should recommend that the FDA seriously consider discontinuing beagle dog studies for progestins?

DR. TAGATZ: How many drugs which were not approved for marketing in the United States have been in general use in Europe or outside of this country? What is the epidemiological experience regarding human cancer with these drugs other than DMPA.

Now, that is the crux of the matter.

DR. SOBEL: I would defer to our European colleagues on that and would ask them to indicate the nature of the epidemiologic data.

DR. DICZFALUSY: When it comes to the specific question with C-21 steroids and whether or not they have been used in other countries, the answer is yes. In both West and East Germany they are using chlormadinone acetate. They have been followed up carefully and we have access to their epidemiological studies from the Ministry of Health.

We know that in the People's Republic of China both chlormadinone acetate and megestrol acetate have been very widely used and, as you may recall, the pill No. 2 of the People's Republic of China is megestrol acetate.

MR. HALL: Chlormadinone acetate has been used for some 20 years in West Germany, with good epidemiological surveillance. I think about 40 percent of the oral contraceptives in that country contain chlormadinone acetate.

They have now joined the WHO long-term epidemiological study.

DR. SOBEL: May I make a plea to the Committee, since these data are shortly forthcoming, to open this question at a future meeting when the data are fully available, and decide at that point.

DR. AKSEL: I just wanted to know if the Committee feels that, based on what they have heard over the last two days, the involvement of the dog in the safety studies of oral contraceptives has been worthwhile?

My feeling has been no.

DR. ANDREWS: You would like this just as a show of hands without a recommendation?

DR. AKSEL: Right.

DR. ANDREWS: Can we respond to Dr. Askel's request about that, a show of hands of how many people think that this has been of benefit?

The one thing I might urge is that the FDA consider not mandating the beagle as a model and possibly having flexibility in the future. The British require rat, mouse, or hamster. I think possibly flexibility and choice might be something to consider for the future.

DR. DICZFALUSY: Whenever you start studies in a species about which you have limited information, the chances that you will be unable to interpret the results are very high.

MS. WEST: Since I am here as a consumer representative in the spirit of public policy and perhaps legal implications, perhaps it would be useful to go back to why we are here, which is to develop recommendations on animal testing requirements for a new generation of steroidal contraceptives.

In terms of preamble, we are here at the invitation of a regulatory agency who, in addition to the scientific background and experiments conducted by all of you, has the responsibility to report to the Congress, who also, because of either their concern, lack of information, or whatever, has interfered with both your operation as well as the operation of the drug companies, especially since the 1962 hearings.

My involvement on the consumer level deals with some public policy issues, including cost to the consumer, cost to the drug company, and the cost in time that we all face as we are involved in these problems as well as the safety and efficacy of the drug.

What I have learned in these two days is the need for some change and to consider our dependence on animal studies that by necessity have a fairly narrow focus.

It would appear that we need a better balance between human clinical results and those from animal testing, at least as it has been done during the last 20 years. One further suggestion I would make in additional to our responses to the six questions is that the FDA take a look at the legal problems involved in making both published and unpublished data available.

There was a lot of discussion in the last couple of days about not being able to compare data because of unpublished results. Now, as an attorney, I don't think it is unrealistic to re-examine the regulatory role of the FDA and to take a new look at the legal implications in interpreting the patent laws of this country.

Concern has been expressed about confidential or proprietary data which cannot be shared. Since I have been privileged to participate in a number of medical and pharmaceutical symposia in America, and have been in those facilities, I am sure that there is a great deal of data and information which is not presently shared because of legal concern and implications.

In the interest of public policy, cost, and more responsive regulatory process I suggest that we consider some of the legal implications of data sharing.

When we were discussing registry, my concern was mandatory versus voluntary. There are registries going on in cancer, finger printing of children, and in all sorts of other areas, and I just wonder if we should look at some of these broader legal issues.

DR. ANDREWS: That is a very appropriate comment. Would you move that we recommend exploring legal ways to share scientific information?

MS. WEST: Yes, absolutely

(The motion was duly seconded)

(No response)

All in favor, signify by saying "Aye."

(Ayes)

DR. BRENT: I don't know if it is a major issue or a minor one, but we have not touched on one subject at all. In the early days of oral contraceptives one of the concerns was the effect on the progeny of women who had taken oral contraceptives.

Most of the epidemiological studies that looked at the offspring of women who had been on oral contraceptives has been negative. We have not touched that issue at all with regard to new steroidal contraceptives, and I gather that the conclusion is that there would be no difference no matter what the new contraceptive would be with regard to its effect on the cytogenetics of the ovum or of reproductive capacity.

The second thing which is an issue, deals with when a woman who has been on oral contraceptives gets pregnant. We have not touched that issue, either, with regard to the exposure of women. Again, I think that the vast amount of information is negative - but we have not touched on this as being of any importance.

DR. ANDREWS: I think the epidemiological studies we have to date have not shown adverse effects. I also believe continuing postmarketing surveillance of any new drug would continue to address that. I don't think we made any firm resolution or recommendation of how long these surveillance studies should continue. We suggested flexibility and consideration, but I didn't feel we could give a specific number.

If there are no further comments I would like to thank all of you for your participation. It has been very educational to me and I hope it has of service to the FDA. Thank you very much.

We are adjourned.

ORGANIZING COMMITTEE

C. Wayne Bardin,
Center for Biomedical Research, The Population Council

Victor R. Berliner,
Division of Metabolism and Endocrine Drug Products, Office of Biologics Research and Review, Center for Drugs and Biologics, Food and Drug Administration.

Gabriel Bialy,
Center for Population Research, National Institute of Child Health and Human Development, National Institutes of Health.

Richard P. Blye,
Center for Population Research, National Institute of Child Health and Human Development, National Institutes of Health.

Henry Gabelnick,
Center for Population Research, National Institute of Child Health and Human Development, National Institutes of Health.

A.T. Gregoire,
Division of Metabolism and Endocrine Drug Products, Office of Biologics Research and Review, Center for Drugs and Biologics, Food and Drug Administration.

Peter Hall,
Special Programme of Research in Human Reproduction, World Health Organization.

Mortimer B. Lipsett,*
National Institute of Arthritis, Diabetes, and Digestive and Kidney Diseases, National Institutes of Health.

Harold A. Nash,
Center for Biomedical Research, The Population Council.

D.J. Patanelli,
Center for Population Research, National Institute of Child Health and Human Development, National Institutes of Health.

James Shelton,
Population Division, Agency for International Development.

*Deceased

Solomon Sobel,
Division of Metabolism and Endocrine Drug Products, Office of Biologics Research and Review, Center for Drugs and Biologics, Food and Drug Administration.

PARTICIPANTS AND CONTRIBUTORS

Sezer Aksel, M.D.
University of South Alabama College of Medicine
Mobile, Alabama

William Andrews, M.D.
Department of Obstetrics and Gynecology, Eastern Virginia Medical School
Norfolk, Virginia

C. Wayne Bardin, M.D.
Center for Biomedical Research, The Population Council
New York, New York

H.W. Berendes, M.D.
Epidemiology and Biometry Research Program, National Institute of Child Health and Human Development, National Institutes of Health
Bethesda, Maryland

Richard P. Blye, Ph.D.
Center for Population Research, National Institute of Child Health and Human Development, National Institutes of Health
Bethesda, Maryland

Robert Brent, M.D., Ph.D.
Department of Pediatrics, Jefferson Medical College
Philadelphia, Pennsylvania

James H. Clark, Ph.D.
Department of Cell Biology, Baylor College of Medicine
Houston, Texas

Thomas Clarkson, DVM
Department of Comparative Medicine, Bowman Gray School of Medicine
Winston Salem, North Carolina

Partha Das Gupta, M.D.
Central Drug Standard Control Organization, Ministry of Health and Family Welfare
New Dehli, India

Egon Diczfalusy, M.D.
Reproductive Endocrinology Research Unit, Karolinska Sjukhuset, (Swedish Research Medical Council)
Stockholm, Sweden

John A. Donohoe, Ph.D.
Chief Pharmacologist, Drug Evaluation Section
Canberra, Australia

William Easterling, M.D.
University of North Carolina, School of Medicine
Chapel Hill, North Carolina

Richard A. Edgren, Ph.D.
Director of Scientific Affairs, Syntex Laboratories, Inc.
Palo Alto, California

Klaus-Wolf von Eickstedt, M.D.
Institut fur Arzneimittol des Bundesgesundheitsamtes
Berlin, Federal Republic of Germany

Kenneth Fotherby, Ph.D.
University of London, Royal Postgraduate Medical School, Hammersmith Hospital
London, England

William Filler, Jr., M.D.
Department of Obstetrics and Gynecology, University of California,
Irvine, California

Uwe Goebelsmann, M.D.*
Professor of Obstetrics and Gynecology, UCLA College of Medicine
Los Angeles, California

A.T. Gregoire, Ph.D.
Division of Metabolism and Endocrine Drug Products, Office of Biologics Research and Review, Center for Drugs and Biologics, Food and Drug Administration
Rockville, Maryland

Ralph Heywood, DVM
Huntingdon Research Centre, Huntingdon
Cambridge, England

Michael Humpel, Dr. Rer. Nat.
Schering AG
Berlin, West Germany

Kamal Ishak, M.D.
Hepatic Pathology Department, Armed Forces Institute of Pathology
Washington, District of Columbia

Benita S. Katzenellenbogen, Ph.D.
Department of Physiology, Biophysics and Chemistry, University of Illinois
Urbana, Illinois

Robert H. Knopp, M.D.
Northwest Lipid Research Clinic
University of Washington, Seattle, Washington

Ronald M. Krauss, M.D.
Donner Laboratory, Lawrence Berkeley Laboratory, University of California
Berkeley, California

*Deceased

Jan Kuzma, Ph.D.
School of Health, Loma Linda University
Loma Linda, California

Mortimer B. Lipsett, M.D.*
National Institute of Arthritis, Diabetes, and Digestive and Kidney Diseases, National Institute of Health
Bethesda, Maryland

Ron Nelson, M.D.
Department of Obstetrics and Gynecology, White Memorial Medical Center
Los Angeles, California

Max H. Parrott, M.D.
8120 S.W. Barnes Road
Portland, Oregon

Johanna F. Perlmutter, M.D.
Department of Obstetrics and Gynecology, Beth Israel Hospital
Brookline, Massachusetts

Solomon Sobel, M.D.
Division of Metabolism and Endocrine Drug Products, Office of Biologics, Research and Review, Center for Drugs and Biologics, Food and Drug Administration
Rockville, Maryland

Bruce Stadel, M.D.
Center for Population Research, National Institute of Child Health and Human Development, National Institutes of Health
Bethesda, Maryland

Donald J. Sutherland, Ph.D.
Bureau of Drugs
Vanier, Ontario, Canada

George Tagatz, M.D.
Department of Obstetrics and Gynecology, University of Minnesota
Minneapolis, Minnesota

Stanford Wessler, M.D.
Department of Medicine, New York University School of Medicine
New York, New York

Frances West, J.D.
Division of Consumer Affairs, State of Delaware
Wilmington, Delaware

Gerhard Zbinden, M.D.
Institute of Toxicology, Swiss Federal Institute of Technology, University of Zurich
Schwerzenback, Switzerland

*Deceased

INDEX